Understanding hard to maintain behaviour change

Addiction Press aims to communicate current ideas and evidence in this expanding field, not only to researchers and practising health professionals, but also to policy makers, students and interested non-specialists. These publications are designed to address the significant challenges that addiction presents to modern society.

Other books in the Addiction Press series

Theory of Addiction
Robert West and Jamie Brown
9780470674215

Clinical Handbook of Adolescent Addiction
Edited by R. Rosner
9780470972342

Harm Reduction in Substance Use and High-Risk Behaviour
Edited by R. Pates & D. Riley
9781405182973

Injecting Illicit Drugs
Edited by R. Pates, A. McBride & K. Arnold
9781405113601

Neuroimaging in Addiction
Edited by B. Adinoff & E. Stein
9780470660140

Treating Drinkers and Drug Users in the Community
T. Waller & D. Rumball
9780632035755

Understanding and Treating Addictions: Psychological Assessment and Intervention
Edited by A. Copello
9781405124171

Addiction: Evolution of a Specialist Field
Edited by G. Edwards
9780632059768

Understanding hard to maintain behaviour change

A dual process approach

Ron Borland PhD

The Cancer Council,
Victoria, Australia

WILEY Blackwell

Addiction
Press

Library of Congress Cataloging-in-Publication Data

Borland, Ron.
  Understanding hard to maintain behaviour change : a dual process approach / Ron Borland.
    pages cm
  Includes bibliographical references and index.
  ISBN 978-1-118-57293-1 (pbk.)
  1. Behavior modification. 2. Change (Psychology) 3. Habit breaking. 4. Habit. I. Title.
  BF637.B4B67 2014
  153.8'5–dc23

                                                                              2013034134

A catalogue record for this book is available from the British Library.

CONTENTS

PREFACE

I have had the great fortune to work for a small organisation that has had a huge impact, not only in tobacco control, but also in skin cancer prevention and other areas of cancer control. Under the inspired leadership of Nigel Gray and David Hill, the Cancer Council Victoria has been a leading light in the development of evidence-driven approaches to health promotion, in particular, the use of mass media and other mass communication tools to drive both environmental and personal changes to reduce behavioural risk factors for cancer. For more than 25 years, I have been contributing to this effort, researching aspects of tobacco control and sun protection, including evaluating the impacts of mass campaigns. For the past 15 years, my work has focussed on smoking. This continues to be satisfying because all the successful efforts to reduce smoking (however small) add healthy years to people's lives. When I started to work in this area, there was implicit confidence that we would quickly get on top of the problem. As smokers came to realise how bad it was and the social desirability of smoking was reduced, most smokers would quit and the problem would largely go away. However, in countries such as Australia, and increasingly elsewhere, the agenda for change that was adopted in the early days of tobacco control efforts has been pretty much completely implemented, but we are still only about half way to our goal.

As I have researched the issue, including being involved in some of the early evaluations of concerted efforts to control tobacco use, I have become increasingly impressed (and concerned) by what a resilient habit smoking is. Not only has it proved difficult to get smokers to quit successfully, it has challenged much of what I had been taught as a psychology student about the nature of learning and unlearning and how they relate to persuasion and choice. I soon realised that this was not a unique challenge. The research I did on sun-protection behaviours highlighted the challenge of maintaining an under-cued set of behaviours, and of the need for constant campaigns, not just to remind people of the need to protect themselves, but also to maintain motivation to do so. Looking over the fence into other efforts to control problematic behaviours, I see similar challenges. Consistently doing enough of certain activities, such as exercising, is beset with similar problems. Many people find it extremely difficult to maintain weight loss, even though many can initially lose some. The difficulties of maintaining seemingly simple behaviour changes all point to this being a set of wicked problems, that is, ones for which the immediately obvious solution turns out to be dangerously over-simplistic.

Most failures to change complex behaviours are not for want of trying. Simple attempts to explain these failures as being due to lack of willpower are not particularly useful. Nor is it productive to disparage those who fail. Drug addicts are notorious for telling therapists that they really want to stop using, only to be found shooting up soon after. Contrary to the views of some, I see this not as lying, but as showing the difficulty of maintaining a consistent position when the environmental cues and the associated cravings for the drug vary so greatly from a doctor's clinic to the streets associated with use. Any useful new theory should be able to shed novel insights into the complexities and seeming inconsistencies of behaviour in these difficult areas.

The work of an applied scientist is of applying theory to solve problems and any theory testing is secondary. Throughout my career I have been frustrated by the limitations of existing theories and the lack of integration of theories used in one aspect of my work to inform other aspects. Working in the real world with complex problems that involve diverse aspects of human thought and behaviour, I have wanted a comprehensive theory that helped integrate understanding: a theory to understand a set of problems, rather than trying to view a problem through the distorting lens of a set of only partly applicable theories.

This book represents an attempt to build up a comprehensive theory of why some forms of behaviour change don't fit the mould of being easy and are difficult to institute and/or maintain, in the hope that it will lead to more effective interventions. It is informed by Alfred North Whitehead's aphorism 'Seek simplicity and distrust it'. My aim is to keep things as simple as I can while taking into account the complex dynamics of human behaviour. Most of the elements of the theory are borrowed and/or adapted from other theories. What is unique here is the ways in which these components are put together and in the ways some of the elements of existing theories are rejected or modified.

My efforts to develop an alternative conceptualisation to the mass of overlapping and mutually inconsistent theorising around behaviour change have been a far from linear process. Some of my early ideas have been abandoned or modified in the face of evidence. However, the rate of need for change has gradually slowed (but not to zero) and I now have less discomfort in having to 'fix' my ideas. I believe the core ideas presented here can be defended and will remain pretty much as postulated, while some of the minor elements are less well grounded and thus may need to change as evidence accumulates. I encourage readers who find the basic ideas useful to let me know about failings and inconsistent evidence. This is not the last word.

ACKNOWLEDGEMENTS

This book has influences reaching many aspects of my life. The strong underpinnings of the theory in the ideas of Pavlov and Vygotsky owe much to my early mentor MB Macmillan, and the ideas from communication and systems thinking to Robyn Penman. David Hill, my long-term boss and mentor at the Cancer Council Victoria, has been a constant source of inspiration and advice and has shaped my thinking in innumerable ways. I am indebted to my research team from over the years for support, suggestions and helping me show how some of my early ideas were wrong. The emergence of the ideas in this book has benefitted from discussions over the years with many people, but particularly with Arie Dijkstra, Robert West, Geoff Fong and Mike Cummings.

Related directly to the present volume, particular thanks are due to James Balmford and David Young for incisive comments on drafts and to other members of my team for chasing references and other bits and pieces. I am also grateful for comments on a preliminary draft from Susan Michie, Steve Sutton and Jill Francis, in particular. I am indebted to those who pointed out the burgeoning thinking about dual-process theories within psychology of which I was unaware, which has allowed me to align my thinking with elements of that work. Finally thanks to my family, my wife Virginia Lewis, who not only put up with me but read and commented positively on key elements, and to Ross and Harry who at least humoured me.

Chapter 1

AN OVERVIEW OF THE THEORY

Most behaviour change is unproblematic. People's behaviour changes all the time, both in response to an ever-changing environment and their increasingly refined responses to it as they learn and adapt. This book is about trying to understand those aspects of human behaviour that aren't readily brought into concordance with environmental conditions and individual desires. It develops and elaborates a theoretical framework, called *CEOS theory* (I will explain the acronym later), which is designed to be a new and comprehensive way of thinking about how people change habitual behaviours. This involves understanding the constraints on and the potential of volitional attempts to change behaviour patterns that are under the moment-to-moment control of non-volitional processes.

The theory also focusses on the different processes involved in the initiation and maintenance of behaviour change. It is primarily designed to understand behaviours that are hard-to-maintain (HTM behaviours); that is, ones that while seen as desirable by the individual are not spontaneously adopted or are hard to sustain and/or are seen as undesirable and hard to reduce or eliminate in the long term. These behaviours include stopping smoking, eating healthy foods to maintain a desirable weight, exercising regularly and controlling alcohol consumption. CEOS theory also encompasses easy-to-change behaviour, where it is similar to many existing theories because there is less need to consider the conflict between volitional and non-volitional forces within the individual.

The focus of this book is on health-related behaviours. The big question it attempts to answer is: Is it possible to help people to enjoy and value healthy lifestyles, to the point where there is no longer any real effort involved in avoiding unhealthy and embracing healthy behavioural alternatives? Where this is not possible, can we develop strategies to help people maintain healthy options, at least most of the time, and to minimise unhealthy choices and to break unhealthy habits, even if it requires ongoing vigilance?

Key ideas and observations that have informed the need for a new theory include the following:

- People sometimes don't act in ways that are objectively in their best interests even when they want to change; for example, they continue to smoke or continue a high-fat low-exercise lifestyle even though they want to be fit and healthy.

Understanding hard to maintain behaviour change: A dual process approach, First Edition. Ron Borland.
© 2014 John Wiley & Sons, Ltd. Published 2014 by John Wiley & Sons, Ltd.

- Even when people try to adopt healthy behaviours, these new forms of behaviour are difficult to maintain and are thus characterised by high rates of failure. The causes of these failures are not well understood, and attempts to reduce relapse rates have a bleak record.
- Recent research has established that the determinants of deciding and trying to change are different from those of maintaining behaviour change, at least for smoking [1, 2]. (See Chapter 2 for more details.) Some of the things that motivate smokers to try to quit, and which quitting improves, are associated perversely with reduced chances of success. It is not yet known whether similar perverse relationships are present for other HTM behaviours.

CEOS is a biopsychosocial theory, in that it postulates that behaviour is co-determined by the interaction between biological factors, modifiable aspects within the individual (psychological factors) and aspects of the environment, especially social factors. Which of these influences is most important for any particular kind of behaviour, or as is the case here, which make it difficult to maintain desirable behaviours, is an empirical question.

Within the individual, engagement with the environment is maintained by a complex multi-level processing system that relates environmental inputs to need states of the individual, leading to behaviours designed to reduce those needs [3, 4]. Emerging from the higher levels of this system is the unique human capacity to represent the world outside of the moment and to operate on conceptualisations of it using language and rules. This representation of the world can encompass aspects of the individual doing the representing, and thus becomes self-referential, and it has the power to influence behaviour in novel ways. The capacity to influence behaviour based on a conceptual understanding of the world is a top-down process, unlike the bottom-up process of dynamic adaptation to the environment that characterises other aspects of behaviour.

The core-characterising feature of CEOS theory is that these two processes (Figure 1.1) constitute two fundamentally different ways of relating to the world, and many of the problems of human behaviour can be better understood by considering them as co-occurring and in some cases competing systems within the individual. The base system that is reactive to environmental conditions I call the Operational System (OS) because it is the system that operates directly on the world to maintain homeostasis. The term is used in computing to cover those routine functions that are automated, that is, are done without executive (external governing) input. The emergent, reflective, self-referencing system that acts on conceptualisations of the world I call the Executive System (ES) because it operates in much the same way as the executive of an organisation works; that is, by setting the goals for an organisation that can only be achieved if the organisation is sufficiently prepared to work towards them. The name CEOS is an acronym for Context, Executive and Operational Systems, which are the core elements of the theory. CEOS is one of a class of dual-process theories [5, 6], which make similar, but not identical distinctions between volitional and non-volitional processes.

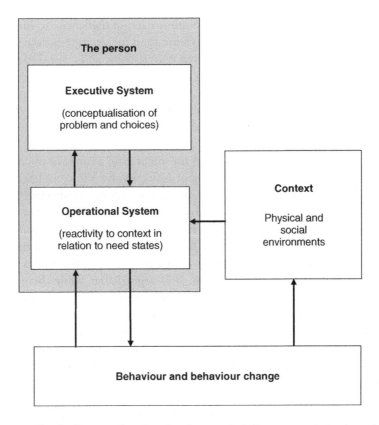

Figure 1.1   Simple diagram showing the three main influences on behaviour change.

The OS is where all behaviour is generated and controlled. The OS is reactive to the environment of the moment, its current states and inputs from the ES. It adapts through associative mechanisms typified by habituation and conditioning. By contrast, the ES uses inputs from the OS and from language-based representations of the world to evaluate ongoing behaviour, and to either resolve conflicts between OS tendencies to act or pursue articulated goals that emerge from its conceptualisation of the world or of possible futures.

Reframed in dual-process terms, the challenge that this book addresses is why, once the ES decides that behaviour needs to change, it is sometimes so difficult to enact that change and to maintain it. CEOS postulates that this is because the OS tends to favour or revert to well-learnt routines when not being explicitly directed to do otherwise, and indeed will not respond to ES directives unless suitably primed. Priming involves acting to generate affective associative links to ES ideas so they also become action tendencies within the OS, and thus if strong enough, compete with other operational action tendencies to be enacted. This priming is necessary because the ES cannot act without the OS accepting the behavioural schemata or script from the ES as 'its own'. The capacity of ES processes to inhibit action tendencies is easier to achieve than building the strength for action tendencies to impel action as inhibition requires lower levels of activation than for exciting action.

Emerging out of the characteristics of the two systems, and central to this book, CEOS postulates that different processes are involved as a person progresses from unconcerned acceptance of one behavioural pattern to the stable adoption of a more desirable alternative; in particular, the determinants of the initiation of change are quite different from those involved in maintenance and this is most clearly manifested in HTM behaviours.

CEOS is a framework (or meta-theory) for integrating a range of micro-theories that help us understand the key component tasks involved in complex behaviour change and how they interrelate. As such, it encompasses descriptive theory (taxonomy), theories of mechanisms and theories of how to intervene. As part of the theory of how to intervene, it includes a model of how a person might best conceptualise a problematic behaviour to optimise his/her chances of successfully changing it.

The theory is designed to explain why some behaviours are hard to reduce or eliminate and others are hard to sustain. It is argued that while there are some similarities with both hard-to-reduce behaviours (such as smoking) and hard-to-sustain behaviours (such as dietary change), there are some important differences, particularly in the role of cues and the role of negative experiences.

The theory was developed with the persisting problem of tobacco smoking as the primary focus. As a result, most of the examples used come from the challenges associated with smoking cessation. However, it has been conceptualised to apply to all HTM behaviours.

Before beginning to elaborate, I provide some background on the conceptual and empirical underpinnings, which together justify the need for a new overarching framework.

Context

Science-based approaches to understanding HTM behaviours are by no means the first societal efforts to encourage us collectively to do what the society sees as desirable – it is one of the enduring projects of human civilisation, involving governments, religions, communities and families. A lot can be learnt from the successes, part successes and failures of the past.

Dual-process theories are also not new. Their origins go back to antiquity [7]. They include the Buddha's analogy of the rider and the elephant and Plato's analogy of the driver and the chariot. More recently in the early days of modern psychology, James [8] made a distinction between experiential and analytic processes, Pavlov [9–11] identified his first and second signalling systems as mechanisms for these two kinds of processes to work, and Freud conceived of the structures of the Ego and Id as the framework within which this interaction occurred, mediated in his case by the Superego [12]. These are all dual-process models of one kind or another. They are all about trying to understand why humans sometimes have trouble doing what they think is best, sometimes described as taming our animal selves.

Within empirically grounded (scientific) psychology, these ideas were rejected by the influential behaviourist movement (e.g. Watson and Skinner) [13–15]. Behaviourist models postulate bottom-up processes by which environmental conditions interact with motivational (drive) states of the organism to determine behaviour. However, as the limitations of behaviourism became apparent for explaining higher cognitive processes, they were replaced by a cognitivist movement that largely ignored lower level processes, implicitly or in some cases explicitly, assuming that these could be controlled in a top-down way by higher cognitive processes. It is the observed limitations of rationality-based cognitive theories that have led to CEOS, and to experimental social and cognitive psychologists re-exploring the role of lower level processes in influencing human cognition and, less researched, behaviour. I was unaware of some of this experimental work until quite late in the development of the theory (and there may be more of which I remain ignorant), but it is reassuring that it is all consistent with the broad theory proposed here, and in a couple of cases has allowed me to refine elements of it. Canvassing the experimental literature has also renewed my concern about the parochial nature of much research and the tailoring of theory to the micro, rather than looking for theories with applicability beyond any specific research stream. I believe that it is important to begin by thinking about human behaviour in totality, and to build models within each domain of enquiry that are consistent with those that are more broadly applicable. CEOS is not the only attempt to do this, other examples include the PRIME theory of West [16, 17], which does not take a dual-process approach, the dual-process approaches of Strack and Deutsch's [18] RIM model, particularly as elaborated by Hofmann *et al.* [19] and the Nudge theory of Thaler and Sunstein [20], which focusses on communication strategies and environmental change to influence behaviour. The relationship of these models to CEOS is illuminated at various points in this book.

Limitations of the existing theories

We need a new overarching theory of HTM behaviours because existing theories have major limitations, either in scope or in their conceptualisation of the central problem.

Three sets of theories have dominated attempts to change problem behaviours: theories of addiction that focus on biological mechanisms, including learning theories that are concerned with the malleability of biological determinants of habits; expectancy-value theories that emphasise the rational appraisal of the balance between the costs and benefits of behaving, given the existing social and environmental contexts; and social determinant models that postulate that mal-adaptive behaviours are the result of imperfect social structures (i.e. problems with the environment). Each of these focusses on one aspect of the totality, and it is apparent that each is too limited to deal with the complexity. See West [16] for an excellent review of many of these theories, including identification of their limitations). To get a better idea of the applicability of these theories, consider the three case studies given in Box 1.1 before you read on.

Box 1.1 Case studies of obesity

Consider three cases studies of the same problem – serious obesity – and from the information given; see what you think is responsible and what sort of strategies you might consider to help the women concerned. All three are excerpts from the stories of severely obese women of early middle age, each of whom live with her husband and children.

Case A: This woman comes from a family that is also obese. She had a happy childhood but ate lots of snack foods and sweet drinks. The area of the country in which she comes from has a history of poor diet and has the highest levels of obesity in the country.

Case B: This woman lives with her family in a different town to her parents and socialises mainly with her husband's family and friends, with whom she gets on very well. She is the only obese person in her friendship network. However, both her parents and several relatives are also seriously obese. She eats a very similar diet to her husband who is normal weight.

Case C: This woman had a stressful adolescence, whatever she tried at she failed and she came to see herself as someone who could not manage herself. She became severely obese in her adolescence and has been unable to keep weight off since. She is very reliant on her husband for advice and often unwilling to take independent action. Most of the people around her are not overweight, including her husband.

As you read Case A, you are likely to be drawn to the social context. Living in those conditions, how could this woman be anything other than obese, clearly the environment is the problem. However, for Case B, this story does not mesh, as she lives with slim(ish) people and doesn't seem to be doing anything wrong; perhaps hers is a case of a biological predisposition. Then, take Case C, who clearly has self-esteem problems and probably has low self-efficacy for change, and perhaps is a candidate for a psychologically based approach.

Now, what if I were to tell you that all three are parts of the same woman's story. Could it be that elements of all three approaches (theories) are right?

This example brings to mind the parable of the blind men and the elephant. A group of blind men are taken to the zoo and get to meet an elephant close-up. One gets to feel the trunk, another the leg, a third gets to run his hands down one side, and a fourth gets to feel the tail. When comparing their experiences afterwards, they all have completely different ideas of what an elephant is (like a wrinkly snake, a tree trunk, a wall and a rope), and in a narrow sense all are part right, but all are wrong in totality. We can learn from each perspective, but need to have a view of the whole to fit them together. If we then want to focus on one part, we can better understand how it fits into the whole.

At one extreme, social determinist models seem to assume that addictions and other undesirable behaviour patterns are a symptom of societal malaise, and that they will disappear if we reform the society. They point to the powerful influence of societal structures, and the differing rates of health problems in different societies to argue their case [21]. Along with West [16], I see that the main limitation of these theories is that they cannot readily account for, let alone predict, the demonstrated influence of individual level factors. Why do individuals (seemingly) exposed to the same social context turn out differently? Social determinist models often accept a role for biological factors, if only to explain individual variability, usually implied to be pathological, but often consider any form of psychological or behavioural processes to be of limited importance [21, 22]. A more productive way of theorising social factors are social ecological models [23], which leave a place for intrapersonal factors, although they do not generally pay much attention to them. Social factors are particularly important for problematic behaviour patterns that are widespread, but only provide a partial explanation of HTM behaviours as they typically continue to occur in the face of increasing social pressure to change. A complete model needs to be able to encompass these factors and the social–ecological models can be readily integrated into the ideas presented here (see Chapter 4).

Biological models of addiction fall into several types, including disease models that postulate the breakdown or lack of some important biological mechanism that makes the individual susceptible to under-regulation of the problematic behaviour and natural variation models that postulate a continuum of vulnerability. For example, the balance between inhibitory and excitatory pathways in the brain is a major determinant of individual differences [24, 25]. Additionally, there are theories about the extent to which the behavioural manifestations of biological factors are modifiable. This book is about those problems that are at least partly modifiable by the actions people take, even if they only mitigate rather than completely solve the problems. For example, an obese person may be able to become less obese, but never gain normal weight. I suspect that in other areas, the fixed biological component of variability in behaviour or outcomes is lower than it is for obesity. I am also of the view that we should never concede that there is nothing we can do, or it will become a self-fulfilling prophesy. Where some modification is possible, then it is important to focus on what can be learnt to maximise the desirable change.

Learning-based theories focus on the relationships within the person's microenvironment, and on immediate contingencies, to explain both the process of development of bad habits and the difficulty of reversing them, with biological factors postulated as key determinants of the variability of effects. There are also some differences between these theories as to whether the focus is on learning new skills or on overcoming inappropriate habits (an issue on which I will have more to say later).

Interactions between biological and environmental factors are recognised as important in some areas, most notably weight control, where notions about people's metabolisms being set or reset for feast or famine being a major determinant of propensity to obesity are receiving strong empirical support, not only by identifying genetic mechanisms by which this occurs [26], but also by showing how early experience, including in-utero, can lead to these settings being changed [27]. These kinds of phenomena may set limits on what sorts of behaviour change are possible, and they certainly affect the relationship between behaviour and its consequences. For example, a person whose metabolism is set to famine needs to constrain his/her diet much more to achieve a normal level of weight than a person with a body set for feasting.

The final set of theories focus on cognitive processes and have been the most influential within the field of health psychology. They are typically grounded in human rationality, for example, expectancy-value theories, which see behavioural choice as a joint function of expected consequences of acting and the values attached to each of the anticipated consequences. Relevant theories here include the theory of planned behaviour [28, 29], the theory of trying [30]; the Health Beliefs Model [31–33]; the Transtheoretical Model (TTM) [34, 35]; and more recently, ASE, now renamed I-Change Theory [36, 37], HAPA Health Action Process Approach [38]; and the Rational Addiction model [39], which is highly influential in some areas of economics (see West [16] and Webb *et al.* [40], for other relevant theories). All the above-mentioned theories view intention to change behaviour as in part determined by the decisional balance between the costs and benefits of change, or alternatively of the existing behaviour pattern.

A favourable decisional balance does not automatically lead to behaviour change. For example, many smokers and overweight people know that changing the relevant behaviours is in their best interests, yet they have not changed. Neither is lack of motivation a sufficient explanation, as many have tried repeatedly to change. Something else is going on. Bandura [41–43] tackled this problem with his conceptualisation of self-efficacy, that is, the person's sense of his/her capacity to enact the change.

All of the above theories include versions of self-efficacy, with some focussing on it having a role beyond intentions in the move to action and in maintenance of change. HAPA theory [44] is the most sophisticated, in that it postulates different forms of self-efficacy for initiation, maintenance and recovery from setbacks. The need for any form of self-efficacy implies processes that operate independently of deliberative decision making but which are modifiable by self-regulatory activities, that is, self-efficacy mechanisms, but Bandura does not elaborate much on what these are, and neither do any of the other theories. Bandura [43, 45] does at least provide some ideas as to how behaviours can be formed, with his identification of the importance of vicarious learning or modelling as means by which the skills to engage in new tasks can be developed independent of or in conjunction with trial-and-error attempts to perform them. However, in most cases, acquisition of the necessary behaviours is not the issue; much relapse back to old behaviours happens after some time, after the new behaviours involved can be thought to have been mastered (at least to a basic level of competence). A learning-based theory would suggest that this failure to maintain change is due to overlearning of the inappropriate behaviour pattern as a result of immediate positive contingencies (e.g. the pleasure of puffing on a cigarette or eating a cream cake). Such an explanation suggests that the immediate consequences of action might play a more important role than delayed consequences, a point picked up by Hall and Fong [46] and common to basic economic theories of behaviour: value is discounted as a function of time. This suggests that decisional balance approaches need to consider the temporal dimension of the consequences that are weighed up.

Cognitive theories have also tended to focus on the determinants of choices or the initiation of action, often operationalised as intentions and plans, and assume that all that is required for the maintenance of change is more of the same; that is, they are based on the assumption that the influences on behavioural choices are the same as those affecting long-term maintenance of those choices. The TTM and HAPA are notable exceptions here, but their elaboration of what is required for the maintenance of behaviour is far less developed than for what is involved in the initiation of behaviour.

Another important and related development has been a focus on self-regulatory or self-control processes following the work of Carver and Scheier [47, 48], Baumeister and colleagues [49] and more recently Hall and Fong [46]. These theories focus on what needs to be done to control impulsive behaviour, but are rather less developed about how to change the nature of the impulses and thus the likelihood of behaviour, except via self-control-related mechanisms. In this regard, they can be thought of as alternative conceptualisations of Bandura's [43] ideas around self-efficacy.

Further, most cognitive theories ignore the role of emotional factors. The most notable exception is Leventhal's perceptual-motor theory, now elaborated as the common-sense model [50, 51], which has been influential in understanding reactions to illness, but has been undervalued in health behaviour change. Leventhal focusses on the implications of how emotions are evaluated, an important issue for understanding the maintenance of HTM behaviours.

More recently, theorising has emerged out of research on distortions of optimal decision making that takes emotion and other factors that affect rational decision making seriously [52–57]. For example, framing of possible outcomes in terms of gains or losses affects the choices individuals make. People tend to take risks in search of low-probability high gains (e.g. lotteries), but are averse to risking large losses (thus they use insurance) [56]. One approach to understand these non-conscious influences has been to postulate non-conscious implicit versions of conscious attitudes and beliefs. However, it is known that non-conscious evaluative processes can operate faster than conscious ones [58], suggesting that implicit beliefs are not functionally equivalent to the consciously elaborated ones, as if they were, one would expect the same amount of processing to generate them and thus there should be no speed advantage.

Thinking has changed to acknowledge the evidence that the unconscious processes that affect decision making operate in quite different ways to conscious reasoning, and thus to postulate dual-process models [6]. As noted earlier, the ones most similar to CEOS include RIM theory [18], later versions of Prospect theory [56], and the related, but more comprehensive Nudge theory [20] that focusses on use of communication and environmental change strategies to help reduce biases in decision making created in part by emotional or reactive influences distorting rational choice processes. Dual-process theories seem to divide [5] into those that focus on how unconscious processes shape reasoning, and those more concerned with parallel competing processes, for example, Petty and Caccioppo's [59] distinction between systematic and heuristic processing. The former is closest to the duality proposed in CEOS. The importance of competing processes in relation to strategies for persuasion is discussed in Chapter 5.

The theories that focus on unconscious influences on reasoning parallel CEOS, and in some cases elements from them have been borrowed, especially when focussing on aspects of decision making. A key difference between CEOS and many of these theories is that they focus on the ways non-conscious processes interfere with conscious decision making, while CEOS is more interested in the limits and possibilities of executive processes to change undesirable behaviours, given that they are primarily under the control of operational processes.

The empirical work on which dual-process theories are based includes studies on biases in reasoning about computationally known outcomes/events (e.g. problems in logic). As we will see, there are reasons to believe that some of the heuristics that distort decision making in these cases may actually increase the adaptive value of choices in situations when outcomes are probabilistic. For example, feeling of discomfort can indicate that decisions have not taken into account important factors or mis-weighted them.

Cognitive theories are quite good at predicting decisions to try to change and the initiation of change, but they do less well when used to predict longer term outcomes. There is increasing evidence that some key determinants of the initiation of behaviour change can, at least for quitting smoking, play quite different roles in maintenance [2], For example, in one study, colleagues and I found that wanting to quit, one of the strongest prospective predictors of making quit attempts, was inversely associated with maintenance among those making attempts [1]. That is, the more you want to quit, the more you will try, but the less likely you will be to succeed on any given attempt. Findings like this make it critical to consider the possibility that initiation and maintenance of behaviour involve quite different processes. We need better theories of maintenance.

The most detailed attempt to understand maintenance is Marlatt's [60–62] theory of relapse. It has been complemented more recently by Rothman's [63] distinction between expectancies being the primary influence on initiation, while experiences affect maintenance, and Piasecki and colleagues' [64] tripartite model in which physical withdrawal, stressors/temptations and cessation fatigue make time-shifted contributions to relapse risk. Marlatt and associates take a system-oriented approach, which is largely consistent with the approach taken here. They see environmental cues as key determinants of relapse, along with internal processes, most notably what they call the Abstinence Violation Effect, whereby negative affective evaluations around a single instance of the old behaviour generate relapse. The empirical evidence for this latter effect is not strong; so, there is a need for different mechanisms to explain the fact that lapses commonly trigger full relapse. Beyond this, their theory is largely descriptive, spelling out likely determinants of relapse, rather than specifying how they operate.

Negative experiences clearly predict relapse [65]. However, many of those who change report feeling better overall and net benefits of change [65–67], yet relapse [68, 69]. It appears that relapse has more to do with negative feelings associated with the new behaviour than the overall tenor of experience. Piasecki *et al.*'s [64] three factors are all important, but a range of other factors are missing, such as what leads to greater withdrawal.

The limitations of taking any one of the above-mentioned theoretical approaches in isolation are becoming most apparent in the area of tobacco control, perhaps because this is the area with the most research. Environmental factors are clearly important. For example, the prevalence of smoking has declined markedly over a period of decades in countries that have systematically tried to discourage use, such as Australia [70]. However, theories that focus on social determinants are moot when it comes to understanding individual differences in quitting success, or more generally why some people continue to smoke and others have given up, except to the extent that they belong to identifiable social groups who are disadvantaged in ways relevant to the persistence of smoking. Help either in the form of quit smoking medications or effective cognitive behavioural counselling results in higher success rates. Further those seeking help tend to be more successful than those who are proactively recruited to try to quit [71]. Both these suggest that elements of motivation and skill are both important. Unfortunately, at this point, our ability to predict relapse is otherwise poor.

Most smokers want to quit and nearly all acknowledge the adverse health effects and that they would be better off if they did not smoke. Their continuing smoking is not for lack of trying to quit. On an average, smokers make around one failed quit attempt a year and at least as many more plans to quit are aborted [71]. The most recent attempt is for a majority not their longest; thus, there is no clear tendency for attempts to get longer before finally succeeding [72]. Inconsistent with learning-based theories, quitting smoking does not seem to be something that people get better and better at before finally succeeding. Further, as noted earlier, aspects of motivation to quit, which are strongly predictive of making quit attempts, are inversely related to success among those who try [1]. These findings are hard to explain. It could be that those most motivated to quit are using relatively ineffective strategies, or they are smokers for whom quitting is genuinely more difficult: if they want to that much and keep on trying and failing; it is very plausible that the task is too hard, they are and heavily addicted. Both explanations point to these smokers needing more effective help.

The above-mentioned analysis suggests that failure to change can be thought of as due to the strength of operational processes supporting the addictive behaviour (genetic or acquired, often thought of as the core of addiction) being stronger than self-regulatory capacity (some combination of poor strategy and lack of self-control) and perhaps interactions between the two. This raises the question of whether a person's beliefs about his/her level of addiction can provide feedback to increase the strength of operational processes that underpin the addiction, and similarly whether different forms of thinking could lead to reductions.

Core elements of CEOS

CEOS has a major focus on the role of non-cognitive (or non-language-based) functions as well as on cognitive functions. It deals specifically with the reality that prolonged periods including multiple attempts are potentially required for the stabilisation of behaviour change, things cognitive theories neglect and which are critical to understanding change. It also considers the way volitional forces interact with non-volitional ones, concepts adapted from self-regulation models [47, 48]. CEOS is designed to be both a theory of self-regulation in the face of difficulty, and of how agents can act to modify both contextual and conditioned factors to reduce self-regulatory demands and automate, as far as possible, desired behaviour patterns. At the core of CEOS is the idea that the person is best conceptualised as consisting of two interrelated systems that jointly, in conjunction with environmental contingencies, determine human behaviour (Figure 1.1). As noted earlier, the two systems that are at the core of CEOS are the OS and the ES. Some key features of the two systems are listed in Table 1.1.

Within the individual, the OS is the locus of action. The OS is reactive to the environment and functions through associative mechanisms typified by conditioning paradigms. It is hierarchically organised and faster acting when it does not need to engage higher levels of the hierarchy in decision making. It can operate independent of conscious awareness, and indeed it operates more efficiently this way. It is primarily influenced by environmental contingencies in relation to its internal settings: innate, acquired and dynamically changing (e.g. hunger and desire for stimulation) and of relationships between the organism and the environment (e.g. perceived threats). I prefer not to describe it as impulsive [18, 19] as this implies that it acts in ways that are not in the person's best interests. The OS has developed to be adaptive, but it does not operate by logical analysis.

Table 1.1 Core-defining characteristics of the two systems

Operational System (OS)	Executive System (ES)
Primary determinant of behaviour	Decisions to behave only result in action if consistent with OS action tendencies
Bottom-up processing	Top-down processing
Processing occurs automatically, much out of consciousness	Conscious of OS inputs, memories, goals, beliefs and some steps of processing
Reactive to environment	Can be reflective, proactive and deliberative
Generates action to reduce discrepancies between current and target need states	Can also act to achieve progress towards linguistically encoded goals for the future

The ES uses inputs from the OS and from language-based representations of the world and can apply rule-based logic in pursuit of articulated goals. It is largely conscious, and is, or can be, goal directed and rule governed. In evolutionary terms, the ES emerged out of higher level functioning of the OS. It analyses inputs from the OS, memories of events and ideas. Its original function was to resolve conflicts within the OS, acting as a higher order part of the OS. The capacity of language has transcended that original goal, thereby enabling alternative paths to be pursued (to those evoked by OS processes). The ES uses conscious deliberation via language to build stories (both explanations and justifications), which it can use to decide on actions which, in turn, act as stimuli for the OS to act. It generates action tendencies in one of two ways: either referenced to goals that have either emerged from the stories and expectations it has produced and/or from processing to resolve competing action tendencies that are referred up from the OS. The ES is the locus of whatever self-regulatory capacity the individual has [47, 49]. The primary role of the ES is as a problem solver, not a long-term monitor and self-regulator. It works best when it can 'delegate' long-term tasks back to the OS (i.e. automate them), including the institutionalisation of behaviour change.

All behaviour is implemented through the OS, and all but some of that which is experienced as volitional is actually initiated by it. The ES, in an analogous way to the CEO (Chief Executive Officer) of a large company, only sets the broad agenda. The ES acts through the OS; so, lower level action tendencies need to be compatible for ES-generated action tendencies to result in behaviour. The ES has no independent capacity to generate action, but can act to inhibit or stimulate action tendencies of the OS, which combined with other inputs on the OS, can tip the balance in determining what the person will do; that is, the ES can try to get the person to act or not, but is dependent on the OS being responsive to determine whether its intentions are enacted. This corresponds with the company CEO who exercises some control over what the company does, but only within limits he/she, if wise, knows not to exceed. The company has to be ready to act on CEO directives or a process of convincing the organisation of the need for the change is required. The analogy becomes strained because the OS controls what the ES perceives in ways the company cannot for the CEO. The CEO has some capacity to perceive independently (i.e. go out and form independent views, something that is common when a new CEO is brought into an organisation from outside).

The formation (or existence) of independent views by the CEO is, however, in some ways analogous to a person adopting a new story to try to explain his/her current situation and thus what he/she need to do. Part of the utility of this analogy is that systems theory has demonstrated direct equivalences between comparable elements at different levels of systems [73]; so, seeing the operation of the OS through the eyes of how an organisation operates allows us to see, through an analysis of these mechanisms, analogues of aspects of OS functioning that are hidden within the individual, that is, are not directly accessible by our ESs. Thus, the analogy may also encourage a more systematic understanding of similarities and differences between the functioning of organisations and individuals.

Viewing the relationship between the OS and ES using different analogies can provide different insights. An alternative analogy is of the rider (ES) on the elephant (OS) [7]. The rider needs to work with the elephant as he/she cannot force it to act as he/she wants. Thus, he/she has to cajole and reward the behaviours he/she wants until the elephant comes to want to respond to the prompts of the rider as if this is what it wants. This analogy may make it easier to think about the collective outputs of the OS, but the organisational analogy is more useful for helping to think through the mechanisms by which the OS works and influences the ES. One area where the elephant analogy falls down is that the OS has greater direct influence over the goals of the ES than the elephant does over the rider. The elephant influences the subsequent actions of the rider through its behaviour, while the OS both does this and also influences the ES directly through internal signals it passes up about its internal states and what it attends to in the environment. The elephant has less influence over what the rider perceives.

Conceptual underpinnings

The central reason for reconceptualising human behaviour as the interaction between two systems rather than of one complex system is the extraordinary nature of the change in potential that occurs once behaviour can be directed towards the attainment of future goals, instead of being confined to optimisation of action in the present. Goals are ideas about the future that can guide action. They can range from simple choices, through to life goals [74].

CEOS is grounded in a form of emergent materialism [75], in that it postulates that virtually all behaviour and all experience has biological underpinnings, but that the complexity of the organism results in novel properties emerging (Box 1.2). These novel properties are encapsulated in the emergent functionality of the ES. There is a brief discussion about the biological limits on what may be possible for the ES to achieve towards the end of this chapter.

CEOS postulates that sensory inputs affect behaviours, including volitional behaviours, independent of their representation in consciousness as well as via conscious awareness [58]. Consciousness is only required for ES-directed activity. Some OS-controlled activity is monitored by the ES, and at other times, the OS is primed to trigger the ES to attend by such things as the novelty of the situation, uncertainty about appropriate action or specific situations the ES has cued the OS to alert it to. Where ES input is available, it can act to override OS tendencies or make a decision that resolves OS uncertainty, but to generate behaviour, it needs to prime the OS to generate appropriate action tendencies.

All advances in knowledge and most human cultural activities are attributable to the ES (experienced as our selves). Even artistic endeavours require ES direction informed by OS impulses (Box 1.3). A person's identity is the way they are represented in the ES's conceptualisation of self in the world. Humans have the capacity, through language, to build a conceptual model of the world in the form of stories about it (things scientists call theories) [76] that has given them the capacity to mould many aspects of the world to their ideas. These conceptualisations (or stories) can be relatively invariant in the face of the ever-changing flow of experiences generated by the interaction between environmental conditions and internal states. They can also shift suddenly under conditions where one story is abandoned in favour of an alternative. The ES has the capacity to guide action in ways that reflect these stories, rather than in ways that are determined by the situation and the related conditioned responses, or innate action tendencies, that is, the factors determining OS-based action. Consciousness is essential for ideas to form, and for them to exhibit continuity in the mind and, moreover, this continuity is necessary for executive capacity to emerge. Consciousness creates the conditions for genuinely goal-directed behaviour because it allows the development of a model of what might happen in future, considered in the present moment, and the goal becomes the main proximal determinant of action [74]. The existence of goals gives the appearance of the future determining the present, but the goals actually exist in linguistic space and precede the actions they stimulate. Or as Bandura [77] put it:

> The capacity for intentional and purposive action is rooted in symbolic activity. Future events cannot be causes of present motivation and action. However, by being represented cognitively in the present, conceived future events are converted into current motivations and regulators of behaviour. (see p. 248)

Box 1.2 Emergent materialism

Emergent materialism [75] postulates that virtually all behaviour (except pseudo-behaviours like falling which can be determined by physical forces alone) and all experience has biological underpinnings, but that the complexity of the organism results in novel properties emerging. Experience is an emergent property of biology, while behaviour is mainly an emergent property of the interaction between biology and environment (context). Behaviour, however, can also be produced directly by biology (uncued behaviour), or purely as a result of physical forces (e.g. falling, the direct effects of being hit or pushed), although we often do not consider such events as behaviour. While experience needs to be able to be explained in terms of biology, this can only happen after the event. As such, for any predictive analysis of experience (beyond general tendencies), a higher level of analysis is required – specifically one that references experiences and their relationships with other aspects of the world people interact in. This is why it is wrong to argue that once biological correlates of some behaviour or experience are discovered that psychological explanations become redundant. Understanding the biological underpinnings may allow our thinking to become more refined, and certainly more grounded, and it can lead to biologically based strategies for changing functioning, but ultimately it cannot provide a complete explanation of why people behave as they do.

Box 1.3   An author's reflection

This book is (necessarily) written from the perspective of the ES, the subsystem through which people consciously reflects on their lives. Our challenge is to understand (inevitably using volitional processes) the roles of the non-volitional processes on which the volitional system is built and elaborated because it is the OS that constitutes the main limitation on our (ES) capacity to act as we would ideally like to do (along with tangible environmental constraints). Because a subsystem cannot completely stand outside itself, it means that we cannot have direct knowledge of the genesis of our consciousness. Further, the ES does not have an unbiased or uniformly privileged view of the OS. Godel's theorem demonstrates that any self-referential model or theory is necessarily incomplete; that is, there are some things that are true that cannot be explained by the theory. I take this to mean that as self-reflective beings, there will always be some uncertainty in the ways we relate to the world.

Even if we could collect all the information we identified as being needed to solve a problem, collecting it would change the world; so, even then our knowledge would either be incomplete or out of date. We are fated to live with uncertainly, but we should at least be able to roughly map out the limits of what we can know, and increase its fidelity with the underlying reality, even though it will never be complete. Increased understanding cannot be achieved by reasoning alone, it requires continuous engagement in a process of experimenting with reality to complement our theoretical understanding (a scientific approach or its day-to-day analogue of reflective action). If we are to better shape the way our ES engages with the world (i.e. self-regulate), part of our increased understanding needs to be of the sorts of influences OS processes and levels of functioning can have on executive functioning, both those signalled to the ES and those that have effects in other ways. This understanding is needed for thinking about the kinds of ES processes and environmental influences that could be modified to influence OS processes in ways that enhance the probability of desired actions.

Thus, ES goals (i.e. consciously formed ones) can have functional effects, becoming a part of the context-determining action. It should be stressed that goals are only one form of influence on behaviour: environmental conditions and OS processes also contribute to determine what behaviour will eventuate. When our subsequent behaviour is congruent with ES goals, we think of that behaviour as freely chosen, as compared to the situation when competing impulses sum to produce action that is inconsistent with ES goals, which we experience as an absence of control. We act by creating stories that elicit virtual environments and virtual objects within them (goal objects) that stimulate our OS to act in ways consistent with the story instead of responding to the balance of forces in the real world. However, this only happens when the emotional impetus on the OS to act in this way is stronger than the impetus coming from the external environment in interaction with internal need states.

The OS operates differently; it is a combination of trait-like response tendencies and variable need states that generate impulses to act in conjunction with conditioned or inherent reactions to external inputs. The apparent goals of the OS are emergent properties of contextual factors interacting with the state of the organism. OS *goals* do not orient behaviour or act as a driver of behaviour; they are merely an ES-generated post hoc description of what happened.

The generation of behaviour

HTM behaviours are behaviours where there is a major divergence between the reactive tendencies of the OS and the relevant goals of the ES. That is, the ES has decided a goal is desirable, but the OS is not sufficiently cued to enact the relevant behaviours in at least some of the situations where it is required. This results in a contest between the ES (what we think we should do) and the OS (what our bodies in context want us to do). The ability to choose *should* over *want* defines self-regulatory capacity, which involves capacity to both maximise the likelihood of making the most adaptive choices, and to implement and sustain the behaviours that result from those choices.

CEOS differs from the Social Cognitive Theory of Bandura [43] and other behaviourally oriented theories, in that it explicitly postulates reciprocal influences within the person (i.e. between OS and ES), as well as between the person and the environment as determinants of behaviour, making behaviour change a shifting function of four broad sets of interacting determinants (rather than Bandura's three) (Figure 1.2). These are:

(a) the nature of the behaviour change required (the challenge), that is, the specific behaviours to change that are chosen. This choice can range from a discrete behavioural choice such as quitting smoking, to a more complex lifestyle change (e.g. eating a healthy diet);
(b) the context or the environment (particularly social, but also physical) in which the behaviour is to take place and how it is changing;
(c) operations of the OS (characteristics of the person, both innate and acquired, such as sensitivity to stimuli and past conditioning); and of
(d) the ES, via the person's conceptualisation of the behaviour change challenge in relation to what is desirable, something influenced both by his/her analysis of implications of the behaviour and of what they want for themselves (their conceptualisation of themselves as part of their life story).

The other elaboration of this model from Bandura's triangular model is of the specific role of behavioural pre-requisites; that is, tools and other objects in the environment that are consumed or used for some forms of action. Thus, one can't smoke without a cigarette (or other similar product) or eat without food. Tools need

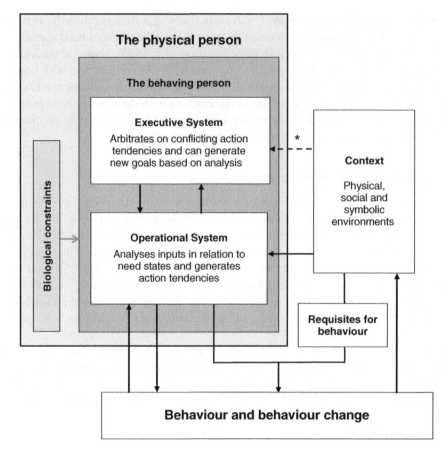

Figure 1.2 A more detailed version of Figure 1.1, which emphasises the impacts of biological constraints and acknowledges the interactive implications of needing or using things in the environment to act with (requisites).

* This link is actually through the OS; it parallels the sensory reactive pathway through the OS, but as it is functionally different. It is depicted this way to highlight the fact that symbolic aspects of the environment (e.g. written or spoken language) only affect the OS once they have been decoded by the ES. NB: This does not apply to physical manifestations of the signals, which influence operational processes directly.

not be necessary, they can just facilitate action, for example, eating utensils can facilitate eating.

The way a person's executive thinks about a problem behaviour, including the compatibility of his/her account with the underlying and changing reality (both environment and OS), is important in determining whether they can change volitionally or not. Other factors include the choices they make and the priority and level of commitment to their chosen goals. These affect the extent to which their script or plan for action correctly identifies the key tasks required for change to occur. To date, most of the theorising for behaviour change has focussed on an understanding of the influences of the environmental context on behaviour, while the ways the OS responds have been relatively ignored (see Chapter 3). One important contribution of CEOS is to correct this imbalance. In this, it shares similarities with a range of theories that focus on mindfulness and/or are concerned with how we interpret our emotional experiences [50, 78].

The key tasks of behaviour change are to identify desirable changes and to work to implement and maintain them. This involves some mix of modifying the environment to change the pattern of cues towards the desired behaviour, reconditioning the OS to be more supportive of change, reframing thinking to support change and more generally enhancing self-regulatory capacity.

Capacity of the ES

The duopoly between OS and ES is an emergent property of a multi-level control system [3], with the lower referenced to the environment of the moment (the OS). The ES emerges out of the higher levels of this system (with capacities for long-term memory) to represent aspects of its internal functioning and to conceptualise what should be, could be, or was. The ES requires large amounts of OS processing to generate the small number of ideas that it can hold in consciousness at any one time and relate them both to each other and to other inputs from the OS (i.e. relevant perceptions, feelings and action impulses). This is because the ideas the ES needs to manipulate in thought are built up from higher order OS processes, a much more complex task than registering and reacting to what is in the environment. When the OS has a high level of other demands on it, some of this capacity can be diverted to dealing with more immediate priorities, limiting capacity for analysis of what is desirable in the longer term, or what is logically consistent.

Both the OS and ES can adapt and change, albeit in different ways, and both are subject to exhaustion if overused (either too much and/or too long). Processing capacity can also be diverted away to other priorities by mechanisms of attention, which can range from lower level processes sensitive to the relevance of environmental stimuli, or via ES choices. Either or both can result in reduced capacity for processing information relevant to any given task. Capacity limitation in the ES is more likely to be apparent than that of the OS that underpins it, in part because it is supported by the part of the OS that requires the most information-processing capacity. Limits on information processing constrain the capacity of the ES to exercise self-control, increasing the risk of relapse. Maintaining commitment to a goal in the face of changing environmental conditions and associated emotional reactions can be difficult when conditions trigger attentional mechanisms that take up processing capacity. Further, there is no fail-safe mechanism for ensuring the resumption of resistance once diversions have been dealt with. This analysis is consistent with subjective experiences: when distracted from any complex task, it is often difficult to pick up from where you were afterwards, indeed unless re-cued, the train of thought can be forgotten.

The more things there are to attend to, the less executive capacity that gets allocated to any one thing or the less time allocated, both of which will reduce the capacity to make decisions. Considerations of goals and commitments are particularly vulnerable to being neglected as they usually lack the benefit of being triggered into consciousness directly by operational processes (environmental cues or feelings), instead being reliant on triggers from other executive processes. The reality is that we spend most of our time attending to the priorities that demand our attention. Among other things, this explains why, once a goal for action has been established; efforts at behaviour change tend to be episodic rather than continual. The challenge is to create conditions so that we focus on our goals at appropriate times. This is particularly important for the maintenance of behaviour as relapse is likely unless self-control mechanisms are initiated in those situations where there is a net tendency to resume an unwanted behaviour.

Initiation versus maintenance of behaviour

CEOS postulates that ES processes are primary for the initiation of change (except those solely in response to a changed environment), but the OS plays a much more important role in the maintenance of change, both directly and by influencing ES choices.

After change is initiated, the ES remains important for the maintenance of goals and for self-management. It can both exercise self-control and create conditions to assist in the retraining of the OS to be better prepared to act in goal-congruent ways. Before change, the task is primarily cognitive (ES); to have the person persuade themselves to make the change and choose an appropriate time to start. By contrast, the main task after change is to maintain the new behaviour pattern. This involves actively persevering in the effort, at least until the OS is recalibrated to minimise the likelihood that cues (environmental and/or internal) will trigger a relapse to the previously highly OS cued behaviour. ES processes can change settings (reference points around which it and the OS operates), including thresholds to trigger its engagement (attention) when undesirable action tendencies occur that may require more than OS processes to inhibit. The very contemplation of change can evoke emotional (OS) reactions, and this can act as an additional force to inhibit further consideration of change. OS processes can block consideration of change or act as barriers to immediate action when the idea is considered. This OS reactance needs to be overcome for ES-directed action to occur. The need for the OS to coordinate the generation of behaviour explains why, even though people may want to change when asked and may make frequent decisions to act, they tend to make far fewer attempts to change than might be expected. For example, smokers, even those who are highly motivated to change, make decisions to quit much more often than they follow through and actually initiate quit attempts [71, 79]. They have been unable to provide sufficient impetus to overcome OS reactance.

CEOS also postulates that the level of motivation or net reasons for action that are sufficient for the initiation of action are sufficient to maintain behaviour, indeed the motivational threshold for relapse is lower than for initiation. However, net motivation fluctuates markedly, largely as a result of OS reactions, and it is this fluctuation that creates the main proximal determinant of relapse along with fluctuations in self-control. Unfortunately, these two processes tend to co-occur, as it is in moments of stress that urges to resume some behaviours are greatest, and the stress also diverts self-control capacity from either resisting the undesirable behaviour or initiating a new behaviour to deal with the source of the problem, thus making relapse more likely.

The relationships between the two systems

CEOS does not conceive of OS actions as distorting the way the ES thinks, unlike some other theories; for example, Prospect theory [56], rather it focusses on the ways the ES needs to act to create a context to get the OS to enact its decisions. The ES has evolved as a mechanism for improving the adaptiveness of OS actions, but can still be unduly influenced by OS processes. However, rationality-based ES processes can also be misled and can lead to inappropriate actions as well. This raises the issue of how the individual decides when to go with what the rational argument concludes is appropriate, when to go with gut feeling, and how to decide between competing arguments or stories.

The ongoing dynamic of the interrelationships between the two systems means that teasing out what leads to the most adaptive outcomes is something that is only ultimately achievable through observations of outcomes. We as a culture have learnt to trust certain ideas, and then if circumstances mean they lose their predictive capacity, to shift to new ideas. However, this process is slow and error ridden. Along with reactions and advice of others, OS reactions are a key element of signalling possible problems in our ES-based analysis. However, this signalling can give the wrong message in cases where the OS is creating impulses towards undesirable responses. While OS reactions can and do sometimes leads us astray, it is important to reiterate that for the most part the OS does a good job.

The ES has the capacity to generate action tendencies or scripts that are designed to achieve goals that are oriented towards the future, while the OS only acts for the moment. This means that the main conflict is often between the contingencies of the moment and the potential of the future. This suggests that approaches to decision making, which focus on the balance between the pros and cons of behaviour, are missing something important. For any given set of conditions, the OS produces a net action tendency towards one behaviour (except in cases of extreme conflict), and, similarly, executive functions can come up with a rational appraisal of the net costs and benefits of options in the long term (outcome expectancies). CEOS postulates that it is the balance between the immediate consequences and the longer term outcome expectancies that is the core of decisional balance. This framing implies that immediate consequences will have some priority over longer term consequences, and explains some of the effects of temporal discounting, along with conceptualisation of the value of outcomes when they are delayed.

Story creation within the ES

CEOS has a focus on conceptualising problems in ways that optimise strategies for change, that is, to increase the likelihood of success and/or reduce the difficulty of the task.

Humans have the capacity to imagine the future and reflect on the past. We organise these ideas and thoughts into stories. Stories are the vehicle for our capacity to transcend our environment in useful ways, including our extraordinary creativity. The roles of stories are elaborated throughout the book, but at this point it is sufficient to say they play roles in providing explanations of what has happened, including justifications for past behaviour, and in evaluating and reflecting on past efforts and their consequences. Also critical here is the capacity to create a 'change story', that is a story that provides both a justification for change (an imagined future) and a plan of action as to how it can be achieved. A compelling justification for goal-directed action is important for generating associations necessary to create adequate OS priming for the behaviour to occur, and eventually, to support the conditions that maintain the change. The plan or script for action is critical for spelling out what to do and when to do it.

The stories and goals people come up with can be their own creations, but they are often ones that their culture has encouraged them to adopt. The range of stories within a pluralist society is often greater for HTM behaviours as it tends to include stories justifying inaction as well as those supporting action. Sharing and discussing stories is one means by which they can be refined and validated as useful. Evaluation of the extent to which stories inform about the normativeness of behaviours is also important in influencing decisions about change (see Chapter 4).

Stories vary in their applicability to specific contexts. Because of the ever-changing reality in which people have to operate, stories, particularly old stories, can lose their relevance and thus utility, both as explanations and/or as scripts for change, potentially resulting in inappropriate choices and failure to achieve goals. This means there can be a need to modify stories as circumstances change, but for HTM behaviours those circumstances include resistance to change; so, there are risks that changes might including rationales for inaction or relapse (see Chapter 3).

Biological constraints

The functions hypothesised for the OS and ES must have biological underpinnings. These are beyond the scope of this volume to specify; however, I believe that nothing postulated in the theory is inconsistent with what we know about biology. The main reason for not discussing biological underpinnings is that all behaviour, including volitional behaviour, has biological underpinnings; so, demonstrating a link to biology does not, of itself, say anything about the plasticity of behaviour.

It is assumed, as a starting point, that all human behaviour is potentially malleable, but that the determinants of some behaviours are more strongly physiologically constrained than for others and that the levels of constraint vary across individuals (due to genetics and/or irreversible past experiences). Thus, the ease of behaviour change varies, and at the extremes, there may be cases where for all practical purposes, physical interventions to change biological processes are either necessary or more efficient than behavioural interventions. It is possible that advances in genetics and cognitive neuroscience will increasingly specify differences between individuals that are innate/acquired, and which are impossible or difficult to change by behavioural means. This variability can include general tendencies to behave (e.g. levels of inhibitory processes) and behaviour-specific constraints. However, until limits on flexibility are established, it remains sensible to assume that forms of change that at least some people are capable of are achievable by all (or most), and to try to identify more effective behavioural strategies to achieve change among those who find it most difficult.

The perspective taken here is to theorise in ways that push the limits for behavioural interventions. Physiological interventions are considered where they shed light on underlying behavioural mechanisms or potentially complement behaviour change strategies. Biological solutions are particularly important in the area of drug addiction, as substitutes for more harmful forms of drugs, or to reduce the experienced pleasures of recreational drugs. Biological interventions are becoming an increasingly part of the solution for obesity, including surgical interventions like lap-band surgery to reduce the size of the stomach, and liposuction. Whether these interventions represent a failure of our attempts at behavioural solutions or necessary interventions to deal with otherwise unmodifiable problems remains an open question.

It is not just behaviours that may be amenable to behavioural interventions, some medical conditions can be reversed behaviourally. For example, eating too much and becoming obese can affect metabolism, resulting in diabetes, which used to be thought to be irreversible. However, lifestyle change in the form of a better and more constrained diet can reverse key features of diabetes [80, 81].

Variability in capacity is not the only biological constraint on behaviour change. Variability in susceptibility to adverse consequences of behaviour is also important, as it is an important potential source of variation in motivation to make changes. For example, there is an increasing evidence that biological factors, both innate and those which can be set or reset in utero or with early experience, can determine whether the body tends to conserve excess energy inputs as fat or to expend them [82], thereby affecting weight gain independent of calorific input. It is also possible, although as far as I know not proved, that behavioural aspects of food seeking and consumption could be similarly influenced by these biological mechanisms. Thus, a famine-programmed person may also be more sensitive to food-related cues; not only being prone to eat more, but also to put on more weight per unit of input. This would help explain why in a culture of excess (for food), some people end up extremely fat while others don't.

However, people need to know if they are at higher risk, something that may require biological indicators being found, if action is to be initiated prior to manifestation of the problem. Biological variability can also influence capacity to self-regulate psychoactive substances. For example, someone whose cognitive capacities are most disrupted by any given level of a drug will become impaired more quickly and thus have less capacity to regulate their consumption, and thus may be more prone to intoxication, and associated adverse effects.

The variability both in susceptibility to adverse effects and in capacity to change behaviour means that one size fits all solutions are unlikely to work. Where biological factors strongly predispose, there will be greater limits on the capacity of behavioural factors to produce change.

Elaboration of CEOS theory

CEOS theory, through its component parts, is designed to explain moment-to-moment influences on behaviour, and to predict the nature and form of longer term changes. Understanding lies at three levels of organisation: (i) theories of the reactive organism acting in its environment; (ii) theories of how stories, underpinned by language, create a new set of referents for behaviour, and how these compete with OS-generated action tendencies to influence behaviour; and (iii) how actions of individuals and other agents interact to create social norms, and a process of social change that typically occurs over a longer time-scale than change within individuals. The primary focus of this book is on the middle of these three, ES functioning, but with a strong focus on how it interacts with OS functioning. There is less focus on longer term societal change, but there is a focus on the implications of the changing nature of the population who engage in HTM behaviours. See Young et al. [83] for an analysis of how the broader, more normative system operates and the role of individuals in working for change.

The central feature of CEOS is the distinction between the OS which is reactive to the environment, and the ES which is built on the OS, but also uses conceptual analysis of what is desirable and feasible to influence behaviour. Key secondary features of CEOS, constructed on the basis of research evidence, are differences between the determinants of the initiation and determinants of the maintenance of behaviour. Further, as a result of the predictability of repeated failures, as the prevalence of the behaviour problem changes, the characteristics of the population engaging in that behaviour must be changing. The rest of this book elaborates on aspects of the theory and its implications.

The next chapter (Chapter 2) spells out characteristics of HTM behaviours, both hard to reduce and hard to sustain, and how they differ from other behaviours and each other. These two complementary forms of HTM behaviours represent the two kinds of discord between operational and executive processes.

Chapter 3 elaborates on the conceptual advantages of the distinction between the OS and ES. It explains how the non-volitional OS works by rapidly processing information from the environment and (more slowly) information on internal states, resulting in the generation of action tendencies, and/or information being sent up to the ES in the form of perceptions, feelings and urges. The OS is the primary determinant of behaviour. Its operations can be modified through conditioning and to a limited extent by some forms of executive inputs. A key insight is that negative affect drives behaviour, even when non-contingent; however, only contingent positive experiences influence subsequent behaviour via operational processes.

Chapter 3 also explores how the ES works and its various roles and functions. The ES can analyse the implications of the moment in relation to future possibilities, and uses stories to motivate the OS to act appropriately and try to organise behaviour towards conceptually formed goals. It focusses on two aspects of self-regulation: self-control and self-reorganisation (recontextualising). The chapter finishes with a detailed comparison of CEOS and RIM [18], a dual-process theory that shares some common features, but potentially theoretically interesting differences.

Chapter 4 considers the role of the environment, and how and when societal and environmental changes can be used to influence personal change and the limitations of this for HTM behaviour It also considers the kinds of environmental changes that can be generated by societal forces.

Chapter 5 drills down into the key conceptual aspects of executive functioning. It considers the importance of the way issues are framed, in terms of both what is considered relevant, and within that, the framing of information that influences its interpretation. It highlights the importance of organising ideas in a quasi-hierarchical manner to simplify analysis, and of cognitively simple arguments that avoid negations as these are processed differently by the two systems. It makes a key distinction between goal formation and the development of scripts to enact change, and focusses on what influences the desirability and perceived feasibility of change and how these facts vary from goal formation to script development and enactment. It argues that decisional balance for action is a balance between long-term outcome expectancies and the net experiences of the moment, in the context of the priority for action in relation to other life issues.

Chapter 6 considers the structure of the change process, focussing first on individual attempts to change, then considering how these accumulate over time to change the nature of the population of those who have not yet changed. It separates out the processes of goal formation from the development and implementation of specific attempts, of which there are typically many. Goals only influence behaviour when brought to mind; thus, there is a need for mechanisms to ensure they are cued to occur at appropriate times, especially for HTM behaviours that are not naturally cued. Determinants of behaviour change differ for persuasion, initiation of action and maintenance of change. Determinants are organised around factors, influencing the desirability and feasibility of the behaviour change. Important concepts developed include the importance of the prioritisation of actions, the nature of commitments to act, and the nature of different kinds of evaluation/feedback loops.

Chapter 7 considers strategies for behaviour change: providing better or more timely information for Executive processes; otherwise improving the efficiency of executive functioning, in particular, using implementation intentions; using executive processes and/or external agents to facilitate reorienting operational processes to be less strongly cued towards unwanted behaviours and more strongly cued to desired ones; and changing the environment; so, the pattern of cues is more conducive to desired behaviours.

The final chapter (Chapter 8) brings together considerations for research, including implications for measurement and key researchable differences in CEOS's predictions compared with other theories.

Summary

This chapter introduces CEOS theory, a theory designed to understand why some behaviour patterns are hard to maintain. At the core of CEOS is the idea that the person is best conceptualised as two interrelated systems that jointly, in conjunction with environmental contingencies, determine human behaviour. These two systems are a more basic OS that responds adaptively to the contingencies of the moment (both internal needs and environmental conditions), and an ES that allows volitional actions in response to articulated goals. The theory focusses on how we can use volitional processes to reshape behaviour away from the contingencies of the moment, and as such is a dual-process theory. This framing helps to understand why the determinants of the initiation of behaviour differ from those of maintenance, and why the latter task is so difficult. CEOS is designed to be a theory of self-regulation in the face of difficulty by self-control and/or self-reorganisation.

References

1. Borland R, Yong HH, Balmford J et al. Motivational factors predict quit attempts but not maintenance of smoking cessation: Findings from the International Tobacco Control Four country project. *Nicotine & Tobacco Research*. 2010; **12**(Supplement 1): S4–S11.
2. Vangeli E, Stapeleton J, Smit ES et al. Predictors of attempts to stop smoking and their success in adult general population samples: A systematic review. *Addiction*. 2011; **106**: 2110–2121.
3. Powers WT. *Behavior: The Control of Perception*. Aldine de Gruyter: Chicago, 1973.
4. Powers WT. *Behavior: The Control of Perception*. 2nd expanded edn. Originally published 1973. Benchmark Publications: New Canaan, CT, 2005.
5. Evans JS. Dual-processing accounts of reasoning, judgment, and social cognition. *Annual Review of Psychology*. 2008; **59**: 255–278.
6. Smith ER & DeCoster J. Dual-process models in social and cognitive psychology: Conceptual integration and links to underlying memory systems. *Personality and Social Psychology Review*. 2000; **4**: 108–131.
7. Haidt J. *The Happiness Hypothesis: Finding Modern Truth in Ancient Wisdom*. Basic Books: New York, 2006.
8. James W. *The Principles of Psychology*. Dover: New York, 1950.
9. Pavlov IP. *Conditioned Reflexes: An Investigation of the Psyiological Activity of the Cerebral Cortex*. Dover: New York, 1960.
10. Razran G. Ivan Petrovich Pavlov. *International Encyclopedia of the Social Sciences*. Macmillan: New York, 1968.

11. Gray JA. *Pavlov's Typology*. Elsevier: Amsterdam, 1964.
12. MacMillan M. *Freud Evaluated the Completed Arc*. Elsevier Science Publishers B.V.: North-Holland, 1991: 430–506.
13. Watson J. *Behaviorism*. Revised edn. University of Chicago Press: Chicago, 1930.
14. Skinner B. *Science and Human Behavior*. Macmillan: New York, 1953.
15. Kimble G. *Hilgard and Marquis' Conditioning and Learning*. 2nd edn. Appleton Century Crofts: New York, 1961.
16. West R. & Brown J. *Theory of Addiction*. 2nd ed. Wiley; Chichester, UK, 2013.
17. West R. PRIME Theory. [http://www.primetheory.com] [updated 27 April 2013].
18. Strack F & Deutsch R. Reflective and impulsive determinants of social behaviour. *Personality and Social Psychology Bulletin*. 2004; 8: 220–247.
19. Hofmann W, Friese M & Wiers RW. Impulsive versus reflective influences on health behaviour: A theoretical framework and empirical review. *Health Psychology Review*. 2008; 2: 111–137.
20. Thaler RH & Sunstein CR. *Nudge: Improving Decisions About Health, Wealth and Happiness*. Yale University Press: New Haven, 2008.
21. World Health Organization. *The Social Determinants of Health: The Solid Facts*. 2nd edn. Wilkinson R & Marmot M (eds.). World Health Organization: Europe, 2003.
22. Stuckler D, Siegel K, DeVogli R *et al*. Sick individuals, sick populations: The social determinants of chronic disease, Chapter 2. In: Stuckler D & Siegel K (eds.) *Sick Societies: Responding to the Global Challenge of Chronic Disease*. Oxford University Press: Oxford, UK, 2011: 26–62.
23. Sallis J, Owen N & Fisher E. Ecological models of health behavior. In: Glanz K, Rimer B & Viswanath K (eds.) *Health Behavior and Health Education Theory, Research and Practice*. 4th edn. Jossey-Bass A Wiley Imprint: San Francisco, USA, 2008: 465–485.
24. Gray JA. *The Neuropsychology of Anxiety*. Oxford University Press: New York, USA, 1987.
25. Carver CS & White TL. Behavioral inhibition, behavioral activation, and affective responses to impending reward and punishment: The BIS/BAS scales. *Journal of Personality and Social Psychology*. 1994; 67: 319–333.
26. Neel JV. The "thrifty genotype" in 1998. *Nutrition Reviews*. 1999; 57(5 Pt 2): S2–S9.
27. Barker DJ. The developmental origins of adult disease. *Journal of the American College of Nutrition*. 2004; 23: 588S–595S.
28. Ajzen I. From intentions to actions: A theory of planned behavior. In: Kuhl J & Beckmann J (eds.) *Action Control: From Cognition to Behavior*. Springer-Verlag: Berlin, Heidelberg/New York, 1985.
29. Ajzen I. The theory of planned behavior. *Organizational Behavior and Human Decision*. 1991; 50: 179–211.
30. Bagozzi R & Warshaw P. Trying to consume. *Journal of Consumer Research*. 1990; 17: 127–140.
31. Janz NK & Becker MH. The Health Belief Model: A decade later. *Health Education & Behavior*. 1984; 11: 1–47.
32. Rosenstock IM. Why people use health services. *Milbank Memorial Fund Quarterly*. 1966; 44: 94–127.
33. Rosenstock IM, Strecher VJ & Becker MH. Social Learning Theory and the Health Belief Model. *Health Education & Behavior*. 1988; 15: 175–183.
34. Prochaska J, DiClemente C & Norcross J. In search of how people change. Applications to addictive behaviors. *American Psychologist*. 1992; 47: 1102–1114.

35. Prochaska J & Velicer W. The transtheoretical model of health behavior change. *American Journal of Health Promotion*. 1997; **12**: 38–48.
36. De Vries H & Mudde A. Predicting stage transitions for smoking cessation applying the attitude-social influence-efficacy model. *Psychology and Health*. 1998; **13**: 369–385.
37. De Vries H, Mudde A, Leijs I *et al*. The European Smoking Prevention Framework Approach (ESFA): An example of Integral Prevention. *Health Education Research*. 2003; **18**: 611–626.
38. Schwarzer R. Modeling health behavior change: How to predict and modify the adoption and maintenance of health behaviors. *Applied Psychology*. 2008; **57**: 1–29.
39. Becker G & Murphy K. A theory of rational addiction. *Journal of Political Economy*. 1988; **96**: 675–700.
40. Webb TL, Sniehotta F & Michie S. Using theories of behavior change to inform interventions for addictive behaviors. *Addiction*. 2010; **105**: 1879–1892.
41. Bandura A. Self-efficacy: Toward a unified theory of behavior change. *Psychological Review*. 1977; **84**: 191–215.
42. Bandura A. *Self-Efficacy: The Exercise of Control*. W. H. Freeman: New York, 1997.
43. Bandura A. *Social Foundations of Thoughts and Action: A Social Cognitive Theory*. Prentice-Hall: Englewood Cliffs, NJ, 1986.
44. Schwarzer R. HAPA theory. [http://userpage.fu-berlin.de/health/hapa.htm] [updated 10th December 2011, 4 July 2013].
45. Bandura A. *Principles of Behavior Modification*. Holt. Rinehart. Winston: New York, 1969.
46. Hall PA & Fong GT. Temporal self-regulation theory: A model for individual health behaviour. *Health Psychology Review*. 2007; **1**: 6–52.
47. Carver CS & Scheier MF. *Attention and Self-Regulation: A Control Theory Approach to Human Behavior*. Springer-Verlag: New York, 1981.
48. Carver CS & Scheier MF. *On the Self-Regulation of Behavior*. Cambridge University Press: New York, 1998.
49. Baumeister RF, Heatherton TF & Tice DM. *Losing Control: How and Why People Fail at Self-Regulation*. Academic Press: San Diego, CA, 1994.
50. Leventhal H & Mosbach P. The perceptual-motor theory of emotion. In: Cacioppo J & Petty R (eds.) *Social Psychophysiology: A Source Book*. Guilford Press: New York, 1983: 353–388.
51. Leventhal H, Brissette I & Leventhal EA. The common-sense model of self-regulation of health and illness. In: Cameron LD & Leventhal H (eds.) *The Self-Regulation of Health and Illness Behaviour*. Routledge: London, 2003: 42–65.
52. Kahneman D & Tversky A. Prospect theory: An analysis of decisions under risk. *Econometrica*. 1979; **47**: 263–291.
53. Kahneman D, Slovic P & Tversky A. *Judgment Under Uncertainty: Heuristic and Biases*. Cambridge University Press: New York, 1982.
54. Kahneman D & Tversky A. Choices, values, and frames. *American Psychologist*. 1984; **34**: 341–350.
55. Tversky A & Kahneman D. Judgment under uncertainty: Heuristic and biases. *Science*. 1974; **185**: 1124–1131.
56. Kahneman D. *Thinking, Fast and Slow*. 1st edn. Farrar, Straus and Giroux: New York, 2011.
57. Nisbett RE & Ross L. *Human Inference: Strategies and Shortcomings of Social Judgment*. Prentice Hall: Englewood Cliffs, NJ, 1980.
58. Zajonc RB. Feeling and thinking: Preferences need no inferences. *American Psychologist*. 1980; **35**: 151–175.

59. Petty RE & Cacioppo JT. *Communication and Persuasion: Central and Peripheral Routes to Attitude Change*. Springer-Verlag: New York, 1986.
60. Marlatt GA & Witkiewitz K. Relapse prevention for alcohol and drug problems. In: Marlatt GA & Donovan DM (eds.) *Relapse Prevention: Maintenance Strategies in the Treatment of Addictive Behaviors*. 2nd edn. Guilford Press: New York, 1985.
61. Witkiewitz K & Marlatt G. Relapse prevention for alcohol and drug problems: That was Zen. This is Tao. *American Psychologist*. 2004; **59**: 224–235.
62. Hendershot CS, Witkiewitz K, George WH *et al*. Relapse prevention for addictive behaviors. *Substance Abuse Treatment, Prevention and Policy*. 2011; **6**: 17. Advanced Access.
63. Rothman AJ. Toward a theory-based analysis of behavioural maintenance *Health Psychology* 2000; **19**: 64–69.
64. Piasecki T, Fiore M, McCarthy D *et al*. Have we lost our way? The need for dynamic formulations of smoking relapse proneness. *Addiction*. 2002; **97**: 1093–1108.
65. Herd N, Borland R & Hyland A. Predictors of smoking relapse by duration of abstinence: Findings from the International Tobacco Control (ITC) Four Country Survey. *Addiction*. 2009; **104**: 2088–2099.
66. Piper M, Kenford S, Fiore M *et al*. Smoking cessation and quality of life: Changes in life satisfactorion over 3 years following a quit attempt. *Annals of Behavioral Medicine*. 2012; **43**: 262–270.
67. Siahpush M, Spittal M & Singh G. Association of smoking cessation with financial stress and material well-being: Results from a prospective study of a population-based national survey. *American Journal of Public Health*. 2007; **97**: 2281–2287.
68. Torres LD, Barrera AZ, Delucchi K *et al*. Quitting smoking does not increase the risk of major depressive episodes among users of internet smoking cessation inverventions. *Psychological Medicine*. 2010; **40**: 441–449.
69. Kahler C, Brown R, Ramsey S *et al*. Negative mood, depressive symptoms, and major depression after smoking cessation treatment in smokers with a history of major depressive disorder. *Journal of Abnormal Psychology*. 2002; **111**: 670–675.
70. Tobacco in Australia: Facts and issues. [http://www.tobaccoinaustralia.org.au/] [accessed 28 August 2013].
71. Borland R, Partos TR, Yong HH *et al*. How much unsuccessful quitting acitivity is going on among adult smokers? Data from the International Tobacco Control 4-Country cohort survey. *Addiction*. 2012; **107**: 673–682.
72. Partos TR, Borland R, Yong HH *et al*. The quitting rollercoaster: How recent quitting history affects future cessation outcomes (data from the International Tobacco Control 4-country cohort study). *Nicotine and Tobacco Research*. 2013: 1–10. doi: 10.1093/ntr/ntt025. Epub March 2013.
73. Miller JG. *Living Systems*. McGraw-Hill: New York, 1978.
74. Carver CS & Scheier MF. Action, affect, multi-tasking, and layers of control. In: Forgas JP, Baumeister RF & Tice D (eds.) *The Psychology of Self-Regulation*. Psychology Press: New York, 2009: 109–126.
75. Corning PA. The re-emergence of emergence : A vernerable concept in search of a theory. *Complexity*. 2002; **7**: 18–30.
76. Kelly G. *The Psychology of Personal Constructs*. Norton: New York, 1955.
77. Bandura A. Social cognitive theory of self-regulation. *Organizational Behavior and Human Decision Processes*. 1991; **50**: 248–287.
78. Brown KW, Ryan RM & Creswell JD. Mindfulness: Theoretical foundations and evidence for its salutary effects. *Psychological Inquiry*. 2007; **18**: 211–237.
79. Hughes J, Solomon L, Fingar J *et al*. The natural history of efforts to stop smoking: A prospective cohort study. *Drug and Alcohol Dependence*. 2013; **128**: 171–174.

80. O'Dea K. Marked improvement in carbohydrate and lipid metabolism in diabetic Australian aborigines after temporary reversion to traditional lifestyle. *Diabetes*. 1984; 33: 596–603.
81. Taylor R. Banting Memorial Lecture 2012: Reversing the twin cycles of Type 2 diabetes. *Diabetic Medicine*. 2013; 30: 267–275.
82. Bell C, Walley A & Froguel P. The genetics of human obesity. *Nature Reviews Genetics*. 2005; 6: 221–234.
83. Young D, Borland R & Coghill K. Changing the tobacco use management system: Blending systems thinking with actor-network theory. *Review of Policy Research*. 2012; 29: 251–279.

Chapter 2

CHARACTERISTICS OF HARD-TO-MAINTAIN BEHAVIOURS

This chapter describes some of the observable characteristics of HTM behaviours. It spells out what is unique to HTM behaviours and similarities and differences between the two main kinds: hard-to-reduce or resist (HTR) behaviours such as some forms of drug use, and their functional opposites, hard-to-sustain (HTS) behaviours such as exercise routines. It also considers the common situation where change involves a mix of both types of behaviour. The consequences of behaviour vary as a function of how immediate they are, which affects the ways they can potentially feedback to influence longer term maintenance.

We tend to study problematic behaviours more than simple ones, and focus our research on the hardest cases. Except for marketers, easy-to-adopt behaviours can take care of themselves. The level of understanding we seek for difficult cases tends only to be enough to develop effective interventions for change, or to get to a point where the behaviour has reduced enough in prevalence to no longer warrant concern. Thus, the amount of research can be taken as an indicator of the difficulty of the problem.

Types of behaviour to change

The term *behaviour* can refer to anything from discrete instances of a behaviour to behaviour patterns, which once established become habits. For example, *exercise* could refer to anything from walking a few steps, to a regular long walk, or a complex routine of walking, jogging, weight training and swimming. Similarly, *smoking* can refer to anything from a puff on a cigarette to a long-term, say 20 per day, habit. Habits are recurring patterns of behaviour consisting of a constrained range of specific actions organised into routines, which are predictable, situation-specific sequences that have limited variability. Looked at retrospectively, habits can be inferred from the history of actions, while prospectively it is the assumption that the past pattern of occurrences predicts future patterns of behaviour that leads to the imputation that something is a habit. HTM behaviours are ones where there is difficulty in either or both habit formation or habit change. To understand this, both

Understanding hard to maintain behaviour change: A dual process approach, First Edition. Ron Borland.
© 2014 John Wiley & Sons, Ltd. Published 2014 by John Wiley & Sons, Ltd.

individual instances of the behaviour to change (especially for initiation), as well as on how routines are sustained, eliminated or otherwise changed (the maintenance of change) need to be considered.

Habit formation is very different from factors determining the occurrence of single instances of behaviour. The former is about being cued at the right time and about persistence, while the latter has more to do with individual decisions and the ability to act. This means theories that are useful for predicting discrete behaviours have no a priori credence for explaining the formation or modification of habits.

Behavioural routines vary in their desired frequency and actual frequency. A person might smoke 20 or more cigarettes per day, while for exercise it would be rare to have more than two or three episodes of extensive physical activity in a day. Both the number and length of episodes of behaviour will have implications for change. Finding 30-min periods to fit in exercise is likely to be easier than fitting in 1 h sessions, but fitting in one episode is easier than two; so, different ways of shaping behaviour might suit people with different constraints on their lifestyle.

Behaviours vary in the functions they serve. The main functions of interest here are self-maintenance functions (e.g. eating and keeping fit) and behaviours that are engaged in for the pleasure of doing them or of their immediate consequences (e.g. drug use and watching entertainment). Among HTM behaviours, hard-to-reduce (HTR) behaviours all have some element of intrinsic value in their immediate performance, while HTS behaviours typically lack intrinsic value (at least initially); their main benefit lies in the future, for example, in protecting health and well-being in the longer term.

Where an undesirable behaviour is engaged in for its intrinsic value, for example, the pleasure of smoking a cigarette and the satisfaction of sitting mindlessly watching TV, there is a need to either find a replacement or convince the person that the value gained is expendable, either because it is not worth the costs and/or it precludes other benefits being gained from forgone alternatives.

Where the behaviour is focal, like the time spent on a recreational exercise regime, then the time spent has to be found from other activities, or in the case of giving up an activity, for example, going outside to have a cigarette, the time spent needs to be filled. In the first case, it is preferable to find time by reducing or eliminating low-value activities, and in the second time is ideally filled by high-value replacements. Where the behaviour to increase is not intrinsically valuable in its own right, there is a need to find value in it or create negative value with the alternatives, else self-control will be required to persist. With sufficient time and practice, the reassurance of a routine might have to suffice if nothing else can be found.

Two other major functions of behaviour are instrumental, that is, involved in manipulating the environment (e.g. to achieve a goal) and social, that is, behaviours designed to maintain or change social relationships. Research [1, 2] is showing that these indirect aspects of behaviour play less of a role in the maintenance of HTM behaviours than has been thought. At least for smoking, these desirable aspects are not strongly linked to relapse, although they can complement and thus facilitate certain HTM behaviours. There are also potential gains from combining two or more goals around the same behaviour. Thus, walking or riding a bike to work can both help achieve physical activity goals and transport needs. Similarly, combining two or more activities together can have similar benefits; for example, many people organise physical activity within social contexts. This example is one where the complementary activity, having others involved, has the additional benefit of providing external cues and incentives to maintain the physical activity (e.g. your friends expect you to join in). Combining behaviours can be risky if it leads to changes in the effects of the complementary behaviour that are undesirable, and thus act as a force for the resumption of the old behaviour. For example, if your friends decide they prefer to socialise sitting down, or if you end up rewarding yourself at a local bar and drink too much.

One critical aspect of habits is the nature of the cues that elicit them. Cues can come from the environment, from behaviour itself, or from ideas appearing in consciousness. A cue is defined as a contextual element that elicits some tendency to engage in the behaviour. Automated behaviours may occur without conscious intent, whereas new behaviours require the cue to trigger executive processes to generate a decision to act. For behaviours to reduce or eliminate, the executive action needs to be to inhibit response tendencies generated by cues.

One factor that affects the availability and frequency of environmental cues is the predictability of a person's day-to-day routines. Some people have quite fixed routines, albeit with clear differences between work and leisure days, while others have much more varying patterns, with routines covering only part of their day. As the aim for desirable behaviours is to institute them into the person's overall routine, the stability of that routine, especially those parts where the behaviour is to be embedded, will influence the availability of cues to help control action, that is, having cues that can trigger thoughts supportive of action at times when the unwanted behaviour is also being cued.

Behaviours also vary in the complexity of the routines they produce and in the extent and manner by which they are cued into people's lives. Thus, eating tends to be highly cued (e.g. around scheduled meals), but timing of periods of exercise may be less cued. For behaviours related to diet, it is the establishment of routines that is critical as there is no problem with any specific action (e.g. episodes of eating specific foods); it is the pattern of eating routines that needs to be shaped to limit inappropriate intakes (i.e. moderate intake of some foods). For some behaviours, such as beginning to exercise, the initiation of the routine will often be enough to ensure a high likelihood that the behavioural goal will be achieved, although natural stopping points (e.g. when completing laps) do constitute risk points. For many behaviours, however, initiation does not affect the probability of successful completion in this way; having the low-fat salad for starters does not increase your likelihood of avoiding the high-fat dessert, indeed sometimes it is taken as a reward! Other behaviours require ending routines earlier (e.g. drinking less and eating less), and here the tendency of a routine to lead to a chain of responses becomes part of the problem, and alternative routines need to be developed and stabilised. For unwanted behaviours, cues to act need to be transformed into cues to resist.

What makes some behaviours hard to maintain?

HTM behaviours are an exceptional form of behaviour pattern. They trouble us because they (because of their presence or absence) create risks to our health, well-being and/or to the societies to which we belong. The problem is that our OSs are not programmed to generate and/or sustain such behaviours in the ways our conscious selves desire and/or the societies in which we live (including families and social networks) consider desirable. Because HTM behaviours cause problems to us, they are highly salient and thus scientists tend to study them and some people implicitly assume that all behaviours have similar characteristics. This is not so.

The matrix in Figure 2.1 depicts the reality that most behaviour is unproblematic. We can do most of our day-to-day activity without much effort, we can adapt to new possibilities such as the internet and mobile phones with little problem even though they fundamentally change the way we live. It is only when the impulses of the OS are at odds with the goals of the ES that HTM behaviours occur (e.g. the OS reacts in a positive way, while the ES sees it as undesirable, or vice versa).

The immediate consequences of behaviour (pleasure or pain) directly affect the likelihood of behaviour recurring through conditioning mechanisms controlled by the OS. However, for delayed consequences to influence subsequent behaviour requires executive processes to make the link. This is the situation for HTM behaviours: the behaviour is seen as desirable or problematic because it is associated with future outcomes and not immediate ones. These delayed consequences can range from relatively short-term (e.g. the negative feelings that occur some minutes after finishing smoking a cigarette) to long-term effects (e.g. improved

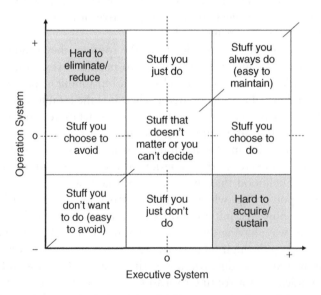

Figure 2.1 The implications for behaviour of different strengths and directions of impulse to action from OS (experienced desire to act) and ES (in this case rational appraisal of the costs and benefits of acting).

long-term health), and this obviously affects when they can be experienced. Consequences can also vary in concreteness; thus, 'getting lung cancer as a result of smoking' is more concrete and easier to understand than 'having better lung function than you would have done if you continued to smoke'. Where benefits are probabilistic or have not yet happened, there tends to be more focus on the effects of behaviour that have been experienced. If the behaviour is found to have positive consequences, it should be more likely to be able to be maintained. The problem we face is that with HTM behaviours, this is often not the case, or if it is, these consequences are delayed beyond the capacity of operational processes to form contingent associations. Because it is impossible to both condition associations with the absence of something and much more difficult to conceptualise absence (such as effects of not smoking), the effects of not doing something are likely to have less impact on subsequent behaviour than the effects of doing something (such as effects of exercising).

HTM behaviours are those that fit at the top left and bottom right extremes in Figure 2.1, where there is a maximum discord between operational and executive evaluations of the desirability of a behaviour. Under-cued desirable behaviours include taking up an exercise regimen and adopting sun-safe behaviours while over-cued undesirable behaviours include smoking, problematic alcohol or other drug use, problem gambling, inappropriate sexual behaviour and over-eating. For undesirable behaviours, a key issue is whether the problem is any level of the behaviour or just excessive levels, while for desirable behaviours, it is whether the behaviour is novel or represents an extension of an existing activity.

A goal of behaviour change is to add sufficient intrinsic value to desirable behaviours to move them into the 'choose to do' segment and even to the 'want to do' segment, while for hard-to-reduce behaviours, it is to add negative valence to move them into the 'choose to avoid' or 'want to avoid' segments. That said, in some cases, coming to enjoy things too much can cause problems on the other side of the spectrum, for example, effects on physical health from overexercise. Thus, some caution is needed in choosing appropriate goals.

One simplification inherent in Figure 2.1 is that it does not reflect the possibility that a tendency to act can also be affected by the positioning of the alternative(s) in the same space. Where one alternative is more positive (or less negative) for the OS, it may be easier to engage in regardless of how it is evaluated by the ES (Figure 2.2). Similarly, for two ES-desired options, the one that involves the least resistance from the OS should be easier to engage in and/or maintain. This is why we often seem to make compromises that make the task easier even if it undermines some of the long-term benefit.

This framework also explains the lure of delay. In theory, a short delay should have only a small negative effect on the benefits of acting for behaviours where the main negative consequences are long term, but it has a large immediate positive effect of avoiding the immediate undesired consequences. When considered in the present, the desire to avoid the pain in the future is weaker than it is to avoid it now, because it is further way, while the strength of the perceived benefits of action is largely unaffected; so, it appears that there will be no real loss but a potential gain

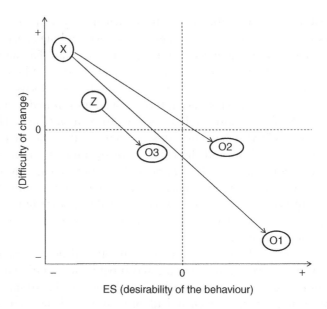

Figure 2.2 Behaviour change conflicts. The desired change in behaviour is from Behaviour X to O1 (e.g. quit smoking) (as this spans the most horizontal distance). However, this is maximally difficult (vertical distance). The difficulty creates incentives for choosing an easier change goal; that is, for Behaviour X it is to O2 (e.g. cutdown rather than quit), giving up some benefit.

A second alternative is to do something even easier, choose another behaviour (e.g. behaviour Z, and change it to O3), even though it might not do much, it is easy to do.

from delay. It is only when the 'next time' is reached (i.e. the delay has expired) that the strength of the avoidance tendency is back to its original level, and the same dilemma faces the person they had seemingly avoided by delaying.

Not explicit in Figure 2.1 is that the strength of the ES assessment of the value of a behaviour, of itself, has limited motivational power, unless it is imbued with affective force (i.e. the OS is engaged). Only in the absence of any competing OS impulse will ES decisions be sufficient to trigger desired actions by themselves. The strength of the reasons for acting is theorised to have the capacity to generate affective force to support change, by stimulating affective mechanisms. This affective force is necessary to compete with strongly affectively charged OS-generated tendencies to act otherwise.

Conflict is created when there are strong competing tendencies for action. Conflicts between OS- and ES-generated action tendencies are only one form of conflict. Conflicts within the OS are the classical approach–approach and avoid–avoid conflicts studied extensively in animal psychology [3, 4]. They are typically resolved by recourse to higher level processing to tilt the balance of a decision one way or the other. Where this does not work, it is manifest as neurosis. For those conflicts that lie predominantly within the ES, that is, where a difficult conceptual choice must be made, it doesn't matter what choice is made unless there are differential consequences associated with factors that are not considered.

Furthermore, it should be clear that the value of a behaviour to a person does not remain stable; value changes as a function of context, need and the person's conceptualisation of the issue. The change in value is of two kinds, moment-to-moment changes due to phasic changes in context and need, and longer term changes that are due to some combination of systematic changes in the context, conditioning and the person's conceptualisation of the issues.

Emerging out of this analysis is the insight that if the behaviours that replace an undesirable behaviour are hard to sustain, it will make the task of change harder regardless of how hard it is to resist the unwanted behaviour. Similarly, if the forgone behaviours for a desirable behaviour change are hard to resist, then again it will be a net contributor to relapse. The matrix in Figure 2.2 can be used to compare options for a behavioural choice. Typically, conflicting choices will be where the options vary in different directions on the two axes, for example, overall more desirable to ES, but less immediately appealing. A complicating factor is that the strength of desire for behaviours is fluid, especially ones with strong OS determinants; so, overall ranking of preferences can shift with the context, something that is a real problem for HTM behaviours.

In summary, the central problem of HTM behaviours is that while a rational appraisal of the merits of a current behaviour may conclude that change is needed, there are net experienced benefits of engaging in that behaviour. If behaviour change is to occur, this discrepancy in value either need to be overcome or changed.

Hard-to-reduce/resist/eliminate behaviours

Hard-to-reduce behaviours are behaviours that occur more often than is desirable. The reason for reducing or eliminating such behaviours is the likelihood that they are doing harm, or at least putting the person at undesirable levels of risk for inadequate benefit. The main hard-to-reduce behaviours include various forms of drug use, including smoking, excessive alcohol use, addictions to various other drugs, licit and illicit; inappropriate sexual behaviour; gambling; and eating too much (either overall, or for some food types) – what Orford [5] calls excessive appetites.

Key characteristics of HTR behaviours include the following:

- The experience of behaving is immediately positive, meaning that their performance is inherently reinforcing, albeit sometimes after overcoming initial negative experiences.
- There are commonly positive anticipatory responses, which are generated through classical conditioning, such that precursors of rewarding experiences of behaving come to trigger the positive experiences. For drugs, the conditioned experiences include coming to look forward to the often initially negative experiences of use (e.g. of the act of inhaling smoke, or amazingly, of putting a needle in your arm).
- Adverse consequences are rarely immediate, they can be either relatively short-term (e.g. negative consequences of intoxication or drug withdrawal) and/or long term (to health and well-being).

- Failure to initiate the behaviour in the presence of cues results in a desire to act, which in the case of addictive behaviours, can be quite compelling.
- Attempts to resist the behaviour are experienced as effortful and commonly fail, and for many, this occurs repeatedly.
- Even after prolonged abstinence, a single instance of the behaviour can trigger a rapid resumption of the habit.

Some behaviours such as smoking create risks of harm at any level of use; so, the goal needs to be its elimination. For others, for example, alcohol use, which have few if any net adverse effects at moderate levels of consumption, control to avoid excessive use becomes the goal. This means attention need to be given to implications of differences between a goal to effectively eliminate a behaviour, and one to reduce it to some controlled level (e.g. responsible drinking), and whether and when controlled use is possible for something that should not occur regularly (e.g. can an ex-smoker smoke an occasional cigarette, without it triggering full relapse).

It is generally accepted that at least for addictions, it is more difficult to control use than to achieve complete abstinence. This is the basis of the approach of organisations like Alcoholics Anonymous (AA). Part of the reason for this is that in any ambiguous context, the possibility of use is likely to stimulate motivation to use, which can overwhelm rational appraisal of whether it is acceptable. That a commonly used strategy for dieting is to cut out some foods completely also highlights the difficulty of controlled use, at least for some people. The tendency of lapses in behaviour to lead to relapse is important, and possible mechanisms are discussed in Chapter 6.

Behaviours can be problematic because they occur too often or tend to occur as binges, something associated more with acute harm (e.g. as a result of intoxication). Intoxication creates its own problems as it compromises rationality, thus limiting rationality-based strategies for regulating behaviour.

CEOS should also be able to encompass issues around avoiding the development of risky habits. I suspect the principles of resisting hard-to-resist behaviours are similar for initial uptake as for re-uptake, although re-uptake is typically much faster. Skill acquisition can act as a barrier, albeit minor, to performing undesirable behaviours. Thus, those who have tried the behaviour are at additional risk as they have some degree of the skill required. However, as there is little skill involved in most HTM behaviours, a single episode can be enough for the person to feel comfortable performing the behaviour, and thus be at increased risk of continuing to use enough for a habit to develop.

Addictions versus other HTR behaviours

Drug dependence has some distinctive features that separate it from other HTR behaviours. It is sustained, at least in part, by direct physiological reactions to the drug. These direct effects become rewards for precursor behaviours or thoughts which in turn become additional reasons for use of the drug. Another unique aspect of some drugs is the intoxication that occurs with some (but not notably with nicotine use). Intoxication does reduce the body's capacity to act and impair behaviour and thinking; so, intoxication can disrupt behavioural attempts to control use. This places stronger likely limits on the potential of controlled use for intoxicating drugs over those that are not intoxicating.

Tolerance builds up to most drugs; that is, there is a reduced response to a given dose, including the desired effects in situations associated with use [6]. One puzzling aspect of drug use is that although it should maximise tolerance, drug users exhibit strong preferences for using in regular contexts and typically develop ritualised anticipatory responses, even though the direct effects of the drug should be greater if used in a novel situation without the anticipatory rituals. This strongly suggests that over time it is the conditioned responses to the drug that become the major determinants of use. If this is so, then in this respect, drug use may not be very different to behavioural addictions such as gambling.

A major determinant of addiction is the experiences of use, independent of the drug itself. Addiction develops to some forms of drug administration more readily than others, and typically only occurs (at least initially) in situations associated with some forms of use. For example, using morphine for severe pain is less likely to result in addiction if removing pain is the sole reason they use [7, 8], rather than use for the euphoric effects or relief from negative mood states. For tobacco, nicotine replacement therapies such as transdermal patches deliver similar amounts of nicotine as from smoking, but are not particularly addictive: very few continue to use nicotine patches long-term because the use of patches does not provide the same experience due to the much more rapid uptake of nicotine from smoking.

The negative effects of withdrawal from habitual drug use occur too long after actual use to be linked to use by operational processes, so does not act as a natural disincentive to use. Rather, because drug use temporarily removes negative affect, withdrawal creates conditions that encourage use.

Most drug addictions would appear to be maintained by two kinds of effects: the role of the drug in reducing negative affect, regardless of whether they are associated with abstinence (use to stop feeling bad), and the positive experiences of use (use to feel good). In many cases, there are elements of both and separating out their relative contributions may be difficult. It is likely that removal of negative effect will be strongest in the early days after change, mainly because of the experience of drug withdrawal, but it can recur if contextual conditions cue the likelihood of use enough to stimulate the body to prepare for drug use. Once expectations of use become less important then anticipation of gain is more likely to be the driving motivation to resume the old behaviour. Drug addictions may be associated with stronger experienced negative effects of acute abstinence than occurs for other HTR behaviours [9]. This may be because an externally delivered dose of a psychoactive drug directly affects physiological processes by actually increased levels of these drugs and their metabolites in the brain, something the body needs to respond to as it disrupts normal homeostatic functioning, while behaviour affects levels of drug neuro-chemicals indirectly via the signals it sends, and is part of normal functioning. As a consequence, the resultant anticipatory changes in physiology are likely to be larger for drug use than for other behaviours.

The example of smoking

In this section, I analyse smoking in more detail and spell out some of the characteristics that make it so hard to change.

Cigarette smoking as a habit is a complex set of routines. For each cigarette, there is the act of finding a pack, then getting it out and preparing to light it. For roll your own tobacco, there are the intermediate steps associated with rolling the cigarette. Then the cigarette is lit and the smokers take their first, usually deep, draw on it. Most smokers hold this in for a couple of seconds before blowing the smoke out, sometimes in patterned ways (e.g. blowing a smoke ring). After a few seconds to a minute or so, they take another puff, and over the next 5–10 min take around 10 puffs before discarding the butt, usually after extinguishing it. Much of this activity is highly routinised and many smokers treat the performance, particularly up to the first puff, as a ritual. The average smoker repeats this routine 15–20 times a day. In past years, before restrictions on smoking and before smokers were concerned about health effects, it was not uncommon to smoke 50 or more. Including the period between puffs, a 20 per day smoker spends around 3 hours per day smoking. Smokers tend to smoke more when stressed and when drinking alcohol [9–12], and in these situations, if smoking is allowed, might smoke virtually continuously for hours.

The action sequence leading up to the reinforcement associated with each puff (particularly the first one of a cigarette) is critical for the long-term maintenance of the habit, although chains of reinforcers are likely to mean that the behaviours will continue for some time even in the absence of the base reinforcer. Thus, smokers will continue to smoke denicotinised cigarettes for some time and, at least initially, get most of the same subjective positive experiences (rewards) from them [13, 14].

There is great individual variability in smoking patterns. Some people only smoke occasionally, while most do so daily, with daily consumption varying from 1 per day to over 50. Smokers can smoke for many reasons: to relax, manage stress, concentrate, while socialising with smokers, or regularly to relieve the negative effects of abstinence.

It is generally accepted that most smokers who consume more than around 5 per day are addicted to a significant degree [15] (i.e. they find it hard to quit), with those smoking less having fewer signs of addiction. For some people, smoking is a highly enjoyable activity, which they are reluctant to give up, even in the light of evidence that it is harming them, while for others it is a chore they feel chained to and would gladly quit if they thought they could.

In past times, smoking could be readily integrated into day-to-day activity, but as smoking has been increasingly prohibited in indoor settings (including homes), smoking has become more of a focal activity rather than occurring concurrently with other activities. Where they can, many smokers still seek company when smoking, and thus smoking still plays a social role, but this secondary benefit has declined greatly from what it was. Offering a cigarette or asking for a light are no longer desirable ways to strike up a conversation.

Smoking is not just a result of being cued by environmental conditions. If it were, restrictions on smoking would reduce consumption by the cigarettes that could no longer be smoked. However, studies find some compensation, with extra cigarettes being smoked where they can [16], and some smokers taking extra breaks to find places to smoke. While there is an overall reduction in consumption, it is also possible that some of the cigarettes smoked are smoked harder, allowing smokers to regulate their nicotine intake [17].

For many, smoking is an extremely difficult habit to break. In one population-based study of ours [18] in four countries that have been taking tobacco control seriously for an extended period (United States, United Kingdom, Canada and Australia), we found on average of around 40% of smokers report making a quit attempt each year, and they report a bit over two attempts on average, thus allowing for forgetting, we estimate that smokers are making at least one unsuccessful quit attempt per year (i.e. one that lasts at least 1 day), and at least as many aborted attempts [18]. This suggests that by the age of 40, the average smokers may make 25 failed quit attempts. Further, some smokers make frequent decisions to quit, but succeed in initiating an attempt only on a minority of occasions [19]. In our study [18], we also found that nearly half of the smokers reported some quit-related activity in the last month, confirming that there is lots of thinking and rather less action. In this context, it is not surprising that many smokers report (retrospectively) that their last quit attempt was spontaneous or occurred without any pre-planning [20, 21]. Many seem to be primed to quit whenever the circumstances favour it for long enough for them to fully implement an attempt.

There are now a range of interventions that can help smokers to quit. These include both pharmacotherapies and cognitive-behavioural interventions. The evidence is clear that a combination of the two provides roughly additive effects, suggesting these two forms of help assist in different, but complementary ways. The most effective package would appear to be the drug varenicline or a combination of two forms of nicotine replacement products (typically the transdermal patch and an oral form) in combination with some advice, with success rates over twice those of controls only getting advice [22]. However, even with the most effective mix of help, only a minority are successful in quitting in the medium term (6–12 months), and around half of these will eventually relapse [23].

All this suggests that tobacco control efforts have been quite successful in motivating smokers to try to quit, but less successful in helping them become permanent ex-smokers. Recent research has identified differences between predictors of making quit attempts and of maintenance [24]. For example, colleagues and I explored the predictive power of seven motivational variables including reported wanting to quit, concern about adverse health effects and recently prematurely butting out cigarettes as a result of thinking about the harms [25]. All seven were positively related to making quit attempts over the following year, with extent of wanting to quit and prematurely butting out independent predictors. However, among those making attempts, all these variables were negatively associated with success, and the two most strongly associated with relapse were the two strongest predictors of making attempts. In short, the more you want to quit, the more you will try, but the less likely you are to succeed (if you try). We have looked to see if this perverse effect is found in other countries, most notably China where tobacco control is in its infancy, and thus many smokers have not made repeated failed attempts. For the measures we had, motivators did indeed predict making attempts, but were largely unrelated to success among those who tried (Li *et al.* in preparation). This is consistent with the original finding being due to a population of smokers who would have quit if they could (i.e. are highly motivated and keep trying), but for the most part, are unable to do so.

While there are lots of failed and aborted attempts, most smokers have been able to survive for at least 1 month on a previous attempt [18], although for most, their longest attempt is not their most recent [26], suggesting that there is little or no improvement in capacity or skills to stay quit.

Because quitting is difficult, some smokers hold beliefs that have the effect of minimising the problem. These include agreement with assertions such as 'If smoking was as bad as they say it is, the government would have banned it', 'I have the kind of constitution that means I won't get the problems others do', 'The medical evidence that smoking is harmful is exaggerated', 'Smoking is no more risky than lots of other things people do' and 'You have got to die of something, so why not enjoy yourself and smoke'. Holding these beliefs would clearly make it easier to justify smoking. However, the role they play in discouraging quitting is not so clear. Some, at least, appear to be associated with a reduced likelihood of making quit attempts, but not consistently with quit success [27]. However, there is some evidence that these beliefs also tend to change with interest in quitting, perhaps being more indicators of current thinking, than true barriers to action [28].

Saul Shiffman, a pioneer in the field of relapse prevention, has used what he calls ecological momentary assessment, that is, use of electronic devices to prompt quitters at random times to report current experiences and also to record experiences immediately after any temptation crisis, regardless of whether they smoked or successfully resisted. Using this strategy, his team was able to compare random reports that occurred shortly before crisis situations with those that did not, and also among crises, to explore differences in antecedents as a function of outcome. They also explored what happened in slips in relation to whether the person recovered abstinence or relapsed completely. This research has confirmed the importance of increased negative affect as a major determinant of slips and subsequently relapse. Heightened negative affect seems to play a causal role in both precipitating a crisis and in its resolution, and if negative affect stays high, in leading to full relapse [29]. These effects are for acute changes in negative affect, not to relatively stable moods. This research also shows that negative affect is not involved in non-stress-related relapses.

Shiffman's work [1, 29, 30] shows that self-efficacy plays a more stable role in relapse overall, with high self-efficacy predicting success. They found no evidence of for changes in self-efficacy before lapses, but after lapses self-efficacy declined, but only if this decline persisted, was it associated with subsequent relapse. Only among those overall low in self-efficacy do lapses tend to reduce self-efficacy. This work has also demonstrated that use of coping strategies led to fewer lapses, and that the occurrence of coping varied within individuals, with negative affect being one factor to inhibit coping.

There is also evidence that overall levels of stress affect the success of quit attempts. Siahpush [31–33] has studied the role of financial stress; that is, concerns about difficulty in paying bills on time or having to miss out on essentials for want of money. Unsurprisingly, he has found that being financially stressed is a motivator for wanting to quit (after all it saves a lot of money). However, this does not clearly translate into more quitting, and among those who try, it is associated with reduced chances of success, even though those who successfully quit become less financially stressed. A similar kind of perverse effect may occur for depression. People with depression are just as likely to want to quit and try, but less likely to succeed, even though success has been associated with reduced levels of depression in some studies [34, 35]. The mechanisms of these effects have not been addressed, but it seems likely that it is the increased frequency of episodes of acute stress/negative affect, which is the likely cause, rather than the underlying stress or dysphoric mood [9, 29].

Research on the dynamic determinants of relapse has focussed on the early days when relapse is most common. There is increasing evidence that some of the determinants of relapse change over the first weeks of an attempt. High levels of addiction, as assessed by the heaviness of smoking index, a combination of time to first cigarette of the day (reverse scored) and cigarettes smoked per day, are strongly predictive of relapse [36, 37]. This appears to be because it predicts relapse strongly in the first weeks of a quit attempt [38], but is not predictive beyond around 1 month [2, 39]. Having lots of smoking friends has a similar curvilinear relationship with relapse. By contrast, the frequency of strong urges (measured after quitting) and number of close friends who smoke are surprisingly not clearly associated with relapse in the first weeks of a quit attempt, but by 1 month post quit, become strong predictors in the expected direction [2]. These changes may be associated with exhaustion of self-control or of the quitter moving quitting from the focal activity in their lives into just something they need to keep on doing while dealing with other life priorities [2, 40]. It would appear that obvious barriers to sustained change like cravings and having lots of smokers around trigger coping early on, but if they persist, may speed up exhaustion of self-control, and because they are cues to smoke, require effort to resist.

While our ability to predict who will successfully quit and to help smokers stay quit is rather limited, that quitting outcomes are predictable based in part on personal characteristics means that the population of smokers is likely to be changing to one where a greater proportion are unable to quit even in the context of a social environment that is increasingly supportive of quitting. This changing nature of the population could mean that interventions that were successful in the past may be less effective in future, especially when used on smokers with a long history of failed attempts. We don't have good estimates of the proportion of ever-smokers who are unable to ever quit. On the basis of self-report of ever being a smoker and using prevalence estimates from people in their 50s (a time before too many smokers have died), it would seem that perhaps around 40% of ever-smokers have been unable to quit. Whatever the number, if it is of this magnitude, it means all our efforts to assist quitting are failing a significant minority of smokers.

Hard-to-sustain behaviours

HTS behaviours do not occur as often as is desirable and attempts to encourage them encounter difficulties. They include exercise regimes, sticking to healthy eating patterns, sun-protective behaviours, and safe-sex practices. More broadly, it includes any behaviour that the person has trouble fitting into his/her normal routines (or in some cases, lack of routines), and thus typically involves some disruption of existing routines or a requirement for a routine where none currently exists. Similar issues also apply to behaviours that have a role in replacing undesirable behaviours, even though they may not be of benefit in their own right. In the next section, I consider the case of partial substitutes, that is, concurrently giving up something and replacing it with something desirable, although often less so.

Typical features of HTS behaviours include the following.

- There is no immediate positive experience of initiating the behaviour.
- Anticipatory responses are either absent or negative.
- There are no or inadequate cues to commence.
- Positive consequences occur sometime after commencing or completing an episode of behaviour (e.g. feeling good during or after exercising) and/or are otherwise only effects on long-term health and well-being.

For some HTS behaviours, initiation is the main problem as once started they tend to be self-sustaining, while for other more complex and varying behaviours, like making healthy dietary choices, more complex routines and rules need to be learnt.

Some HTS behaviours are conditional, that is, only being required in some circumstances. Thus, sun-protection behaviours such as applying sunscreen are only relevant during periods of likely high UV exposure. The existence of high UV levels is not naturally cued; so, there is a need to develop cues and routines that are arranged around salient cues, such as the season of the year; for example, the rule, always protect yourself when going outside in the summer months. Choosing inappropriate cues can be problematic. For example, not using sun protection in high UV periods when it is cloudy. The cloud may temporarily reduce the UV level, but if the cloud disperses, then the risk re-emerges. It is likely that different sets of strategies will be required to optimise behaviours of these different kinds. It may require cues to engage in the decision-making process, rather than cues to initiate the behaviour.

Some HTS behaviours take up dedicated time; so, some previous activities will need to be forgone; for example, exercise replaces sedentary behaviours. If the forgone behaviours are missed, this can act as a barrier to sustained change, and thus it can be useful to explicitly work out where priorities lie.

Changing to HTS behaviours has an advantage over change from HTR behaviours in that raising the topic can act as a cue to act, thus the more these behaviours are talked about the better. This is not the case with HTR behaviours because mentioning them evokes the undesirable behaviour, and often more strongly; so, minimising the discussion may be beneficial there (see Chapter 3).

It is worth pointing out that CEOS was developed primarily as a result of studying the complexities of quitting smoking. Thus, the implications of the theory for HTS behaviours are less empirically grounded.

Examples of HTS behaviours

Exercise regimes typically require finding time to engage in recreational exercise, although some people can incorporate a level of exercise into their work (e.g. manual labour) or travel routines (e.g. cycling or walking to work). Some forms of exercise involve getting fit to perform at desired levels; so, require a level of build-up. Further, some of those at most need are very unfit and sometimes overweight, adding to the difficulty of achieving levels of exercise that will improve their health and/or getting to the point where the exercise is sufficiently self-rewarding to at least not be a major barrier to persisting.

One common way people use to maintain interest in exercise regimes is to focus on performance, something that works for the athletically gifted, but not for the main group who should be exercising, the average types whose performance is never going to be worth bragging about. High-level performance is beyond the reach of most, and personal targets can seem inconsequential when others have far higher ones.

In principle, most forms of exercise can be done without any special equipment; however, it is common to get special equipment. For some, special equipment acts as an additional set of incentives to persist, but it might discourage others. For example, people who don't feel good in lycra or who don't want to outlay the cost of special equipment before they are sure they will persist, cost can be significant barriers to adaption.

Creating a structure to support any new behavioural routine is important, as it is easier to cue the initiation, and at least some of the barriers to performance (competing behaviours) have at some level been addressed. Some people join gyms or groups to provide structure and others exercise with friends both for the social benefits and for the way others can mutually support persistence.

Exercise is something that for some becomes a pleasant form of recreation in its own right. If you begin to miss exercise when it does not occur, you have the cues that can facilitate long-term maintenance, but can be at risk of overuse-related problems. Most behaviours are easy to adopt for some; the focus of this book is on when they are hard.

Eating a healthy diet is a HTS behaviour that provides a more complex set of challenges than exercise. Unlike exercise, eating a healthy diet does not require a lot of skill (to eat it), nor is it something about which performance matters. The challenges are in the choices that are made and any negotiation required to implement those choices. What we eat is strongly influenced by those who prepare our food for us, whether it be in our homes, in restaurants, or in processing plants. Much of the skill required lies with the food preparer and to a lesser extent with the gatherer. Where there is information on ingredients, it can be used to influence the choices made. Except where a person lives alone and prepares all of his/her own meals, these social determinants of what we eat require some form of negotiation involving the end-user – the eater. The skill lies in negotiating towards healthier choices.

Episodes of eating are much more strongly cued than exercise. Meals are typically scheduled, albeit with some flexibility of timing. Snacks are a different matter, as they only occur for some, and having breaks without food is not only possible, but common. That said, there is still much that the individual can do, both to influence the context and in choices that they make around what is available.

Diet also involves reducing key behaviours, for example, limiting intake of high-fat foods. This involves resisting temptations to eat more immediately satisfying foods (sweet and fatty) and/or keeping serving size at appropriate levels. In this sense, it is the ultimate balancing exercise, but where the centre of the balance isn't clearly marked, and an arbitrary goal may need to be set as a target for behaviour, for example, daily calorie intake.

Combinations of both kinds of behaviour change

Many kinds of behaviour change involve both giving up things that were previously valued or which were otherwise strongly habitual, and taking up alternative activities. This is likely the case for any behaviour that takes up significant amounts of dedicated time, or where some alternative or partial substitute is involved. Where there is a less problematic total substitute, behaviour change should be easy.

A good example of the need for both kinds of behaviour change is weight loss. For example, sustained weight loss appears to be a function of 'engaging in high levels of physical activity (1 h/day), eating a low-calorie, low-fat diet, eating breakfast regularly, self-monitoring weight and maintaining a consistent eating pattern across weekdays and weekends' [41].

Here, we have a mix of doing more of some things and less of others, and the relative difficulty of the tasks involved also varies. Even if we assume that eating breakfast regularly is not too hard, and that monitoring weight is not a great impost, it is clear that for most exercising for at least an hour a day, eating a low-calorie low-fat diet and maintaining a constant eating pattern across weekdays and weekends are all far from straightforward to achieve. The dietary changes involve eating one class of foods (low-calorie ones) and avoiding or reducing consumption of another class. In an area of such complexity, it is easier for the person to opt out of the more difficult to achieve elements of the package, thinking the remainder might be enough to provide most of the benefit.

Where there are a range of effects, it is also easier to misattribute effects. Thus, people may attribute all the perceived benefits to the aspects they like, and all the bad things to the aspect they like least, thus providing a context to justify abandoning part of the package.

Guidelines, like the one above, don't provide much advice about the risks of occasional deviations. From the perspective of behaviour change, the key issue is the extent to which an occasional deviation from a routine increases the risk of relapse back to less desirable routines. On the other hand, there are social costs of having too rigid routines when they conflict with the activities of others, for example, not visiting others because of concerns about inappropriate diet or not adjusting exercise routines when visitors drop in. What is ideal for an individual to maintain desired behaviours, may not be for their social group (family and friends).

Having to do more of some things and less of others may be characteristic of areas where the goal is some kind of outcome, other than the behaviour itself. For example, it is very much the case for sun protection (put on sunscreens, shirts and hats, but avoid being in the sun during high UV periods). Similarly, if the aim is to have a healthy pattern of physical activities (rather than just getting enough exercise), something now recognised as important [42–44], then avoiding too much sedentary activity becomes part of the mix. The time taken for a new behaviour does reduce the chances of engaging in some other behaviours (like sitting watching TV if the new behaviour is going for a walk), but does not preclude them altogether. Clearly, where there are a range of options for achieving a goal, we need to consider the ease and potential benefits of each option.

Some form of combination of doing more of some things and less of others may be the norm for behaviour change, except for behaviours that always occur as a complement to other behaviours. This is because most forms of behaviour change either take time away from other possible activities or free up time for other activities. Thus, in all these cases, it is potentially possible to reframe change from a focus on one form of change to a dual focus on both what is lost and gained. This might be a useful framing in many cases as it can encourage the maximisation of benefits from time freed up and on strategies to replace the least valued activities when extra time is required for the new behaviour. It is important for maintaining change to be noticing and reflecting on the gains, and to understand that there can be additional costs if the person dwells on what he/she has lost. Indeed, actively thinking about what is forgone can lead to it gaining apparent value, and thus make change away from it more difficult.

Replacements and substitutes

When a behaviour is reduced in frequency or eliminated altogether it often leaves a gap, which may need to be filled. The replacement can be a substitute, that is, something functionally equivalent to what it replaces (e.g. low-fat foods for their high-fat parallels) or an alternative that serves different purposes. Some behaviours are part substitutes, for example, nicotine replacement products only replace some of the functions of smoking. For alternatives that serve completely different functions to those they replace, it is important to consider the value to the person of those alternatives; for example, of exercising instead of relaxing, or of staying home instead of going out with friends as a way to control alcohol consumption. Where the forgone activity is likely to be missed, substitutes are likely to be much more effective than alternatives, as no matter how desirable the alternative is, it does not detract from the desirability of what is forgone, and dwelling on the missed experience may interfere with the positive experience of the chosen alternative.

If a perfect substitute can be found, that is, something that serves the same functions but without the adverse effects, it is likely that change will be easy, taking it out of the class of HTM behaviour change. Typically, substitutes are partial, and there are differences in consequences; for example, low-fat food may seem like a good substitute, but if it doesn't taste quite as good, it may be less easy to persist with. Moreover, if it does not inhibit further food consumption, the way full-fat food does, one may end up consuming more, thus reducing or even eliminating the initial benefit. Furthermore, some possible substitutes may not be seen as such. Whether vegetarian meat substitutes are seen as direct substitutes for meat or as an alternative diet depends on how the person views them. The way these issues are framed can have large effects on what people do (see Chapter 5). For example, there are different psychological consequences of seeing a dietary change as giving up high-fat forms of food to taking up low-fat versions, although both are functionally the same.

Substitutes may be particularly useful for drug use, especially where the problems with the drug are its dirty delivery system rather than the psychological effects it produces. In recent years, the possibility of replacing cigarette smoking with use of lower toxin forms of nicotine has excited considerable interest. To date, no other less harmful form of nicotine delivery competes with cigarettes in its ability to deliver nicotine to the brain, although some forms of e-cigarettes appear to be getting closer.

Some drugs such as methadone and nicotine replacement therapy are explicitly designed to be partial substitutes. They are designed to reduce the negative effects of stopping, thus making it easier to sustain abstinence, even though they are also designed to minimise the positive effects of the drug use, thus limiting their appeal as mass recreational products. This model of drug therapy is prefaced on the assumption that prolonged use of the drug is inherently bad, while the search for less harmful substitutes is grounded in an acceptance of the drug use and a focus on minimising the harms.

What is learnt in HTM behaviour change

Most HTM behaviours do not require complex skills, it is better thought of as a vigilance task (see Chapter 6). It is important to differentiate the development of habits from the development of the skills that may be required to perform them. Skill learning is a different process. It can require specific learning and can be fine-tuned by conditioning processes. In the case of HTM behaviours, it is rarely a skill that is an issue – the individual behaviours are relatively easy to perform and can often be performed without specific training, by just trying, or by trying after watching others perform them. Of more importance here is the next part of skill development, the routinisation of skills, that is, the process of becoming comfortable engaging in the behaviour and the transfer of control of the performance to automated (OS) functioning. In some cases, such as physical activities, the person might need to gradually build up the strength and or endurance necessary to complete the desired exercise regime, but once again skill is rarely a big part of this. The challenge is to feel comfortable in the new behaviour and be prompted to do it often enough to achieve the goal.

My research team have recently found that for smoking, a recent failed quit attempt predicts trying more often, but a reduced chance of success on any subsequent attempts [26], inconsistent with a skill learning model. So, we do need to ask the question: when are past failures relevant to future efforts? Has it got something to do with the memorability of the event (a function of recency and magnitude), the attributions that are made about failure, or has it got something to do with self-regulatory exhaustion?

Once a behaviour is learnt, it pretty much stays with us as a skill. Behaviour change is not about eliminating the capacity to perform a behaviour, it is about changing the incentive structure. For a behaviour to eliminate, it is about creating conditions such that the person no longer wants to perform the behaviour, or has the strength to resist engaging in the behaviour. For a desired behaviour, it is about increasing cues and incentives to use. What is critical for behaviour change is the extent to which the desired behaviours come to have or acquire intrinsic rewarding properties or the behaviour is missed if not performed, which is a mild form of avoidance learning. A good example of the latter is seat belt use. I feel uncomfortable if I get in a car without seat belts and the simple routine of putting it on is disrupted. It is easier to maintain something you enjoy, or something you miss when you don't do it, as these can be both cues to engage and rewards for acting.

Repeat performance is necessary for routinising a habit; however, for things we want to happen, there is a need to avoid habituation of rewarding elements or the build-up of negative consequences of behaving. For example, repetitive behaviours can come to be experienced as boring. There are strategies to avoid this, for example, by adding complementary attractive activities, such as listening to music while jogging, or walking with a friend and catching up on local gossip.

Where behaviours never get to be valued in their own right (e.g. putting on sunscreen is one for many), then the person needs to ensure that the cues to act are strong enough to stimulate the decision and enough arguments are there to provide a context for overcoming resistance. This may be facilitated by being provided with frequent reminders about the importance of the activity. In this way, cues to behave become imbued with motivational force.

There are some differences between HTS and HTR behaviours in what is learnt. For HTS behaviours, the novelty and the value of trying are important for initiation, while becoming comfortable doing them and being appropriately prompted is important for maintenance. For HTR behaviours, novelty is not an issue, but it may be an issue for the replacement behaviours. On the other hand, missing the behaviour that was forgone can be a strong cue to its resumption.

It should also be clear that there are likely to be differences in what is involved in the initiation of a behaviour change and its maintenance. Initiating something for the first time (or after previous experiences are forgotten) comes with a sense of foreboding (or anticipation) about the unknown. What will it be like? With HTM behaviours, foreboding is more likely. There may be some initial concern about performance, but more likely it will be fear of missing something you have come to expect to enjoy, or perhaps of anticipated immediate negative consequences such as withdrawal from drugs.

As most HTM behaviours are chronic relapsing ones, most people trying to change are trying in the face of experience of previous attempts. Thus, they should have a clear idea of what to expect. That said, if the stories they told themselves about past failures are inaccurate, for example, exaggerating the negative effects in order to self-justify failure, then their expectancies may be distorted. Once change is initiated, then it is likely that experiences will replace expectations as determinants of persistence, although once again, distorted interpretations can exaggerate negative effects or lead to undervaluing positive effects. Further, expectancies of future changes will remain important as HTM behaviours typically promise benefits that are not realised until well after the behaviour is routinised.

In summary, unwanted behaviours are those that will not just go away, are hard to reduce, and are over-cued, while hard to acquire or HTS behaviours are under-cued, and do not occur often enough. While there are some similarities, there are also important differences between these two classes of problem behaviours. This may mean some differences in the kinds of strategies needed to change them.

Summary

This chapter describes some of the observable characteristics of HTM behaviours. It spells out what is unique to HTM behaviours and similarities and differences between the two main kinds: hard-to-reduce (HTR) behaviours such as some forms of drug use, and their functional opposites, HTS behaviours such as exercise routines. It also considers the common situation where change involves a mix of both types of behaviour. The consequences of behaviour vary as a function of how immediate they are, which affects the ways they can potentially feedback to influence longer term maintenance.

References

1. Shiffman S, Balabanis M, Gwaltney C *et al.* Prediction of lapse from associations between smoking and situational antecedents assessed by ecological momentary assessment. *Drug and Alcohol Dependence.* 2007; **91**: 159–168.
2. Herd N, Borland R & Hyland A. Predictors of smoking relapse by duration of abstinence: Findings from the International Tobacco Control (ITC) Four Country Survey. *Addiction.* 2009; **104**: 2088–2099.

3. Lewin K. *A Dynamic Theory of Personality*. McGraw-Hill: New York, 1935.
4. Miller NE. Experimental studies of conflict. In: Hunt J (ed.) *Personality and the Behavior Disorders*. Ronald: New York, 1944: 431–465.
5. Orford J. *Excessive Appetites: A Psychological View of Addictions*. John Wiley & Sons: UK, 1985.
6. Stewart J & Badiani A. Tolerance and sensitization to the behavioral effects of drugs. *Behavioural Pharmacology*. 1993; **4**: 289–312.
7. Højsted J & Sjøgren P. Addiction to opioids in chronic pain patients: A literature review. *European Journal of Pain*. 2007; **11**: 490–518.
8. Fishbain D, Cole B, Lewis J *et al*. What percentage of chronic nonmalignant pain patients exposed to chronic opioid analgesic therapy develop abuse/addiction and/or aberrant drug-related behaviors? A structured evidence-based review. *Pain Medicine*. 2008; **9**: 444–459.
9. Baker TB, Piper ME, McCarthy DE *et al*. Addiction motivation reformulated: An affective processing model of negative reinforcement. *Psychological Review*. 2004; **111**: 31–51.
10. Piasecki T, McCarthy D, Fiore M *et al*. Alcohol consumption, smoking urge, and the reinforcing effects of cigarettes: An ecological study. *Psychology of Addictive Behaviors*. 2008; **22**: 230–239.
11. Kassel J, Stroud L & Paronis C. Smoking, stress, and negative affect: Correlation, causation, and context across stages of smoking. Review. *Psychological Bulletin*. 2003; **129**: 270–304.
12. Brandon T. Negative affect as motivation to smoke. Review. *Current Directions in Psychological Science*. 1994; **3**: 33–37.
13. Benowitz NL. Nicotine addiction. *New England Journal of Medicine*. 2010; **362**: 2295–2303.
14. Benowitz NL & Henningfield JE. Reducing the nicotine content to make cigarettes less addictive. *Tobacco Control*. 2013; **22**: i14–i17.
15. Shiffman S. Tobacco "chippers" – individual differences in tobacco dependence. *Psychopharmacology*. 1989; **97**: 539–547.
16. Borland R, Chapman S, Owen N *et al*. Effects of workplace smoking bans on cigarette consumption. *American Journal of Public Health*. 1990; **80**: 178–180.
17. Chapman S, Haddad S & Sindhusake D. Do work-place smoking bans cause smokers to smoke "harder"? Results from a naturalistic observational study. *Addiction*. 1997; **92**: 607–610.
18. Borland R, Partos T, Yong H *et al*. How much unsuccessful quitting activity is going on among adult smokers? Data from the International Tobacco Control Four Country cohort survey. *Addiction*. 2012; **107**: 673–682.
19. Hughes J, Solomon L, Fingar J *et al*. The natural history of efforts to stop smoking: A prospective cohort study. *Drug and Alcohol Dependence*. 2013; **128**: 171–174.
20. Cooper J, Borland R, Yong H *et al*. To what extent do smokers make spontaneous quit attempts and what are the implications for smoking cessation maintenance? Findings from the International Tobacco Control Four-Country Survey. *Nicotine and Tobacco Research*. 2010; **12**: S51–S57.
21. Murray R, Lewis S, Coleman T *et al*. Unplanned attempts to quit smoking: Missed opportunities for health promotions? *Addiction*. 2009; **104**: 1901–1909.
22. Cahill K, Stevens S, Perera R *et al*. Pharmacological interventions for smoking cessation: An overview and network meta-analysis. *The Cochrane Library* [Internet]. 2013; (5). doi: 10.1002/14651858.CD009329.pub2.
23. West R. The clinical significance of 'small' effects of smoking cessation treatments. *Addiction*. 2007; **102**: 506–509.

24. Vangeli E, Stapeleton J, Smit ES *et al*. Predictors of attempts to stop smoking and their success in adult general population samples: A systematic review. *Addiction*. 2011; **106**: 2110–2121.

25. Borland R, Yong HH, Balmford J *et al*. Motivational factors predict quit attempts but not maintenance of smoking cessation: Findings from the International Tobacco Control Four country project. *Nicotine & Tobacco Research*. 2010; **12**(Supplement 1): S4–S11.

26. Partos TR, Borland R, Yong HH *et al*. The quitting rollercoaster: How recent quitting history affects future cessation outcomes (data from the International Tobacco Control 4-country cohort study). *Nicotine and Tobacco Research*. 2013: 1–10. doi: 10.1093/ntr/ntt025. Epub March 2013.

27. Borland R, Yong H, Balmford J *et al*. Do risk-minimizing beliefs about smoking inhibit quitting? Findings from the International Tobacco Control (ITC) Policy Evaluation Survey. *Preventive Medicine*. 2009; **49**: 219–223.

28. Fotuhi O, Fong G, Zanna M *et al*. Patterns of Cognitive Dissonance-Reduction Beliefs among smokers: A longitudinal analysis from the International Tobacco Control (ITC) Four Country Survey. *Tobacco Control*. 2013; **22**: 52–58.

29. Shiffman S. Dynamic influences on smoking relapse process. *Journal of Personality* 2005; **73**: 1715–1748.

30. Shiyko MP, Lanza ST, Tan X *et al*. Using the time-varying effect model (TVEM) to examine dynamic associations between negative affect and self confidence on smoking urges: Differences between successful quitters and relapsers. *Prevention Science*. 2013; **13**: 288–299.

31. Siahpush M, Borland R & Yong H. Socio-demographic and psychosocial correlates of smoking-induced deprivation and its effect on quitting: Findings from the International Tobacco Control Policy Evaluation Survey. *Tobacco Control*. 2007; **16**: e2.

32. Siahpush M, Spittal M & Singh G. Association of smoking cessation with financial stress and material well-being: Results from a prospective study of a population-based national survey. *American Journal of Public Health*. 2007; **97**: 2281–2287.

33. Siahpush M, Yong H, Borland R *et al*. Smokers with financial stress are more likely to want to quit but less likely to try or succeed: Findings from the International Tobacco Control (ITC) Four Country Survey. *Addiction*. 2009; **104**: 1382–1390.

34. Cooper J, Borland R, Yong H *et al*. The impact of quitting smoking on anhedonia and depressed mood: Findings from the International Tobacco Control Four-Country Survey. 2013.

35. Piper M, Kenford S, Fiore M *et al*. Smoking cessation and quality of life: Changes in life satisfaction over 3 years following a quit attempt. *Annals of Behavioral*. 2012; **43**: 262–270.

36. Baker TB, Piper ME, McCarthy DE *et al*. Time to first cigarette in the morning as an index of ability to quit smoking: Implications for nicotine dependence. *Nicotine and Tobacco Research*. 2007; **9**: S555–S570.

37. Borland R, Yong H, O'Connor R *et al*. The reliability and predictive validity of the Heaviness of Smoking Index and its two components: Findings from the International Tobacco Control Four-Country study. *Nicotine & Tobacco Research*. 2010; **12**: S45–S50.

38. Yong HH, Borland R, Balmford J, *et al*. Heaviness of Smoking Index only predicts smoking abstinence in the first month of a quit attempt: Findings from the International Tobacco Control Four-Country Survey. *Nicotine and Tobacco Research* (*in press*).

39. Yong HH, Borland R, Balmford J *et al*. Heaviness of Smoking Index only predicts smoking abstinence in the first month of a quit attempt: Findings from the International Tobacco Control Four-Country Survey. 2013.

40. Piasecki T, Fiore M, McCarthy D *et al.* Have we lost our way? The need for dynamic formulations of smoking relapse proneness. *Addiction.* 2002; **97**: 1093–1108.
41. Wing R & Phelan S. Long-term weight loss maintenance. *American Journal of Clinical Nutrition.* 2005; **82**: 222S–225S.
42. Owen N. Sedentary behavior: Understanding and influencing adults' prolonged sitting time. *Preventive Medicine.* 2012; **55**: 535–539.
43. Owen N, Sugiyama T, Eakin EE *et al.* Adults' sedentary behavior: Determinants and interventions. *American Journal of Preventive Medicine.* 2011; **41**: 189–196.
44. Owen N, Healy GN, Howard B *et al.* Too much sitting: Health risks of sedentary behaviour and opportunities for change. *President's Council on Fitness, Sports & Nutrition: Research Digest.* 2012; **13**: 1–11.

Chapter 3

THE ROLES OF THE OPERATIONAL AND EXECUTIVE SYSTEMS

This chapter spells out in more detail the characteristics of the OS and the ES that interact with the external environment to co-determine human behaviour. It is not concerned with the biological mechanisms that underpin the functioning of the two systems, although I believe that all proposed mechanisms and processes in the theory are biologically realisable. The distinction between the OS and ES is designed to provide a theoretical framework to help us better understand the challenges and possibilities of improving self-regulatory processes. From a Public Health perspective, the focus is on self-regulatory processes directed towards adopting and maintaining lifestyles that are increasingly consistent with the kind of lives we believe are desirable, rather than with what we feel impelled to do. This involves acting to achieve imagined futures, rather than being constrained to simply adapt to present circumstances.

The focus of this chapter is on how the two systems work and the functions they serve. Dual-process approaches have been a part of our attempts to understand the limits of humans to act rationally since antiquity [1]. As noted in Chapter 1, within cognitive and social psychology, there has been a renewed interest in this way of thinking, largely as a result of an inability to explain all human behaviour in terms of rational processes. In a similar way, behaviourist theories that emphasise lower level, non-rational processes have also proved inadequate. The OS/ES distinction is one of several similar distinctions that attempt to differentiate between our animal selves and the conscious, deliberative self that we conceive ourselves as being [2–5]. An analysis of the similarities and differences between CEOS theory and one key dual-process theory [4, 6] is provided at the end of this chapter.

Before jumping into the meat of this chapter, a few words about terminology. The English language does not make clear distinctions between the functions of the ES and OS; so, it is useful to spell out the terms I use to describe OS processes and the related terms describing the representation of those processes in the ES. *Consciousness* refers to ES experiences, while *awareness* refers to things that are processed to some level by the OS and influence subsequent activity, regardless of whether they are represented in consciousness. *Experiences* is used more generally to refer to inputs from the OS to the ES, that is, things that become conscious. *Feelings* refers to the experience of states of the OS. *Memory* refers to conscious

Understanding hard to maintain behaviour change: A dual process approach, First Edition. Ron Borland.
© 2014 John Wiley & Sons, Ltd. Published 2014 by John Wiley & Sons, Ltd.

Table 3.1 Pairing of terms for OS processes and their experienced manifestation within consciousness (i.e. ES)

Focus	OS	Conscious experiences
Overall	Awareness	Consciousness/ experiences
Environment	Sensations	Perceptions
OS need states	Need states	Needs/feelings
Outcomes of OS activity	Action tendencies	Impulses/urges
Representation of past experiences	Activation patterns/ associations	Memories
Systematic changes in responding	Conditioning	Learning
Feedback	Feedback	Evaluation

memories, while *activation patterns* refers to those aspects of memory, which may not be consciously experienced, but are manifest in the ways the OS reacts to stimuli. *Learning* or *conditioning* refers to changes in activation patterns due to past experience (see also Table 3.1).

The Operational System

The OS acts in the moment and often acts outside of conscious awareness. It is essentially our animal, non-linguistic self. It does most of the work of keeping us alive and functioning, but much of this goes unnoticed by our ESs. Only a subset of its activities are consciously experienced, those that have been passed up to the ES for processing and those where the ES calls for input. The OS acts primarily in relation to the world as it is sensed in relation to its needs, which can include facilitating movement towards the achievement of goals when ES processes are activated (see later in this chapter).

The nature of the Operational System

The OS is a hierarchical sensory-motor control system designed to coordinate action to meet needs, and a signalling system from physiological processes as to what the homeostatic needs of the individual are from moment to moment. The continuous processing of the stream of sensory inputs creates patterns of associations which,

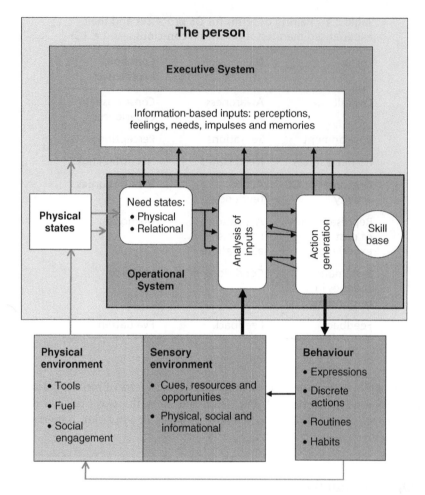

Figure 3.1 A schematic diagram of the Operational System and how it is influenced by inputs from both the environment and the Executive System.

tempered by inputs about current needs, results in a set of action tendencies that *compete* to be realised in the ongoing flow of behaviour. Resultant behaviour then feeds back to influence both the ongoing stream of perception and, more slowly, need states (Figure 3.1).

The individual receives two kinds of input from the environment: informational input including signals from sensory organs (sight, sound, taste, smell and touch), which are fed into the sensory-motor processing part of the system; and physical input including resources such as air, water and food, which directly influences need states. For the conscious ES experiences of the external world, I use the term *perceptions*, while *sensations* refer to the larger set of things that are sensed by the OS, much of which never reaches conscious awareness.

Need states can be either physical (e.g. hunger, thirst, physical comfort, physical exhaustion and sex urges) or relational (e.g. safety and social needs). They represent deviations from ideal or target levels of OS functioning. There are also needs for mastery of the environment, manifested as curiosity, and for maintaining skills and fitness. These can be thought as forms of relational need, in these cases to know the environment better, and to improve one's capacity to act within it. The experiences of need states by the ES are referred to as *needs* when they relate to specific need states, but *feelings* when used more generally to refer to states of the OS, particularly when they include relational and other more complex needs.

The physical state of the organism affects the efficiency of all functioning; thus, levels of exhaustion and fitness can directly influence performance, as can overloading capacity. Levels of physiological systems tend to run down over time, and some behaviours, such as eating, are designed to restore balance and thus directly affect need states.

The OS, as an information processing system, is theorised to be built up as outlined in Powers' [7] control systems theory of behaviour. Behaviour is conceived of as the means of controlling our *perceptions* (*sensations* in the language used here), of both the external world and signals from internal need states, so as to reduce discrepancies or internal error signals between targeted states and those actually achieved. Inputs generate associative networks of activation, which result in action tendencies and/or activation of higher level control systems. Action tendencies are properties of the output or motor aspect of the processing system, commonly referred to as *urges* or *impulses* when conscious. Action tendencies become more complex at higher levels of the system and require activation of their component lower level action tendencies if they are to result in behaviour. More complex action tendencies, especially when being discussed in the context of being implemented, are referred to as behavioural schemata.

Each higher level of the multi-level OS is involved in increasingly complex activities. It is a bottom-up processor, with processing only going as far up the hierarchy as necessary to decide on and coordinate action. The processing load means that higher order processes take longer to resolve than lower level ones; so, invoking higher level processes inevitably slows down decision making and thus action. Powers' model postulates that five levels of organisation are required to fully explain the complexities of representing the external world and responding to it, with a sixth level beginning to take into account the relationship between the actor and the represented world, thus affording the possibility of even more complex behaviours. All levels of the system have some degree of plasticity, in that their sensitivity levels for generating both action tendencies and signals to higher processes can be altered. This plasticity comes from both changes in needs and from experience, which includes short-term changes such as habituation, and higher up the hierarchy, more complex, longer term changes that are manifest as learning.

The information processing aspect of the OS has both excitatory and inhibitory processes, the levels of which determine aspects of personality (e.g. sensation-seeking, overly inhibited), including capacity to exercise self-control [8–11]. They are thus are a major source of individual differences in susceptibility to undesirable behaviour patterns and the capacity to change them. Inhibitory processes are essential for enabling higher order input because they can stop action tendencies from being implemented until higher level processes chose which one(s) should occur. Sensitivities to activation or inhibition can vary across parts of the system, and while they have a fixed genetic component, they can be shaped to some degree by experiences; for example, sensitivity to food-related cues can be shifted, even across generations, by living through a famine.

The hierarchy of input processing and output-generating loops has comparators set at each level to determine whether no action is required (not enough stimulation to generate further transmission of signals), in which case processing stops, or there is some further transmission of signals into the system; to generate action tendencies that are controlled by this part of the system, to inhibit potentially competing action tendencies and/or to activate higher level processes. Under normal conditions, inhibitory tendencies would be expected to inhibit all but the strongest action tendencies, else there would be a lot of impulsive and uncoordinated action. This means that inhibitory signals from higher levels of the system (including the ES) should be able to temporarily suppress all but the strongest action tendencies.

Signals about internal needs act in a different way to sensory information; they act to change the sensitivity of the core sensory-motor processor to sensory stimuli relevant to that need, within whatever limits there might exist for that individual. For example, when hungry, the sensory-motor processor amplifies responses to stimuli associated with food, thus making food-seeking or consuming behaviours more likely. Powers [7] describes this mode of acting as a reorganising system. It is the mechanism for changing the settings by which environmental conditions stimulate particular action tendencies, and/or further processing of input signals; that is, it results in the system being reorganised such that it responds in different ways to environmental cues. Reorganising mechanisms underpin state-dependent learning, that is, the tendency to learn things relevant to focal need states, and the capacity to ignore irrelevant associations, for example, when hungry animals learn to do things that lead to food rewards, but are less prone to learn these associations when sated. Reorganising capacity is characteristic of any higher level system that has downward links to the input processing functions of the level(s) below, not just to the output-generating aspects. Thus, aspects of ES functioning can also act to reset sensitivity levels of various levels of sensory-motor processing. Changes in settings proceed on slower time scales than the information processing that they influence. A simple example from lower level OS processes of a reorganising process is light–dark adaptation; when moving from the light into a darker environment, it takes several seconds for the process of adaption to occur and even longer to reach full sensitivity.

Integrated with the sensory processing capacity of the OS are mechanisms to generate and coordinate action tendencies. Action tendencies refer to dispositions to act, with each specific tendency being partly determined by actions that have previously been associated with reductions in needs. At the lowest level of the hierarchy, they are not 'needs' as we would normally think of them, but rather imbalances that need to be resolved for competent, smooth-flowing behaviour to occur. The most primitive form of action tendency is an evaluative reaction: to approach (positive evaluation), or avoid (negative evaluation) something in the environment.

Action tendencies for any particular behaviour are jointly determined by stimuli from the immediate environment, need states, and the recency and intensity of past instances of the behaviour. At the highest point in the control hierarchy where processing occurs, the balance of associations comes to favour one set of action tendencies over competing alternatives. The dominant one then becomes the behavioural schemata that directs behaviour until that schema is exhausted or interrupted. This domination is achieved by systematically inhibiting alternative tendencies, so that only the strongest signals (e.g. those generated by a sudden threat) are able to disrupt the implementation of the dominant schemata. Where no alternative comes to dominate, the person will be stuck in indecision, until the conflict is resolved by higher level inputs or dissipates because of changing environmental inputs.

The smooth flow of behaviour depends on relevant capacities, for example, motor skills. Capacity is partly innate, but within this constraint, varying degrees of competence can be achieved. Competence is affected by the past history of behaviour (e.g. training can transform latent capacity into realised skill). Capacities can also vary over time, affected by such things as the person's health (both physical and mental) and overall homeostasis (e.g. level of exhaustion). In Figure 3.1, the skill set is linked in a line without an arrow as it is not a separate process, but a reminder that having the necessary skills is essential for behaviour to occur.

Information from sensory-motor processing also feeds back internally to both activate physiological processes that might be required for action, and to influence some need states, particularly relational needs. For example, seeing a smiling friend triggers action towards the relational need of bonding with others. Feedback to activate relevant physiological mechanisms is important for controlling arousal. It is assumed that arousal increases when signals are being sent, but declines in their absence, with physiological arousal being necessary to support implementation of the behavioural schemata. There may also be a form of feedback that changes the probability (either increase or decrease) of a specific behaviour recurring in the short term, independent of influences via needs.

The above-mentioned analysis implies that for any given set of environmental conditions, there are many possible courses of action, and the one chosen at any moment will be that associated with whatever need state dominates. Need states can be conceived of as organised in some loose hierarchy [12] with those more central to survival likely to dominate the generation of behaviour when they are strongly activated. For example, it is hard to think about much else when you are very hungry or freezing cold, but far easier to be distracted from creative activities. Need states also vary in the extent to which they require cues, ranging from those that are strong enough to elicit behaviour independent of specific environmental cues (i.e. they only require that the environment allows the behaviour), through those where action requires minimal environmental cues, to those where action only occurs when restricted environmental conditions are met (e.g. eat only at meals, sex only with partner). Behaviours linked to specific sets of environmental cues tend to have priority for action when those cues are present, given a sufficient level of need. In cases of relational needs, such as threats, the environmental cues generate the need. Important need states for HTM behaviours include those related to consumption, avoidance of discomfort and pleasure seeking. These are all fairly high on the priority list, especially in environments where threats to immediate survival are rare.

The ongoing stream of behaviour also feeds back directly and sometimes indirectly on internal states. There are at least three direct effects of feedback: immediate, for the correction of ongoing behaviour; medium term on continuation and recurrence via effects on need states; and longer term, via changing the relative strengths of associative pathways to action tendencies, that is, via conditioning. This particular kind of direct feedback is critical for the characterisation of HTM behaviours; it stimulates the production of hard-to-reduce behaviours, but has the opposite effect for those that are hard to sustain.

Functions of the Operational System

The OS is designed to help the individual act in, maintain, or create environments in ways that mitigate threats and/or increase the probabilities of the individual engaging in desirable activities. In this subsection, operations of the OS are described in terms of the functions they serve, rather than in the mechanistic language of the previous subsection.

The key tasks of the OS are (i) selecting aspects of the environment to attend to, (ii) processing the information sufficiently to generate action tendencies, and where necessary engaging higher level processes to arbitrate on appropriate action, (iii) coordinating the implementation of chosen behaviours and (iv) adjusting subsequent behaviour based on immediate feedback.

The first function of the OS is to control attention. Only a fraction of the potentially available sensory information is processed to a level that stimulates any kind of action tendency, let alone conscious awareness. Thresholds for reacting to stimuli can change in relation to internal conditions. Changes in attention are influenced by the nature of ongoing OS processing of sensory inputs, plus influences from need states and the ES. The focus of attention can also be changed by moving in and/or manipulating aspects of the environment, that is, changing what is available to sense. Acting to change one's position in the environment can be part of acting instrumentally, to seek out cues relevant to need states or because there is nothing in the present environment to trigger interest, and thus action can be purely exploratory.

The second task is to decide on appropriate action. For any complex behaviour, certainly for HTM behaviours, a complex of action tendencies, some incompatible with others, are typically generated each time environmental conditions cue the possibility of action. Each action tendency is built on an evaluative element, with a primary distinction made between positive stimuli that evoke approach-related action tendencies, and negative ones that evoke avoidance tendencies [4]. Avoidance tendencies can either be manifest in tendencies to try to remove the target or to move away from it. These evaluative tendencies emerge well before conscious awareness of the objects occurs. Processing of inputs needs to go high enough up the hierarchy of control to deal with the complexity of behaviour required,

Table 3.2 Relationships between positive and negative experiences and related behaviour

Experience	Contingent on behaviour	Non-contingent
Positive	Reinforces future instances of the behaviour it follows	No motivational force – stasis
Negative	Suppresses future instances of the behaviour it follows	Motivates a general search for actions to reduce negativity

including the need to resolve any incompatible action tendencies (conflicts). The behaviour chosen will be the one with the most affective force, that is, the one most strongly linked to a need or set of needs, unless it is inhibited by ES processes. If higher level processes act to change the needs activated and/or their strengths, they can affect the relative strengths of competing action tendencies, and thus influence the ultimate choice of behaviour.

While both positive and negative experiences affect behaviour when contingent on it, negative experiences also have a general motivating effect as they represent unmet need states (Table 3.2). By contrast, positive mood states signal a lack of need for action, such as those associated with the successful attainment of some need or goal, or with the anticipation of impending action that will likely achieve some desired end, and therefore only tend to motivate immediate antecedents, not their consequences. This has important implications for HTM behaviours, particularly those that are hard to reduce, as abstinence is often associated with negative feelings that the undesirable behaviour can at least temporarily reduce. For example, smoking is seen as a way of coping with feeling stressed or unhappy [13, 14]. However, as there is no comparable process linking feeling good to not smoking, even though smokers report feeling better after they quit, this is not protective against relapse [15].

The third function of the OS is to enable the smooth implementation of chosen behaviours. Coordinated action is via the highest level of behavioural schemata activated. Arousal is generated and managed through feedback into physiological processes, and information about this is fed up into higher levels of processing, including to the ES where necessary. The coordination of action also involves the concurrent production of expressions that appear to have evolved, at least in part, to alert others to likely actions, and thus facilitate social coordination.

Ongoing processing of feedback is critical to adaptive functioning. Actions that reduce needs are experienced as positive and are reinforced, while those that fail, or worse, exacerbate the target need, are experienced as negative and tend to be inhibited. Feedback about the consequences of our actions with respect to inanimate objects is fairly straightforward to interpret. However, feedback from animate objects, most notably other people, is more complex, as the way they act is influenced by the way we act. Our senses are highly attuned to picking up very subtle reactions of others to what we do (see Chapter 4).

For higher organisms, most notably humans, another important aspect of OS functionality is to provide inputs into ES functioning, that is, conscious experience. How conscious experiences influence behaviour is the topic of the next major section. There is also evidence that the OS can influence ES decision making in ways that are not consciously represented, but because they are not represented in consciousness, they cannot be directly taken into account by the ES, and need to be inferred from biases they create in decision making (see the subsection on Limitations of ES Processing).

The end result of OS functioning is predictable patterns of behaviour, or habits, being learnt and maintained. For the most part these habits are adaptive, but where they are not, strategies are needed to change them.

Modifying OS functions

The main mechanism for changing OS settings in the longer term is through processes of conditioning and extinction [16]. There are two main kinds of conditioning: classical and operant. Classical conditioning is where stimuli that are newly, but regularly, presented just before the occurrence of something inherently rewarding, come to elicit some of the same responses as those produced by the rewarding object itself. This is now generally accepted as being a preparatory response, rather than being in some ways the same as the unconditioned response [17]. The classical case is ringing a bell before food is supplied to an animal, which leads to the bell eliciting a flow of saliva, something naturally generated by the presence of food (for a hungry animal). In the language of CEOS, conditioning is the linking of action tendencies to new cues. Similarly, negative states like fear can be conditioned by pairing a previously neutral cue with a painful experience. Conditioned fears that can be reliably avoided by some form of action are remarkably persistent even if the original aversive stimulus is no longer present, presumably because the animal never gets to experience that this is the case. The animal needs to be forced to stay in the fearful situation for the strength of a conditioned fear to reduce in strength.

The other form of conditioning is operant conditioning. This is where a new behaviour is generated or changed in frequency; if a behaviour is rewarded, it leads to an increase in response frequency. Again, the classical case is of a rat learning to press a bar for food rewards. Similarly, if a behaviour is punished, it reduces in response frequency. If the possibility of punishment is signalled, it leads to avoidance of the situation where the punishment had been delivered.

Behaviours that have positive immediate effects increase in strength, while those that have negative effects are suppressed, and those that produce no meaningful consequences tend to extinguish (i.e. activation of associations declines to the point where action tendencies are weakened to the point they rarely occur). Conditioned associations generate the routines that constitute habits. The habitual component becomes part of the person's lifestyle; it may occur relatively independent of conscious intent, but can be the focus of attention, and some aspects of the performance may come to be valued (e.g. smokers blowing smoke rings), or it may be the experience of performing it that is valued (e.g. the feeling of the smoke on the back of the throat). When the person stops engaging in a habit, these action patterns or the associated experiences are often missed, as they have become rewarding, leading to urges or cravings to resume the behaviour that can persist for quite extended periods, above and beyond any direct effects of drug withdrawal. As we shall see, ES responses can sometimes modulate the effects of these OS-controlled processes.

This analysis leaves out an explanation as to why some behaviours develop stronger conditioned links than others. Much of the thinking in this area is around addictive behaviours, particularly drug use [18]. CEOS theorises, along with others [7, 19], that excessive behaviours tend to arise when there is over-sensitisation of cues to the occurrence of rewarding behaviours, and too-rapid recovery of satiation (that is periods of reduced cue sensitivity following performance of the behaviour). This is similar to Robinson and Berridge's [18] incentive sensitisation model, but framed slightly differently. Along with incentive sensitisation theory, CEOS posits a central role for conditioned stimuli leading to the incentive value being sensitised. However, it does not depend on the effects of the behaviour on the underlying state, so does not include response sensitisation. There is a lot of evidence that sham (or placebo) doses of drugs produce many of the same effects as real doses, at least in the short to medium term [20–22].

This is theorised to occur because the nervous system does not have direct imme-diate feedback loops from the consequences of behaviour; these are mediated by the aforementioned slower signals of changing need states. It is the anticipations, and signals about the actions, that are fedback to modify system functioning. In this way, it is the conditioned experiences that users come to value, often more than the actual physiological effects of the drug. This phenomenon also helps explain why smok-ers have routines for smoking, even though this has been shown to be associated with increased tolerance for the drug [23, 24] and thus smaller physiological effects for any given dose. If they smoked entirely for the physiological effects, one might expect them to be seeking new situations that unambiguously offer opportunities to increase physiological effects, not holding strong preferences for old ones.

To the extent that drug use does not result in permanent changes in the oper-ations of the relevant brain circuits underlying this process, that is, ones that are fundamentally different to those produced by learnt associations, then changes in drug-related behaviour should be able to occur via the same mechanisms as non-drug-related addictions. That said, like all learnt behaviours, extinction is not a wiping of all experience. Skills once learnt are not unlearnt, they are just not per-formed (much) unless there are benefits for acting; so, resumption of old behaviour patterns can occur rapidly when either self-control mechanisms are lifted or rewards are reinstated. Under this model, withdrawal from a drug is not a central motiva-tor of the resumption of the behaviour; it only triggers the behaviour to the extent that it leads to stronger reactions to drug-related cues, or as a negative affective state, something that stimulates greater searching for activities with the potential to reduce the negative affect.

Previously rewarded or intrinsically rewarding behaviours will tend to recur when suppressing conditions are removed, because the associative network associating the behaviour with the reward remains intact. However, unlike the negative consequences (e.g. punishment) meted out in experimental contexts, the anticipated negative consequences of undesirable behaviours, such as smoking, are likely to persist as long as knowledge of the harms remains salient; so, the suppressing effects of executive decisions are also likely to persist as long as the person believes the consequences are real, and these beliefs are triggered at appropriate times.

The strength of the tendency to persist with a behaviour is influenced by the predictability of rewards. Variable ratio schedules, such as those found in gaming (you only win on a random percentage of cases with the overall percentage chance fixed), sustain behaviour more than a constant reward or a fixed ratio of rewards (every so many performances). Similarly, fixed intervals between rewards (e.g. you only get one for the first act after the interval expires) have different effects to variable interval rewards. In both variable ratio and variable intervals, unrewarded cases of the behaviour do not clearly signal removal of the reward, and the behaviour is more likely to recur while the schedule is in place, and to persist for longer if the reward is withdrawn.

Where the association between a behaviour and a reward is broken, and is experienced to be lost, the strength and/or frequency of the conditioned response declines. However, after periods of no exposure to the situation, there is typically some degree of recovery of the behaviour when the opportunity to engage in it recurs, but this declines again rapidly if no reward is forthcoming. This recovery of habit strength is experienced by the ES as nostalgia about old habits. If the person gives in, and if the old rewards are there (or for suppressed ones, the aversive consequences are no longer there), the habit can rapidly re-establish itself.

As is the case for conditioned emotional responses, if the person never gets to experience that the link is broken, then the strength of the association between a behaviour and its consequences may not decline. For example, when a person smokes cigarettes, the act of smoking becomes conditioned to the immediately positive effects of the nicotine (mainly) on the brain. When they quit, this association remains, and thus if circumstances lead to the person smoking again, the conditioned link is likely to lead to the person rapidly returning to regular smoking. There is now considerable evidence that smoking denicotinised cigarettes (i.e. ones with no nicotine) leads to a reduction in positive experiences of smoking and can facilitate smoking cessation [20, 25]. However, to date, this is not widely used as a therapy to help smokers quit.

There are two other aspects of conditioning that are of relevance to the challenges of HTM behaviour change. First counterconditioning, or the linking of an incompatible response to an existing response, resulting in the original response being reduced. Houben et al. [26, 27] found that while linking positive pictures with words related to alcohol drinking increased interest in drinking, those presented with negative pictures actually reported drinking less in the following week. Another example is the use of health warnings on cigarette packs. The warning acts as a stimulus that elicits concern about smoking and does this at the same time as the presence of the pack elicits the conditioned anticipatory reactions to getting a rewarding dose of nicotine. If these new associations are strong enough, they can disrupt or even overwhelm the anticipated enjoyment of smoking and thus reduce the value of smoking. Health warnings on cigarettes are known to lead to thoughts about the harms of smoking, which in turn is related to actually not smoking individual cigarettes. Both of these reactions are associated with increased likelihood of attempting to quit smoking [28, 29]. The problem with this approach is that because smoking does produce positive experiences, if the behaviour occurs without the cue to elicit the countering experience, then the behaviour is likely to recur, that is, the person will smoke as much when not thinking about the harm, but may be more constrained when they are thinking about it.

The second aspect of conditioning is of the competing response, also sometimes known as habit reversal [30]. This is where the person practices a response that directly competes with an undesired behaviour. It has been most commonly used as a therapy to control undesirable repetitive behaviours, such as tics or nail biting. This idea represents an unused potential for undesired behaviours where suitable competing alternatives can be identified.

More detailed analysis of the various forms of conditioning can be found in any textbook on the psychology of learning. West and Brown [31] provide a good overview as it relates to addiction.

Conditioned associations are one reason why addiction to one form of a drug often does not generalise to other forms of the same drug, and this may be enhanced by the rate of uptake of the drug by the brain [32]. The preparatory activities and the cues associated with use of the drug (what it looks like, its smell, etc.) become conditioned stimuli that elicit a positive anticipatory response. If other forms of the drug don't have such properties, then the anticipation will be lost, and the alternative form of use will not be as satisfying.

The ES has some influence over conditioning. Conditioned habits can be overridden or suppressed to varying degrees by ES action, and deliberate practice can speed up the establishment of conditioned links. However, volitional action does not replace conditioned behaviours as is implicitly assumed by some cognitively oriented theories. Conditioning allows for a lot of behaviour to go on with minimal executive oversight. It is only when these reactions are inconsistent with ES goals that we become concerned and seek to engineer change.

In summary, conditioning is the primary means by which the OS adapts to the world independent of the ES. Thus, changing the pattern of conditioned associations is critical to sustained behaviour change, else ongoing self-regulatory activity will be required to suppress recurrence of the undesirable habit, or to trigger desirable behaviours that are insufficiently cued to occur without executive oversight.

The Executive System

This subsection describes the structural and mechanistic aspects of the ES and how it functions as a self-regulatory system. The functioning of the ES as a conceptual system is discussed in Chapter 5. In talking about the ES, it is far easier to talk in purposive terms than using the mechanistic language of patterns of associations leading to action tendencies. Thus, influences that are theorised to occur outside of consciousness are described in mechanistic terms, while executive processes are described in terms of analysis and intentions.

The main role of the ES is to provide higher level direction to the OS. The ES has the capacity to operate via a model of the person (self) in the environment in which he or she operates. This requires more complex models of reality than those built up by the OS, that is, those that control reactive behaviour. The ES operates via a different mode of organisation that is grounded in the highest levels of processing in Powers' hierarchy of control systems. Executive processes require activation of appropriate lower level OS action tendencies to result in behaviour.

Core capacities of the ES

The ES takes inputs from the OS and processes them consciously to influence behaviour (Figure 3.2). It is also influenced by OS processes in ways that are not represented in consciousness. In some ways, it operates in a manner parallel to the OS. *Goals* are forms of need generated by the ES. The term implies a gap, with goal attainment and its resolution. Goals do not refer to OS needs, unless they have been adopted by the ES as deliberate objectives. *Cognitions, concepts, thoughts* or *thinking* are terms used for the equivalent of OS-automated processing; complex action tendencies generated by the ES are called *scripts* or where they are not likely to need ES oversight for implementation, *behavioural schemata*.

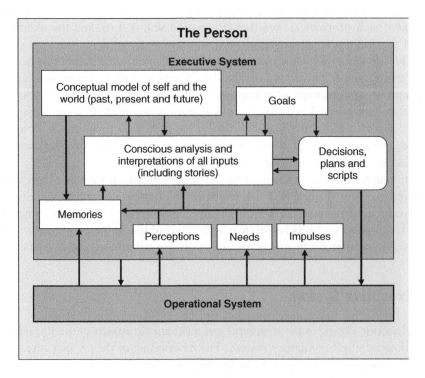

Figure 3.2 Core functions of the Executive System indicating key inputs from the OS.

In addition to the functions, it shares with the OS, the ES is theorised to have a number of unique features.

- Consciousness or the capacity to be aware of being aware, which provides self-reflective capacity. It includes representations of the external world (perceptions); and representations of internal need states (feelings), the latter being necessary to be able to reflect on self (at least in the ways we can).
- Long-term or episodic memory, not just changes in associative networks (the kind of longer term 'memory' the OS has).
- Language and other capacity to manipulate symbols and develop and apply rules.

This remarkable set of capacities is why it is useful to think of the ES as a separate system to the OS. People are not born with some of these capacities, most notably language, rather they develop them in early life and they become fully operational in adolescence [33, 34]. Similarly, in old age, some of the functionality can be lost, as it can through brain injury or disease. It can also be affected by physical states, being more limited when the person is exhausted, under the influence of psychoactive drugs, or when capacity is being drawn away to other functions.

Consciousness

Consciousness, or the underlying processes which it represents, is theorised to be a necessary precondition for the operation of the ES. What is meant by consciousness is awareness of being aware, or the ability to reflect on awareness [35]. I see consciousness as the experience of being the kind of individual who has the higher order symbolic processing capacity that humans so clearly possess. Seen this way, the contents of consciousness represent activities of a different kind to those which do not appear in consciousness, and it is the significance of those differences that we should be attempting to understand. Whether consciousness is just a sign of differences in the nature of processing, or part of the cause of those differences, is both uncertain and not relevant here. For convenience, we will assume that consciousness serves a functional role. This thinking is different to other recent theorising, for example, of Wegner [36], who argues that the lack of total control shows that consciousness is not central to higher processing. Lack of total control is not a reasonable criterion for irrelevance; indeed, in complex systems, nothing has total control. In my view, all that is required for consciousness is capacity to exert influence of a different kind to those operating via OS processes.

Consciousness is experienced as continuously flowing from the present. It is the mechanism by which the past and future are related to the present and is a necessary condition for complex planned action towards future possibilities. It is not clear whether some level of self-reflective capacity is also required for the kinds of insightful problem, solving that some infra-humans are capable of, for example, insightful use of tools by apes, although if it is, it is of a more limited kind. Consciousness is externally operationalised through a person's reports of it, and this requires memories of the events (for long enough for the person to report on them), and language for communicating them.

There are several different types of representations in consciousness. These include representations of the environment (perceptions), internal states (feelings), memories and thoughts. Of these, it is the representation of internal states that is most notable and of central importance to understand behaviour change. Many affective experiences or feelings occur when there is no contested action, or no change in what one is doing. Feelings are theorised to be the mechanism by which aspects of operational functioning are made available to the executive for analysis. They are important for decision making; where no new decisions are needed, then no consideration need to be given to internal needs, and feelings are less likely to appear in consciousness.

We all have the capacity to make conscious decisions about courses of action. Volitional action is defined as action that is deliberately chosen by the ES, and which would not have occurred but for that choice. Such actions tend to be those where there are no competing OS-generated action tendencies, or in the case of HTM behaviours, where the person has used ES processes to stimulate the OS to generate action tendencies consistent with ES plans, thus overcoming pre-existing OS-generated tendencies. Not all conscious action is volitional, some are reflections on behaviours that were not actively chosen, and in some cases can be behaviours the ES would prefer not to be doing.

Memory

Long-term memory is an essential characteristic of the ES. It includes both semantic and episodic aspects [37]. Semantic memory is memory for meaning and is strongly linked to OS processes. Episodic memory is for events and pieces of information, and may not be affectively linked. Episodic memory requires representational capacity, and language is the medium for most of this. Episodic memory gives us the capacity to remember ideas, and to be able to access them independent of environmental context. It is necessary for maintaining an idea of the past, and the basis of being able to plan for future possibilities. All memories, including ideas, generate more associative networks and associated action tendencies. Episodic memories, in particular, generate associative connections, both with other ideas and with action tendencies. The extent and strength of the latter index the strength of desire to act, and are accompanied by emotions, especially when the person is not in a position to act immediately. Some emotions, particularly negative ones are signs that processing is continuing to try to identify appropriate actions. Semantic memories are the experience of associative patterns, which is what memory is at the level of the OS. Associations provide the connotative aspects of meaning, while episodic memories provide the propositional or denotational aspects (e.g. the formal definitions). The connotative aspects include the affective reactions that indicate engagement with patterns of memories and provide the basis for linking to action tendencies.

For hard-to-reduce behaviours, memories represent strong past associations between the behaviour and the related expectations of benefits, and are central to the maintenance of those behaviours. For hard-to-sustain behaviours, it is the lack of such a rich store of memories, or of memories of unpleasantness, that makes it hard to stimulate the desired behaviours.

Language

Language is a symbolic system that allows representation of objects and events and rule-based links between them. Language is temporally de-linked from the reality it represents. Language, and the novel self-regulatory functions that it allows, leads to a new dimension of understanding, in an analogous way to the jump from chemistry to biology: while all biological organisms obey the laws of chemistry, explaining that life in chemical terms is not particularly useful for understanding the behaviour of life forms. In principle, language-based action can be explained in terms of reactive processes, but the level of complexity makes it impractical and of no real utility. For any predictive understanding of behaviour, conceptual determinants of behaviour are best conceived as following rule-based causal pathways that are fundamentally different to reactive, stimulus-based causes, which in turn differ from purely physical causes.

Language allows for the development of systems of rules, such as logical analysis. However, the ES is neither inherently logical nor rational. These skills need to be learnt and then applied. Language also allows stores of knowledge to reside outside of the individual, to be accessed when needed. This is most manifest in the amazing power of search engines like Google.

Language is important both for thinking and in the way people interact with the social environment. Language begins as a social activity, and gradually becomes internalised with development [33]. The ES can also operate via imagination (visual or otherwise), but cannot communicate these directly to others; so, its role in decision making is not well understood. As the OS is primed to allow the physical production of speech or writing, propositional content is delivered via the OS to the world as if it came directly from the ES. However, the emotional meta-delivery remains under OS control, although the ES analysis can have some influence on how the OS delivers messages. Competing OS action tendencies and impulses can act to disrupt speech, leading to dysfluencies and unintended meanings (e.g. Freudian slips).

Volitional, language-based processes are not a complete system of themselves, but rather an influence on non-volitional processes, which continue to drive behaviour directly as well as indirectly through their impact on volitional processes, something most obvious with HTM behaviours.

Inputs to the ES

All the inputs into the ES come from the OS and are built up by OS processes. There are three main forms, namely, perceptions, feelings and urges to act (or the experience of action tendencies; see Figure 3.2).

Perceptions are the OS's interpretation of the external environment produced by its sensory capacities. What is perceived is also affected by attentional mechanisms, which lead us to favour the perception of some things rather than others. These attentional processes vary from sense to sense. At best, attentional mechanisms allow us to attend to what is important, but in some cases, we are tuned to attend to some things that may not be important (any more) and potentially to ignore things that are important. The ES has the capacity to direct the OS to shift attention, but what we perceive is ultimately what the OS allows. For example, we can choose to close our eyes or turn away, but any filtering of what is sensed is carried out by the attentional processes of the OS. That said, for most purposes, the link between the environment and our perceptions can be treated as real. Further, symbolic information can only affect the OS after it has been decoded by the ES; thus, it can also be thought of as being directly accessed (Figure 3.2). These effectively direct influences of symbolic information do not include perceptions of, and thus reactions to, the carrier of the message (e.g. the appearance of the words, tone of voice), which are generated by OS processes, directly interpreted by it and fed up to the ES, rather than having to wait until the words are decoded. These connotations influence the meaning the ES extracts.

The second set of inputs are feelings, including experienced needs. Needs refer to a range of signals to the ES about imbalances in the current state of the OS, while the term feelings tends to be used more when the need relates to the person's relationship to the environment. Experiences of relevance here are mainly negative, for example, anxiety, fear and anger. There are also feelings that are experienced as positive, signalling the resolution of imbalances and hence no further action is required, or that the satisfaction of needs is imminent. Without feelings, people would not be able to take operational factors into account in decision making. Information about needs provides a basic element of self-reflective capacity. It is not clear whether feelings arise directly from signals about need states, or from changing thresholds or settings for associative processes, but for our purposes, this does not matter. The ES also has the capacity to generate new needs through the generation of goals for action, but these only come with feelings when they have been linked to OS-level needs.

The third form of input is of urges or impulses to act in particular ways, which is the experience of action tendencies (or drives) within the OS. I use the terms *urges* and *impulses* to describe the experience of OS-initiated action tendencies and *desires* for those coming from the pursuit of ES goals. Complex or higher level action tendencies are called *behavioural schemata*, where they can be brought under OS control, and *scripts*, where they are more complex and require direct executive input. It is difficult to choose to act while the OS has generated competing action tendencies as these need to be inhibited for the chosen action to occur. For example, consider someone skydiving or bungee jumping for the first time. They do not simply step off the edge into the void, they often act by tricking the OS into not attending to the immediate reality, by closing their eyes or having someone push them. It is simply too difficult for most to overcome direct resistance from the OS to such actions.

Feelings can range from signalling no need for action (e.g. satisfaction), through anticipation of impending behaviours, either positive (anticipation) or negative (fear), to those with no clear path (e.g. anxiety), to ones reflecting outcomes of past action (e.g. various forms of good or bad). In general, uncontested action has no strong affective component, being experienced as flow [38]. Negative feelings are particularly important, as they are signals from the OS to the ES that all is not well, that things are out of balance in some way, and that action is needed to restore the balance.

The OS also generates affective responses to executive inputs, such as stories, memories and the interpretation of experiences, and these can generate feelings or act to heighten or blunt existing feelings. I use the term *emotions* to refer to feelings that have been elaborated by executive processes. What we experience as emotions are complex mixes of raw feelings, action tendencies and cognitive elaborations, especially of needs and desires that are not currently being resolved. Knowing which experiences are direct OS reactions (feelings) and which are modulated by ES interpretations (emotions) is important for managing change (see Chapter 7) as inappropriate heightening of emotions can act to help sustain undesirable behaviours. The two can be distinguished by temporarily suppressing the ES activity, perhaps using techniques of mindfulness [39], and seeing what is left (pure feeling) or by considering what affective force is left in a context where operational forces are not activated, although the latter does not tap the modulation of OS-generated feelings, only the unique contribution of executive processes.

The emotion most prone to executive elaboration is anxiety, or the experience of uncertainty as to what to do. Our ESs are great generators of uncertainty through their capacity to imagine the future. The future is a time of infinite unrealised possibilities, possibilities that our actions can change the likelihood of, but in ways we can never be certain of until after the event. Learning to control anxiety is an important challenge, as exaggeration of uncertainty or the creation of excessive doubt can be a strategy for undermining action to address difficult problems.

Feelings and emotions are signals, not ends in themselves; therefore, changing emotions should not be a goal to be pursued directly, but one that can only be achieved by changing the underlying conditions that produced the feelings. For example, one should not seek to avoid fear, but to avoid the situations that generate fear, or reimagine the situation to reinterpret the fear-evoking aspects as less central.

The other main form of input to the ES is through memories. The OS generates a flow of associations to stimuli that are influenced by past exposures to those stimuli and the reactions that occurred, which is the form of memory operational processes have. Memory for the executive is the conscious experience of the results of this process. Stimuli need not just come from the environment; ideas and other aspects of the conceptual world can also generate affective responses and action tendencies and can also be influenced by past experiences. These experiences can be both propositional and non-propositional. The ES also has some capacity to search memory for relevant past experiences or pieces of propositional knowledge, and in so doing generates new waves of associations, including affective elements, which shape options for action. These analyses can lead to either action and the dissipation of the emotions, or continued inaction and the strengthening of existing emotions and/or the generation of competing emotions.

Both context and needs influence what is pushed towards consciousness, and thus can influence decisions by influencing what constitutes the focus, or content, of decision making. The ES can also influence the likelihood of memories being retrieved by way of its framing of the situation, and the associated desires it generates. To give a simple example, remembering reading a story about a visit to a house turns up different memories if the retrieval is done from the frame of a homebuyer versus a burglar [40]. Similarly, when stressed, and the frame is dealing with stress, different memories of smoking will be recalled than when the context or frame is thinking about how to improve one's long-term health.

It is the OS that is ultimately required to generate the actions that higher order scripts or behavioural schemata specify. The ES needs to find a context that stimulates the OS to act on its plans. When the OS has generated action tendencies that are inconsistent with ES plans, the ES can inhibit such tendencies much more efficiently than it can implement its own plans; stopping action requires less coordination that enacting it.

Stories and the roles they play

A core element of human functioning is trying to make sense of the world in which we live so that we can act more effectively within it. This conceptualising is done through the creation of stories. Stories are used by people to explain what they experience, to identify needs and thus goals for action and strategies to achieve identified goals. The stories I talk about here are the ones related to the person's attempts to make sense of the world and their place in it. I am not talking about purely fictional stories. The term stories, as used here, refers primarily to elaborations of beliefs and rationales for behaviours.

Every story has a framing, that is, a point of view from which it comes and often a set of assumptions that go with it [41, 42]. The frame chosen affects the associations made and thus the likely consequences.

There are three main kinds of story elements: those that simply describe aspects of the world or history (what is, or was and or could be), including people's stories of who they are (Descriptions); those which explain how the world works and why things are as they are, including stories to justify past actions, or to identify goals for future action (Explanations); and stories to help determine future action, including promises and commitments (Scripts). These elements correspond roughly to what scientists call taxonomies, explanatory theories and intervention models, which are judged on their ability to explain, predict and influence events in the world by guiding action and/or justifying inaction. Stories often consist of all three elements. Where we talk generally, we will use the term story, but where the focus is on one element, we will use the more specific term.

The genesis of all stories is social and their continued use is socially reinforced. Stories need to share common referents to be communicated to others. A person's stories are often grounded on assumptions (typically unspecified) about the nature

Table 3.3 The relationship between type of story and story focus on the kinds of questions it addresses

Type of story	Focus of the story			
	Self	Others (US)	Them	Environment
Description	Who am I?	Who are we and what we are doing together?	What other kinds of actors are around, and what are they doing?	What is my situation?
Explanation	Why I am doing or will do, what I do?	Why do we do what we do together?	Why do others do what they do?	How do things work?
Action plans	How do I do it? What am I going to do? How can I do it better?	How will I act with others? How will we act?	How can they do it? How will I act towards them?	How can change occur in the existing environment?

of the world that are widely shared by the society in which the person lives. Indeed, it is often the social confirmation of our analytic stories that convinces us that these explanations can be more useful than just relying on the implications we draw directly from experiences. Understanding the assumptive base of our stories can be important to an analysis of how stories can sometimes lead us astray.

Each of the three main kinds of story can have as its topic the self, other actors, the environment or any combination of these (Table 3.3). Collectively, each of us has a set of stories or potential stories that describe aspects of ourselves, and how we relate to others and the world in general. This set ranges from grand stories about who we are, to specific scripts for doing quite mundane tasks. These can be thought of as hierarchically organised in terms of complexity, and also ordered in terms of areas of applicability (e.g. work and home life).

The set of stories a person holds can vary in the extent to which they are mutually consistent. Inconsistency is easier to deal with when stories are used in non-overlapping parts of the person's life, but when normally separate aspects of a person's life come into contact and the scripts prescribe incompatible actions, it is likely to create problems. Inconsistency can create cognitive dissonance [43]; that is, the feeling of conflict when beliefs about what is appropriate, and rationales for behaviours, are mutually incompatible. People are motivated to reduce dissonance either by bringing behaviour into congruence with beliefs where the beliefs are important to the person's sense of self, by bringing beliefs into congruence with behaviour or where neither of these seem viable, by avoiding thinking about the issue. For example, for smokers who believe themselves to be sensible people who do not expose themselves to unnecessary risks, the story about the harmfulness of smoking should lead them to the rational conclusion that it is desirable to quit, putting them in a dissonance situation. He or she could try to quit, discount the evidence, focus on the difficulty of quitting (I am addicted) or simply try not to think about it as ways to reduce the dissonance. Any of these are preferable to changing their self-story.

Stories of *who we are* are particularly important as they include considerations of our values and aspirations. They can also, but need not, include a model of our OS. Indeed for some people, what their OS wants corresponds with what they want. Because what our OS wants is not always in our best interests, it is desirable if the self-story encompasses both our ES and OS as separate, but related aspects of who we are. Life stories typically include elements of our relationships with others (e.g. I am respected by my friends) and with aspects of their relationship with the environment (e.g. I decide what I will do and not do). The environments in which this story must continue to work includes people and things which can, and do, act in ways that are different to how the person's story specifies the individual should act. This can be a major source of conflict. For an individual who believes a story of individual autonomy, finding oneself unable to volitionally change HTM behaviours can be very personally threatening.

Stories grounded in the person's experience have different characteristics to those grounded in propositional knowledge, with those based on vicarious experience having elements of both. The key difference is the strong emotional engagement in stories based on personal experience. Our capacity to volitionally influence experience-based stories or beliefs is limited. We cannot deny the experience, but we can work to alter the interpretation (i.e. what the experience means) when it appears to be creating problems [44]. The ES can act to amplify or constrain OS reactions. For example, ES-augmented fear of pain can inhibit people engaging in important but mildly painful activities.

An important feature of stories is that they can be about possible futures, which can be thought about independent of the context in which they can be brought about. Multiple stories can be compared with each other. Emerging out of this, stories can specify absence. This gives us the capacity to plan not to do things, an idea that has no referents in the world of the OS, where all action is in relation to what is present.

Critical to CEOS theory is the role stories can play in facilitating change. Using stories to resolve conflict requires the representation of OS-generated reactions. This can involve resolving conflicts between impulses to act, or stories that focus on explaining or justifying these OS-generated impulses, and conceptual models of what is or should be desirable. As a justification, story has intrinsic links to OS processes; it is likely to have motivational force. Any conceptually generated scripts supporting alternatives will need to compete against the justification story if they are to lead to alternative behaviours.

Decisions for action emerge out of stories as a function of decision rules and/or via analysis using a mix of logical implications and affective reactions. Decisions can be about what forms of story or theory to use in deciding on actions, as well as on which actions to take.

Scripts for change need to be simple enough to follow, and explanations simple enough for us to understand why they justify action. However, at the same time, they need to be complex enough to deal with the challenge that is being confronted. They also need to be ones that we can have confidence in, which means we need to see them as credible. Criteria that affect the credibility of stories vary. Stories that relate to us as people, or what we should do, need to be congruent with OS-generated experiences, or they are likely to be rejected. By contrast, the credibility of propositional knowledge that is independent of experience is largely dependent on logical consistency and social acceptance. The ultimate criterion for the credibility of stories is their utility in action, whether this be as an aid to rational analysis or in social bonding. The latter means truth value and predictive utility are not always the most important criteria of story utility. Stories that are not disprovable are particularly useful for social coordination (e.g. role of religious stories); they may have high credibility for some forms of action, even though they may be recognised as beliefs of convenience (myths) rather than as factual analyses.

What the ES can do

The unique capacity of the ES is manifest in its capacity to use language to build up stories that represent models of the world, and through these it can generate goals and plans or scripts to achieve those goals. The ES is the seat of the enormous creativity that has transformed the material world. The focus here is on its capacity to harness some of that creativity to improve the ways we think and act in relation to ourselves, that is, to self-regulate.

The ES has the capacity to conceive of action independent of context, even if it has no capacity to act independently. This means our conceptual models of effect (both that of the individual and of the change agent) are typically individually focussed, and as a result tend to neglect the underlying reality that the genesis of actions by the OS originates in interactions between the state of the organism and cues in the environment.

Arguably, one of the main flaws of most human thought is its tendency to locate causality within entities (e.g. people) rather than in the relationship (interactions) between the person and their environment. The myth arises from referencing actions to personal goals, and seeing them as uniquely personal choices. However, even personal goals (ES) are in reality at least partly determined by environmental, particularly cultural, factors. Homogenisation of culture helps to mask the fundamental role culture can have in determining espoused goals, and thus behaviour. Similarly, considering environments that provide less support for individual autonomy to be in some sense unnatural or artificial is in part grounded in the myth that under normal circumstances goals are chosen by the individual, independent of constraints. That said, there is an element of truth in the myth, as unlike the OS, ES goals do have some capacity to operate across contexts, and thus provide an alternative guide to action to the contingencies of the moment. Understanding this requires a model of the individual acting over time to some extent independent of context.

The ES effectively works via semantic relations, with statements being assigned truth value, while the OS acts thorough associative mechanisms, with associative links formed through processes of contiguity and similarity. Change within the OS is produced via processes of habituation, conditioning and extinction. By contrast, change in the ES occurs through the formation of new or modified stories. The dynamic relationship between the two systems creates the conditions for cognitive factors to influence conditioned habits, which in turn modulate biological potentials.

The ES does not act directly on the world. Like the CEO of a company, it needs to get its OS sufficiently primed such that the behavioural schemata and scripts that it generates stimulate appropriate action tendencies from lower level processes (operational parts of the organisation), and where necessary, is able to suppress competing tendencies.

Central to HTM behaviours is the extent to which emotional reactions accompany ES-generated behavioural schemata or scripts. Where the affective force is strong, it is hard to resist action, but where it is weak, desired behaviours can easily be displaced by behavioural tendencies with more affective force. The ES can act to change the balance of forces for action in a number of ways. It can do the following:

- Use language to create stories that can act to guide behaviour by imagining possible futures and thus allow for the articulation of future goals.
- Analyse and interpret OS inputs, that is, what feelings mean.
- Take different perspectives or framings on a situation. This can include different perspectives on self-functioning that allow reinterpretation of the significance of OS inputs and re-evaluation of past actions. For example, interpreting reducing fitness as a sign of getting old, rather than being due to smoking or lack of exercise obviates the need for any action.
- Act to reorient attention, and thus influence what OS inputs are passed up to it, either by changing internal sensitivity settings, or by reorienting attention to different aspects of the external world (including by moving), thus changing what is available to be perceived (sensed). For example, paying particular attention to the health warnings on a pack of cigarettes to help maintain motivation to quit.
- Act to modulate OS-generated affective responses and reinterpret them in ways that are more adaptive. This includes both dampening reactions and their associated experiences that lead to undesirable behaviours, and augmenting the ones that lead to desirable tendencies.
- Act to stimulate affective engagement within the OS for ES-generated action tendencies by creating real and/or imagined contexts.
- Exercise self-control by inhibiting OS-generated action tendencies, and thus effectively change the balance point between a HTM behaviour and its alternatives.

- Plan and make decisions or choices, including deciding what to do, where, when, how and with what resources.
- Act with respect to negations and absence. Not doing something, or acting with respect to things that are not present in the immediate environment, is a capacity unique to the ES. There are an infinite set of things not being done; so, it is only what is present that affects OS processes directly. This is an extremely important capacity, but one that can lead to ES actions in ways that do not adequately engage OS processes.
- Act as an evaluation system that reviews actions and can change or attempt to change priorities for action on the basis of feedback.
- Make commitments to act using conceptual means (e.g. promises) or by initiating structural changes (e.g. financial bets on success and requests to friends for help) to increase the likelihood of achieving desired outcomes.
- Act on or be influenced by rules suggested or imposed by others.
- Communicating ideas to influence others to act now in ways that may facilitate future actions by oneself, and/or by the other.

Where there is a potentially competing response tendency (generated by the OS), an ES script needs to be able to be linked to equivalent or greater OS impulses if it is to be implemented. For many HTM behaviours, the strength of the competing response tendency varies from moment to moment. Thus, at some points, there is sufficient emotional force to act on plans, at other times the opposing forces become stronger and the plan is disrupted, modified or abandoned. If ES thought processes or scripts are irrelevant to the OS, it may not support them. This is experienced as inability to concentrate, boredom, and so on. That said, most of the challenges for HTM behaviours involve suppressing competing tendencies. Action scripts need not be complex to affect behaviour. Simple *Don't* scripts can inhibit OS reactions (if they are initiated before the behaviour is initiated/completed), but it is far harder to initiate alternative behaviours (see Chapter 2).

Some of the variety of actions, or decisions on action, that will be required from time to time by the ES include arbitrating in cases of competing OS action tendencies; acting in the face of OS impulses and managing them; coming to terms with the experience of counter-to ES action; choosing between competing ES stories; and modifying stories or developing new ones in the face of evidence that existing ones are inadequate.

Unlike the volatile OS impulses to act, a volitional goal is based on some analytic understanding of what is in the person's best long-term interests, giving it greater capacity to be stable across contexts. This means the ES is, in principle, more flexible in its capacity to direct change than the OS, as it can use a model that reinterprets experience, which changes the associative context, and thus can work to disrupt previously conditioned associations or responses. Change in the OS involves a slower period of re-conditioning.

The system as a whole is motivated to minimise conflicts between the ES and OS, and this is manifest in the ES seeking justifications or causative stories that are consistent with the inputs from the OS. There are needs to attend to realities that rational appraisal cannot readily conjure (e.g. aspects of sexuality or gender identity). It is desirable to have congruence between OS and ES, but caution is needed in achieving this by rationalising OS impulses. Acting purely on rational-isations of OS impulses is likely to end up with outcomes that you will regret in the morning. On the other hand, lack of consideration of OS inputs can result in important information being overlooked. People with impaired capacity to read their, or others, emotions do not operate well in social situations, and people who are insensitive to emotions can seem unfeeling to others, undesirable in a criminal, but sometimes lauded in a company executive.

A person has no guarantee that either the ES or OS will generate the most adaptive actions in any given situation. People need to rely on past experiences and/or the experiences of others to give them some indication of what is the correct course of action. These others can be individuals (e.g. friends), or the accumulated wisdom of a society, which includes scientific knowledge on the topic.

CEOS accepts that the optimum personal story (model of reality) for influencing day-to-day action is not necessarily the one that is closest to the objective truth. There is adaptive value in having an optimistic bias for enacting change [45, 46]. Depressives tend to be more accurate at predicting possible outcomes [47] and are less likely to try new behaviours, even when there is a reasonable possibility of success, creating self-fulfilling predictions of failure [48]. Similarly, under some circumstances, acknowledging a possibility can make it more real than it would oth-erwise have been, thus changing the underlying reality. Further, sometimes espoused positions (or expressed intentions) allow others to act in ways that change the prob-ability of the intentions being realised, either through acting in supportive ways or in ways designed to thwart the action. Thus, the need for a poker face in some competitive situations. All these are examples of where honesty is not the best pol-icy, although all but the last example relates to what is desirable for the person to believe, while the last only relates to what is expressed. For some things, such as understanding the nature of a task, accuracy is beneficial, while modest optimism has value in assessing the likelihood of successful execution. This certainly applies to HTM behaviours where success is unlikely on any given attempt; so, persistence is necessary, and that is unlikely to be helped by focussing on the high probability of failure on any given attempt.

It is hypothesised that the OS can influence behaviour change independent of the ES as it continues to generate old behaviours under appropriate cues, and to the extent that it does so, it can interfere with conscious attempts to generate new, more desirable, actions; especially where the two are incompatible. Over time the OS comes to take over the performance of new behaviours or routines. That is, they become automated at least in part, with the most critical part being their initiation, or the initiation of the desire to act. Difficult-to-resist urges to engage in an unde-sired behaviour pattern are evidence that the OS is cued to act in opposition to the desires of the ES. Finding yourself doing things you want to do, seemingly before you choose them, is evidence of OS–ES congruity and of the actions actually being driven by the OS (Figure 3.3).

Apart from these direct OS effects on behaviour, there is an indirect effect that reduces capacity to self-correct. One key function of the OS is to keep us from harm.

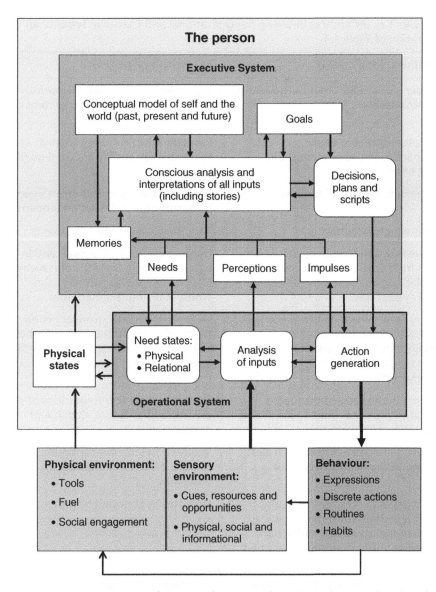

Figure 3.3 A complete model of the main functions of the three elements that directly or indirectly influence behaviour. The lines with the open arrows represent physical effects, and the lines with closed arrows represent information-based influences.

As a result, we are not attuned to acting to protect ourselves when the OS is not signalling threats. This is the dilemma the ES faces when it comes to accept a story (theory) that a behaviour is harmful, but that behaviour elicits no natural alarm bells (i.e. no OS tendency to avoid). This is part of the dilemma of HTM behaviours.

A summary of differences between the ES and OS can be found in Table 3.4.

Table 3.4 Key differences between the Operational and Executive Systems: an elaboration of Table 1.1

Operational System (OS)	Executive System (ES)
Processing occurs automatically and out of consciousness	Conscious of OS inputs, memories, goals, beliefs and sometimes steps of processing
Generates action to reduce discrepancies between current and target need states	Can also act to achieve progress towards linguistically encoded goals for the future
Primary determinant of behaviour	Impulses to behave only result in action if consistent with OS action tendencies
Bottom-up processing	Top-down processing
Generates action tendencies based on inputs from environment in context of signalled gaps between target and actual need states	Generates action tendencies within OS based on inputs from OS, plus memory (especially episodic memory) and symbolically represented rules
Primary determinant of behaviour, coordinates implementation of behaviour that occurs when strongest action tendency exceeds threshold for implementation	Needs to stimulate stronger action tendencies within the OS for its choice of behaviour (than for any competing tendency) if that behaviour is to occur
Operates in the present through associative processes linked to similarity and contiguity	Operates using representations of past, present and/or future. Capable of time discounting
Sensitive to negative affect regardless of contingency to past behaviour	Required to link non-contiguous positive effects of behaviour to outcomes
Operates as a process by which inputs trigger associative networks that lead to differential stimulation of action tendencies until a threshold is reached and action occurs	Operates by choosing between options
Behaviour controlled by targets: aspects of environment, or person in relationship to the environment, that are the focus of behaviour designed to reduce need imbalances, based on innate or conditioned associations	Goals are ways of allowing ideas about the future to influence current behaviour
Provides affective tone to language and the basis for associations that provide connotative meaning to concepts. Distinctions between concepts emerge as a function of associative links and evoked action tendencies	Role of language critical. Essential for denotative aspects of meaning of concepts. Distinctions between related concepts achieved through rules of inclusion and exclusion

(continued)

Table 3.4 (*continued*)

Operational System (OS)	Executive System (ES)
Learning is the result of changing in patterns of associations over repeated experiences	Learning is rule based and can be rapid
High-capacity and parallel processing. Exists largely at birth and is refined	Limited capacity and typically sequential processing. Develops gradually in childhood with language
Must be engaged at some level for any relevant behaviour to occur	Not always necessary for behaviour; so, needs to be evoked when needed
No sense of negation or absence. Associative links are to what is present, thus there are associative links to concepts mentioned, and not to any negating term	Parameterises *Not*. Can deal with absence in current environment using concept of absence. In language, negation dealt with according to rules of logic
Reactive to environmental cues and to aspect of ES concepts via associations	Reflective: Can anticipate and anticipations can acquire affective force via associations with the concepts involved

Limitations of thinking

Potentially, the ES has the sum of human culture available to it; the enormous progress we have made to understand the world and our role within it. However, even where we have access to it, this understanding is far too complex for most of us to understand, let alone to use as a guide for action. Simplifications are required.

The ES is a limited capacity information processor. There are limits to the number of concepts that people can hold in mind (or working memory) at any one time because the patterns of associations that constitute each idea require huge amounts of neural activity. It is a lot of work to think and it distracts from other activities; so, as a limited resource, it needs to be used efficiently. Issues requiring the consideration of multiple concepts can be beyond ES capacity, and strategies to deal with these limits are required. In addition, ES functioning is also affected by OS states independent of conscious OS inputs. One important influence is that, under conditions of stress, other demands can reduce executive capacity, a phenomenon known as perceptual narrowing, thus potentially either swamping the reduced capacity, or irrelevant (to the task) activity taking over. These limits mean that complex decisions are hard to get right, particularly at the times we need them most, when we are under pressure to act in undesirable ways.

The ES only affects the OS directly when it is actively engaged in an issue. This is why people only occasionally try to do things they know they should do, and why appropriate cues need to be created to prompt the ES to be engaged at times when its input could help prevent relapse to an undesirable behaviour. Organisations provide a good parallel to this. When the CEO is focussed on an issue, it is likely the whole organisation will try to act in accord with her wishes (if the CEO has made her intentions clear), resistance will tend to be muted and progress is likely to be made towards the goal if the organisation has the skills and resources to do what is required. However, unless this revised pattern of action comes to be valued in its own right, when the CEO's attention shifts to other issues, the old patterns are likely to re-establish themselves.

The CEO has limited ability to understand their organisation. It is too complex to understand in total at any one time; so, they must focus on aspects. They are also largely reliant on reports (summaries of what is happening created by staff) and limited personal experience. Their challenge is to take all this into account and make decisions that will lead to goals being achieved without causing undesirable effects on other aspects of the organisation's functioning.

The ES has limited control over the information presented to it for decision making. OS inputs can force themselves into conscious awareness (i.e. as perceptions, feelings and urges). The framing of the situation or story being used to understand a situation also influences the accessibility of memories, and the context where the story is used influences the accessibility of story elements to consciousness (including arguments). Influences can be as simple as the experience of anxiety triggering the cognition 'I must do something now'. These inputs *compete* to be part of the limited set of ideas that can be contemplated at any one moment. Relevant aspects of immediate experiences take priority along with emotionally charged memories (when the OS calls, the ES must listen). These un-ignorable inputs can result in potentially critical propositional considerations being squeezed out of consciousness. Where this happens, it can mean that elements of the story used to drive volitional behaviour can be lost and thus its potency to maintain change diminished.

A second important limiting characteristic of conscious cognitions is that people cannot directly generate experiences (e.g. feelings). Experiences are consequences (outputs) of OS activities. Thus, if a person wants a particular subjective experience, then they need to generate actions (or imagine possibilities) for which the experience is a consequence. This can include seeking appropriate environments or retrieving memories of events that had produced the desired experiences. Posing an emotion is one way to generate those feelings [49, 50]. Similarly, thinking about events (imagined or remembered) can lead to the generation of appropriate emotions (the link from conscious cognition back to functional states in Figure 3.3). In an analogous way, we have some capacity to influence the feelings that are consciously experienced by selectively attending to some at the expense of others. This capacity can serve both positive and negative purposes. For example, imagination, often facilitated by communication (especially pictures or other non-verbal material), can be used to create the emotional desire to try to stop doing things we rationally know are harming us or which authorities we respect are telling us are bad. It can also be used to stimulate desired alternative actions. Unfortunately, it can also stimulate undesirable actions, for example, advertising for foods we are prone to over-indulge in can trigger strong impulses to consume those foods.

Rational analysis is not always consistent or as accurate as it might be. Errors in rational appraisal are the result of widely occurring biases, heuristics and fallacies.

These can result in making choices that may not be in the person's best interests. Much of the research on these problems [5, 51] are framed around the assumption that rational appraisal is always superior. This research tradition typically studies closed problems (i.e. those with a known solution), where all the relevant information to make the decision is available, plus analyses of what is used and how, and what is ignored, in the decision-making process. This is a limited conceptualisation.

Many of the problems of living that we face are open or *wicked* problems with no uniquely defined solution, no guarantee that the required information is necessarily available, and typically no constraints on what is not relevant. Decision making takes place in a context of an infinity of possibly relevant events and relationships that are manifest in the person's environment, or are potentially there to 'discover'. Thus, choosing what to attend to needs to be heavily influenced by OS processes. There may also be multiple 'best' answers to problems, with the best solution dependent on the frame or context from which the problem is viewed. Under these circumstances, it is not a given that rational appraisal is optimal. Examples of rationality not being optimal include the greater apparent rationality of sociopaths, and of people who are depressed. Sometimes over-reliance on rational analysis can cause problems. Rationality will only deliver the right answers if you have the right questions and all the relevant information available (and not hidden in a morass of irrelevancy). The interesting questions are when and how it is in people's interests to take account of their intuitions, and when it is likely to lead then astray.

There is a lot to be gained from an analysis of the limits of our thinking, as this is one way we can reduce error. Researchers such as Kahneman and Tversky [5, 51–53] have generated a rich understanding of some of the limitations. Many of these biases arise from the way the problem is framed [41], sometimes also called the choice architecture [54]. These include the following:

- The information that the person considers. This is related to the availability heuristic of Kahneman and Tversky [53]. More salient, and thus more emotionally charged, objects and events influence our decisions more than less salient information. Of course, the salience of the information varies by context, an important reason why preferences change from context to context. The availability heuristic can have negative effects on people; where they overstate risks. People sometimes purchase unnecessary insurance or act on low likelihood, but salient, risks at the expense of more probable, but less salient ones, for example, avoid activities such as climbing or parachuting, but continue to smoke. This bias helps explain why prevention is not given the same emphasis as treatment in the health care system; possibilities prevented never occur and thus have little salience, while diseases do occur and demand action. Society gives less credit for successful prevention than successful cure, but, curiously, anger can be greater over failed prevention than failed cure.
- How the information is categorised. People tend to judge the probability of an event by finding a 'comparable known' event and assuming that the probabilities will be similar. This is known as the representativeness heuristic [53]. Classification of things into ordered categories is an essential part of creating

meaning from what we experience. Where an event or thing does not fit into a pre-existing category, we tend to try to fit it into the nearest class available, as creating entirely new categories leaves us with the problem of working out how to deal with them. By contrast, we typically have a range of options for dealing with existing categories; so, less cognitive work is required. Only when we repeatedly find a misfit, might we be sufficiently motivated to seek a new category. The primary fallacy is in assuming that similarity in one aspect leads to similarity in other aspects. For example, an example of the representativeness heuristic with sequences of events is the *gambler's fallacy*, the belief in runs of good and bad luck. People tend to reject randomness when they see any pattern (e.g. runs of the same outcome), including a tendency to take evidence of a high or low score on some outcome as representing some inherent characteristic, ignoring the possibility of random patterning. Thus, we tend to see sportspeople being on runs for skills such as hitting or goal kicking, even though it can often be shown that these patterns are genuinely random – not the overall likelihood of scoring (some people are more talented than others), but the pattern of hits and misses.

- The reference point used (sometimes called anchoring). People use their current situation as a reference point for recalling the past and predicting the future. Thus, if you are currently happy, you will rate the future more positively and the past more positively than if you are currently unhappy. Most judgments are relative, there are a few situations in which there is an absolute benchmark.
- Making socially acceptable choices. People are heavily influenced by the actions of others and they often make different decisions in social situations to those they might make alone. This is sometimes described as herd mentality. The costs of being wrong alone are far greater than the costs of being wrong as part of the pack. Sometimes choices are not just about what is right, but are also about maintaining social relationships as well, and in these cases there may be a need to compromise.

Biases in choices can also come from other sources. There is a tendency to persist with previous behaviour (habits) even though this course of action may clearly not be in a person's best interests. This is sometimes described as the 'status quo bias' [5]. This occurs when we persist with failed strategies, and when we do not undo choices that have changed their implications to become less beneficial, or even to have unnecessary costs. An example of the latter would be a person who has accepted the new evidence of the harms of too much sedentary activity [55, 56], but who has not done anything to change their own behaviour.

Finally, there is a bias favouring inaction in many circumstances, especially where there are risks or costs of acting. Society sees less responsibility in failing to act than in action: letting 10 people die through inaction is preferable to actively killing one. This represents deep societal values. For example, in the area of tobacco control, there is resistance from many to tobacco control policies that involve using less harmful substitutes that could produce major reductions in the epidemic, but still leave a problem and potentially expose some who might take up the substitutes to increased risk. It is this last concern that is explicitly used to justify opposition.

All of these factors lead to tendencies for us to act in ways that are not necessarily in our best interests, or in the best interests of the society in which we live. One critical question is when these kinds of problems are actually distorting our choices in meaningful ways, and what we can do to minimise their impact, a topic we return to in Chapter 5.

Self-regulation

Self-regulation refers to the ability to institute action based on an analysis of what is in the person's interests, and thus it is critical to successfully achieving HTM behaviour change. It refers to those psychological processes that allow executive control over thoughts, feelings and behaviour [10, 57].

CEOS postulates that there are at least four major functions of the ES, two of general importance and two more centrally relevant to HTM behaviours. The general ones are to resolve conflicts within the OS as to how to act in the moment, and to innovate, that is, to come up with new possibilities or rationales for action. The other two involve ways to pursue different activities to those generated directly by OS processes [31, 58]. The first is to exercise self-control; that is, use ES inhibitory powers to suppress undesirable behaviours or generate strong enough affective links to ES scripts to impel hard-to-sustain behaviours against OS tendencies. The second, which I refer to as self-reorientation, is to change the way the OS reacts. This can be done in a variety of ways including changing the framing so as to reinterpret OS action tendencies and associated feelings as nolonger demanding action, and to prevent positive feedback from ES interpretations (i.e. accentuating the valence of an undesirable reaction), thus making it easier for more desirable alternative habits to be established. Like a boss trying to get their workforce to do something new, the ES needs to create a context where the OS is positively oriented to engaging in behaviour the ES wants to occur (the target behaviour change). That is, act to create conditions that neutralise impacts of environmental cues.

Self-regulation is a limited resource and thus we have limited capacity to maintain effort and engagement, although it can be re-activated when needed. It is also an exhaustible commodity [59], but one which recovers with time. Placing excessive demands, or placing demands for too long, can result in exhaustion leading to either arbitrary choices (such as sticking with the status-quo) or to dominance of OS-cued behaviour. There appear to be at least two types of exhaustion. The first can occur within minutes (the effort of doing a task). The second may not become manifest for weeks (rarely longer) and relates to the effort of maintaining vigilance; so, applies mainly to self-control. Whether the fall-off in self-regulation for any given task is actually physical exhaustion or merely reflects a change in preferences towards other life priorities is unclear, I suspect shifting priorities are much more important than many students of self-regulation seem to assume, but exhaustion can clearly be important.

Resource depletion signals are not always represented with high fidelity to the ES (as feelings of exhaustion). While it can have the physical effect of making the operation of the ES more sluggish and less able to respond to OS pressures, this can be experienced as a sense that ES resistance does not seem as important any more, and thus it is alright to succumb. Further, exhaustion can deplete the capacity of the ES to rapidly counter OS impulses, resulting in the impulses being experienced as being stronger, and less resistible, rather than being due to reduced capacity to resist.

Self-regulatory capacities are conceived as arising out of the balance between the strength of excitatory and inhibitory processes. The strength of inhibitory processes is critical for self-control, and may need to be greater to achieve the same outcome where excitatory functions are stronger. Self-control is critical for making stable changes to behaviour.

The stability of change

Sustaining a decision or action for change is not straightforward. The changing context changes the balance of forces between change and the unwanted current behaviour on a moment-to-moment basis. At some point, this balance is such as to initiate change (Figure 3.4), but unless those conditions persist until the habit strengths of the competing alternatives have reversed in strength, relapse would be inevitable. Self-control is the executive mechanism that provides additional impetus towards a desired behaviour pattern, thus changing the threshold at which relapse back to an unwanted alternative will occur. Because self-control is a limited and exhaustible, resource, self-control mechanisms cannot be relied on to provide long-term changes in behaviour unaided by other processes. That is, unless there is sufficient reorientation of the OS to allow the new behaviour to be sustained in the long term with minimal needs for self-control, relapse will be likely as self-control capacity is diverted or exhausted (Figure 3.5).

As noted in Chapter 2, we find that determinants of success in smoking cessation appear to change somewhere within the first month of quitting, something consistent with this being the limits of focussed self-control [15]. The decline in self-control does not have to be sudden, and in reality is more likely to be intermittent, but it can act as a counterpoint to whatever declines there have been in the relative strengths of the competing behaviours (Figure 3.5). If the balance has not passed the point of equilibrium, relapse will be likely when the next temptation to engage in the old behaviour occurs.

Relationship of CEOS to other dual-process theories

The core rationale for dual-process theories is that there are fundamental differences between higher, largely conscious cognitive processing, and the less conscious or unconscious processing that can influence higher processing, and/or behaviour, independent of higher order desires. Evans [3] notes that the theories differ in where they make the major distinction. In CEOS, it is between conscious deliberation, and

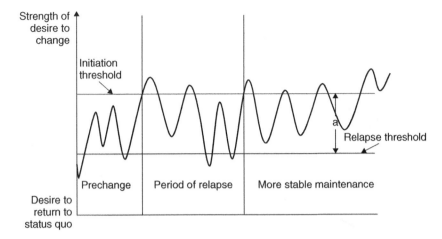

Figure 3.4 Schematic diagram to show why the thresholds for initiation and maintenance of behaviour change need to be set at different levels.

'*a*' denotes the distance between threshold for action, and relapse is a function of the level of self-control committed to the problem.

A schematic diagram of the fluctuating nature of desire to change and the postulation of different thresholds for action and for relapse.

NB: This gap between the two thresholds is important, else relapse would be almost inevitable in the period shortly after change unless there was a major jump in the balance of action.

The initiation and relapse thresholds are depicted as stable here, but in reality they change over time, unfortunately sometimes in concert with changes in the net level of desire to persist.

other processing arising from lower level, associative decision making, while for others it is between rational and non-rational factors.

Gerrard and associates [34] have developed a dual-process model, called the prototype willingness model, that focusses on decision making in adolescents. It is based on Gray's [8] model of behavioural inhibition and excitatory systems in the brain in essentially the same way as CEOS. It, along with other similar theories [60–62] notes that the development of higher level processing is not fully developed until sometime in adolescence, ideas that stem back to Vygotsky [33] and Piaget [63], where the focus was on the roles of language, and capacity for formal operational thought, as determinants of higher cognitive processes.

Prototype willingness theory labels the two paths to action as the reasoned path, which they see as operating similarly to the theory of reasoned action [64], and the social reaction path, which is more image based and uses heuristic reasoning. It argues that the social reaction path provides a partly independent set of influences on behaviour mediated through what they call behavioural willingness, which relates to the extent of being tempted or openness to act in various situations. Prototype willingness is theorised to be generated from two sources: images of the kind of person who engages in the behaviour, with positive images associated with

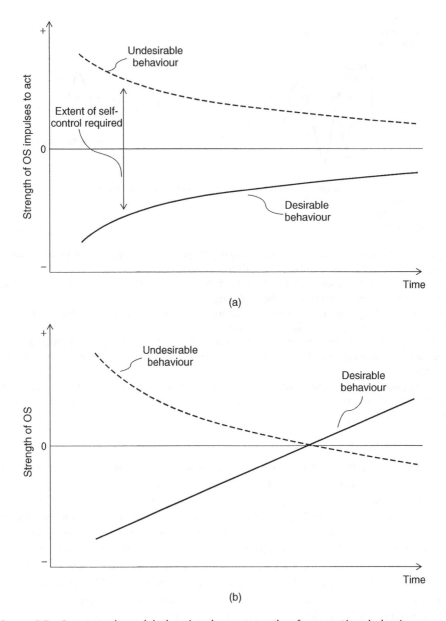

Figure 3.5 Conceptual model showing how strength of competing behaviours may change over time and the implications for self-control. (a) Behaviour change requiring ongoing self-control and (b) behaviour change where the desirable behaviour comes to be preferred, and self-control is no long required. At the point where the two lines cross, the need for self-control disappears. In reality, the lines are not smooth; that is, it is more like the line in Figure 2.3, especially for the undesirable behaviour. As a result, the point of equilibrium may be crossed and recrossed many times before change stabilises.

high willingness to engage; and second, perceived vulnerability to harm, which is a modulator of these images. It is operationalised as 'how willing are you to engage in' the target behaviour, following a description of a typical situation where the behaviour might occur. Prototype willingness is particularly important for engaging in risky behaviours. Gerrard *et al.* [34] provide evidence that it is a stronger predictor of behaviour than intentions up to age 17 or 18.

Translated into the terms of CEOS, willingness reflects the strength of OS-generated impulses to act (albeit sometimes supported by ES processes) that is independent of executive intentions. Willingness needs to be transformed into a decision to act before action will occur. The need for a decision helps to explain why people concerned about their unhealthy habits are not constantly trying to change. The concept of willingness seems to work quite well for the uptake of counter-attitudinal behaviours (i.e. doing things you know you shouldn't), but it tends to confuse when applied to changing unwanted behaviours, where willingness now refers to the status-quo. Thus the theory provides useful insights into the uptake of behaviour, but it has less to say about getting rid of undesirable behaviours, and about the maintenance of behaviours.

The dual-process theory that is closest to CEOS is that of Strack and Deutsch [4, 65, 66] (especially as adapted by Hoffman and colleagues [6, 58, 67, 68]. Strack and Deutsch call their two systems the reflective and impulsive systems, and their model the RIM (Reflective, Impulsive Model). The components and implications of the two theories are similar, and it is not always clear to what extent the differences are truly fundamental, or are more accurately seen as a function of framing. RIM was developed to explain aspects of human reasoning, while CEOS focusses on behaviour and why volitional change is sometimes compromised.

In RIM as in CEOS, the impulsive system (or the OS) is theorised to operate via 'associative links between elements, and is formed according to the principles of contiguity and similarity' ([4], see p. 223), with behaviour elicited through the spread of this activation to form behavioural schemata. In RIM, the reflective system relates elements through semantic relations to which a truth value is assigned, and behaviour is 'the consequence of a decision that is guided by the assessment of the future state in terms of its value and the possibility of attaining it through the behaviour' (see p. 229). This is a narrower framing than for the ES. I see behaviour potentially emerging from any rule-based response to an espoused goal. RIM focusses on rational action, only one of a possible range of sub-classes of ES-directed actions. Others include compliance with rules or expectations (I do what my parents want; or what my scriptures say; or I act to confuse others by doing what is least expected).

According to RIM, the impulsive system is always engaged in processing (either by itself or in parallel with operations of the reflective system), whereas the reflective system can be disengaged. I don't think this distinction is worthwhile. In a simple sense, the OS is always operating in some way, albeit minimally when sleeping. However, if the focus is on any given form of behaviour, then there can be long periods when nothing is happening. The OS is always active when the behaviour is cued as it is an essential element of its performance, while the ES is clearly not involved in some behaviours, so may not be engaged. However, we sometimes have thoughts that don't activate any meaningful OS action tendencies; the OS is only needed to implement a plan, and to the extent that thoughts do not generate any affective engagement, let alone behaviour, OS activity can be ignored.

Both theories accept that the reflective system requires high levels of cognitive capacity, and RIM theorises that its functioning will be disrupted by extremely high or low levels of arousal. CEOS concurs for high cognitive load, but for low cognitive load, the two theories diverge for reasons related to the disagreement on whether OS processes are necessary for ES functioning. In CEOS, low arousal means reduced processing of inputs beyond the lowest levels of the OS; thus the ES may not be sufficiently engaged under low levels of arousal, rather than being disrupted. Under-arousal is experienced as boredom or, if the ES is otherwise active, as an inability to concentrate. Related to this, sometimes the ES can generate behavioural schemata which fail to activate the OS even though there are no competing action tendencies, something experienced as: 'I just couldn't be bothered'. CEOS also accepts that ES processing can be impaired when the OS is functionally exhausted or damaged, in which case the whole system's functioning becomes impaired.

RIM along with CEOS, argues that there is a common path to action (behaviour) controlled by OS processes. We agree that the OS has to implement the component parts of the behavioural schemata that guide action, and unless appropriate action tendencies exist, there is nothing for the ES to activate. If ES-initiated action is to take place, it must involve mechanisms to activate appropriate OS processes and to overcome alternative action tendencies where relevant.

RIM proposes that the reflective system has the capacity to form intentions, which link a behavioural schemata to a likely or inevitable future environmental contingency. The potential to represent the future is the basis for purposive action. CEOS is in general agreement; however, there is no need for interposing an explicit intention between the idea of behaving and its implementation if the behaviour is immediately implemented, intentions are only needed to span a delay. The concept of an intention implies a capacity to evoke it when the appropriate conditions are met. Gollwitzer [69] made a major conceptual leap here in his conceptualisation of implementation intentions, that is, if-then statements of conditions leading to actions (see Chapter 7). I think it is the focus on the conditions for behaving, and thus the likelihood that the thought will be regenerated when the context is appropriate that leads to an increase in the likelihood that the behaviour will be elicited when the conditions occur. This is why it is important that implementation intentions have the form: 'If condition X occurs, I will do Z' [69]. RIM states that 'The mechanism of intending is terminated if the behaviour is executed or if the goal of the preceding behavioral decision is already fulfilled' ([4], see p. 230). I think this may be overly simplistic. For HTM behaviours, the intention needs to persist for maintenance, albeit in a changed form, and as initiation does not guarantee implementation, intentions may persist across past failures to implement fully. Also some intentions are never implemented, and there is a need to accept that some are forgotten, and still others are explicitly abandoned if the challenges of performance are perceived to be too high.

RIM postulates two basic motivational orientations: approach and avoidance. I agree, and this important point has led me to elaborate CEOS more than I had previously. However, I think it more likely that the more basic tendency is to avoid, and higher processing is required to decide whether avoidance of the event is desirable and, if so, whether it can be implemented by fight or flight. Alternatively, the event may be benign and nothing needs to be done; or the event has desirable attributes, and can be approached.

RIM has a compatibility thesis that emerges out of their motivational orientation assumption: 'The processing of information, the experience of affect, and the execution of behaviour are facilitated if they are compatible with the prevailing motivational orientation' ([4], see p. 232). I take a somewhat different perspective. As noted earlier, I agree that the OS has to be 'co-opted' to act for reflective, or ES generated, behaviour to occur, and that is more difficult if the motivational orientation (action tendency) is inconsistent with the ES-initiated action tendency or script for action. In this case, ES processes are required to create suitable associations in the OS. For the processing of information where there is congruence, there may be little need for elaborated processing as there is agreement, and thus no differences to resolve. Thus, it is not that processing is facilitated, but the speed with which a conclusion is reached.

I fundamentally disagree with RIM's proposition that congruence between the two systems facilitates the experience of affect. In CEOS, affect, particularly negative affect, mainly occurs in situations where there is a lack of congruence, where strong OS needs are not resulting in actions that should reduce them, and where strong ES impulses to act are resisted by incompatible OS activation, or the lack of an appropriate context to carry them out. Take sky diving for the first time. Fear is felt, and for some the only way to leave the plane are either to close their eyes and pretend there is a floor out there, or request to be pushed. The conflict exacerbates the emotional response. Uncontested behaviour is the experience of flow [38] and is notable for the lack of affect at the time, but of pleasure when voluntarily interrupted or the script is completed. Both theories accepts that basic affective responses are generated by the OS, and it is their cognitive elaboration (and I would add the feedback into the OS to influence those affective reactions) that culminates in experienced emotions.

Both theories are in agreement on the importance of bi-directionality; that is, behaviour affects processing and vice versa. In particular, Strack and Deutsch [4] review evidence that emotional expressions and aspects of posture influence affective states through internal feedback as well as potentially through external feedback. Both theories agree that there can be homeostatic dysregulation in that 'deprivation of basic needs leads to activation of the behavioural schemata that in the past frequently led to satisfaction of those needs' (see p. 236). I would note that this can include schemata that support exploration of the environment where the conditions to meet the need state are not immediately present.

One important theorem of RIM that emerges out of the different processing modalities of the two systems, is that the cognitive process of negation can only be executed by the reflective system (ES), and thus the impulsive system cannot represent non-gains (missing out on something desirable) and non-losses (not losing something) in terms of propositions, only as patterns of associations that do not include the negated outcome. A similar process applies for non-presence [70]. Thus, RIM predicts that information about negations can have opposing effects depending on whether the information is conveyed through the impulsive or reflective systems, that is, via associative learning or through verbal forms. There is now considerable evidence for this [71]. In Chapter 5, I discuss how this provides a better way of understanding the implications of framing messages and their implications for persuasion than Prospect theory.

There are areas where CEOS has postulates not covered in RIM. CEOS proposes that inhibitory processes tend to dominate excitatory processes, meaning that it is easier to inhibit behaviours than to excite new ones. This provides the basis for self-control mechanisms, and helps explain why it is hard to institute new behaviours that compete with existing routines and helps explain phenomena such as the status quo bias [5]. It also postulates that the OS is more finely tuned to avoidance tendencies as one of its most central functions is to rapidly respond to threats. As HTM undesirable behaviours typically do not signal threat to the OS, they do not carry the affective associations with threat, which means a lack of motivational force to avoid them. This highlights the need for ES mechanisms to generate the conditions to create the appropriate avoidance associations.

CEOS also has a mechanism to explain why non-contingent negative affect is important in influencing maintenance of change, while non-contingent positive effect has no such OS-mediated effects. Sustained changes in OS reactivity are engineered through processes of conditioning and extinction for rewarding (positive) outcomes, but for negative consequences, discriminative stimuli tend to only suppress behaviour, as extinction does not occur unless there is experience that the link between the behaviour and consequence has actually been broken. Finally, CEOS has a strong focus on maintenance of behaviour, whereas RIM tends to only focus on decision making and relatively discrete behaviours; however, the work of Wiers and others [68] is extending the implications of the work to long-term behaviour change.

Overall, it should be clear that the main differences between the two theories are the fundamentally different perspectives on emotions, and that RIM treats its reflective system as essentially rational (an approach common to other theories), for example, Nudge Theory's [54] distinction between Econs (rational beings) and *humans*, while my ES is a rather more complicated beast. Evans [3] notes that there appears to be two main trains of thought, those that are concerned with the differentiation of explicit and implicit knowledge systems, and those concerned with how preconscious processes affect decision making. CEOS and RIM are both more the latter, although CEOS is primarily concerned with behaviour rather than decision making. CEOS also accepts a version of the implicit explicit distinction in the model it proposes for persuasion (see Chapter 5). Thus, the ES has the capacity to be rational, but also the capacity to act in relation to intuitive non-conscious and affective inputs, while RIM tends to place these non-rational influences within its impulsive system. The difference in the way emotions are treated may relate to the difference in emphasis around rationality. It is clearly easier to act rationally when what you think you should do is in line with what you feel like doing. However, if CEOS is right, the main role of emotions is to provide information to the executive as to states of the OS; so, they are not needed as much when there is congruence. Emotions appear during delays, and interruptions, I think to serve the purpose of helping maintain desirable activities, and also on termination, as a sign to 'lighten up, the job is done and you can relax'.

The differences notwithstanding, I find it impressive that there is such convergence between bottom-up theorising coming out of psychology laboratories and my attempt to understand the complexities of smoking cessation and other HTM behaviours from an overall (top-down) perspective. It suggests that the dual-process approach has considerable potency as it has important things to say about behaviour as well as about decision making [66, 72]. I am hopeful that the differences between CEOS and other dual-process approaches might stimulate research.

There is a rich strain of thinking and ingenuous empirical work in the area of decision making on the influences of implicit versus explicit processes [68, 73–76]. This work is showing real promise for not only increasing the understanding but also for the development of potentially useful interventions (see Chapter 7). From the perspective of CEOS, the problem the experimental work fails to address is around the primacy of OS processes and the confusion between OS influences on ES functioning and rational influences. In CEOS, these are hard to separate (for the individual), but important elements of executive decision making, while for most decision-making theories, they are distortions, and thus belong to the impulsive system.

There are now increasing efforts to apply these models to health-related behaviours, with some success. Friese and colleagues [67] have summarised some of this work around strategies for taming the horse (reorienting the OS in my terms), strengthening the rider (more self-control strategies), and giving direction to the rider (conventional cognitive behavioural therapies to enhance executive capacity). Some of the strategies for interventions are described in Chapter 7. There is also interest from other researchers in shaping the environment, especially the communicational environment to nudge behaviour in desirable ways [54], which is the topic of the next chapter.

Summary

This chapter spells out in more detail the characteristics of the OS and the ES that, together with the external environment, are theorised to co-determine human behaviour. The OS operates via associative mechanisms and relates to inputs provided on a moment-to-moment basis, and the ES which has the capacity to create and act on conceptual models of the world and thereby generate goals that can become targets for action. The interaction between the two systems allows us to understand the nature of some of our human limitations.

References

1. Haidt J. *The Happiness Hypothesis: Finding Modern Truth in Ancient Wisdom*. Basic Books: New York, 2006.
2. Smith ER & DeCoster J. Dual-process models in social and cognitive psychology: Conceptual integration and links to underlying memory systems. *Personality and Social Psychology Review*. 2000; 4: 108–131.
3. Evans JS. Dual-processing accounts of reasoning, judgment, and social cognition. *Annual Review of Psychology*. 2008; 59: 255–278.
4. Strack F & Deutsch R. Reflective and impulsive determinants of social behaviour. *Personality and Social Psychology Bulletin*. 2004; 8: 220–247.
5. Kahneman D. *Thinking, Fast and Slow*. 1st edn. Farrar, Straus and Giroux: New York, 2011.
6. Hofmann W, Friese M & Wiers RW. Impulsive versus reflective influences on health behaviour: A theoretical framework and empirical review. *Health Psychology Review*. 2008; 2: 111–137.
7. Powers WT. *Behavior: The Control of Perception* 2nd expanded edn. Originally published 1973. Benchmark Publications: New Canaan, CT, 2005.
8. Gray JA. *Pavlov's Typology*. Elsevier, 1964.
9. Carver CS & Scheier MF. *Attention and Self-Regulation: A Control Theory Approach to Human Behavior*. Springer-Verlag: New York, 1981.
10. Carver CS & Scheier MF. *On the Self-Regulation of Behavior*. Cambridge University Press: New York, 1998.
11. Carver CS. Impulse and constraint: Perspectives from personality psychology, convergence with theory in other areas, and potential for integration. *Personality and Social Psychology Review*. 2005; 9: 312–333.
12. Maslow A. *Motivation and Personality*. Harper: New York, NY, 1954.
13. Baker TB, Piper ME, McCarthy DE *et al*. Addiction motivation reformulated; an affective processing model of negative reinforcement. *Psychological Review*. 2004; 111: 31–51.
14. Carmody TP, Vietan C & Astin JA. Negative affect, emotional acceptance, and smoking cessation. *Journal of Psychoactive Drugs*. 2007; 39: 499–508.
15. Herd N, Borland R & Hyland A. Predictors of smoking relapse by duration of abstinence: Findings from the International Tobacco Control (ITC) Four Country Survey. *Addiction*. 2009; 104: 2088–2099.
16. Kimble G. *Hilgard and Marquis' Conditioning and Learning*. 2nd edn. Appleton Century Crofts: New York, 1961.
17. Rescorla RA. Hierachical associative relations in Pavlovian conditioning and instrumental training. *Current Directions in Psychological Science*. 1992; 1: 66–70.
18. Robinson TE & Berridge KC. Addiction. *Annual Review of Psychology*. 2003; 54: 25–53.
19. Baum WM. Rethinking reinforcement: Allocation, induction and contingency. *Journal of the Experimental Analysis of Behaviour* 2012; 97: 101–124.
20. Benowitz NL & Henningfield JE. Reducing the nicotine content to make cigarettes less addictive. *Tobacco Control*. 2013; 22: i14–i17.
21. Rose JE. Nicotine and nonnicotine factors in cigarette addiction. *Psychopharmacology*. 2006; 184: 274–285.
22. Testa M, Fillmore MT, Norris J *et al*. Understanding alcohol expectancy effects: Revisiting the placebo condition. *Clinical and Experimental Research*. 2006; 30: 339–348.
23. Poulos CX & Cappell H. Homeostatic theory of drug tolerance: A general model of physiological adaptation. *Psychological Review*. 1991; 98: 390–408.

24. Perkins K, Sayette M, Conklin C *et al.* Placebo effects of tobacco smoking and other nicotine intake. *Nicotine and Tobacco Research.* 2003; **5**: 695–709.
25. Walker N, Howe C, Bullen C *et al.* The combined effect of very low nicotine content cigarettes, used as an adjunct to usual Quitline care (nicotine replacement therapy and behavioural support), on smoking cessation: A randomized controlled trial. *Addiction.* 2012; **107**: 1857–1867.
26. Houben K & Wiers RW. Response inhibition moderates the relationship between implicit associations and drinking behaviour. *Clinical and Experimental Research.* 2009; **33**: 626–633.
27. Houben K, Wiers RW & Jansen A. Getting a grip on drinking behavior: Training working memory to reduce alcohol abuse. *Psychological Science.* 2011; **22**: 968–975.
28. Borland R. Tobacco health warnings and smoking-related cognition's and behaviors. *Addiction.* 1997; **92**: 1427–1435.
29. Borland R, Yong H, Wilson N *et al.* How reactions to cigarette pack health warnings influence quitting: Findings from the ITC Four Country survey. *Addiction.* 2009; **104**: 669–675.
30. Azrin NH & Nunn GR. Habit reversal: A method of eliminating nervous tics and habits. *Behaviour Research and Therapy.* 1973; **11**: 619–628.
31. West R & Brown J. *Theory of Addiction.* 2nd ed. Wiley: Chichester, UK, 2013.
32. Samaha AN & Robinson TE. Why does the rapid delivery of drugs to the brain promote addiction? *Trends in Pharmacological Sciences.* 2005; **26**: 82–87.
33. Vygotsky LS. *Thought and Language.* MIT Press: Cambridge MA, 1962.
34. Gerrard M, Gibbons FX, Houlihan AE *et al.* A dual-process approach to health risk decision making: The prototype willingness model. *Developmental Review.* 2008; **28**: 29–61.
35. Dennett DC. *Consciousness Explained.* The Penguin Press: Boston, 1991.
36. Wegner DM. The mind's best trick: How we experience conscious will. *Trends in Cognitive Sciences.* 2003; **7**: 65–69.
37. Tulving E. Episodic memory and autonoesis: Uniquely human?. In: Terrace HS & Metcalfe J (eds.) *The Missing Link in Cognition.* Oxford University Press: New York, NY, 2005: 4–56.
38. Csikszentmihalyi M. *Flow: The Psychology of Optimal Experience.* Harper and Row: New York, 1990.
39. Brown KW, Ryan RM & Creswell JD. Mindfulness; theoretical foundations and evidence for its salutary effects. *Psychological Inquiry.* 2007; **18**: 211–237.
40. Borland R, Flammer A & Wearing AJ. Text memory: Recalling twice, using different perspectives. *European Journal of Psychology and Education.* 1987; **11**: 209–217.
41. Bateson G. *Steps to an Ecology of Mind.* Paladin: Frogmore, St. Albans, 1973.
42. Wilden A. *System and Structure.* 2nd edn. Tavistock: London, 1980.
43. Fazio R & Cooper J. Arousal in the dissonance process. In: Cacioppo J & Petty R (eds.) *Social Psychophysiology A Source Book.* The Guilford Press: New York, 1983: 122–152.
44. Leventhal H, Brissette I & Leventhal EA. The common-sense model of self-regulation of health and illness. In: Cameron LD & Leventhal H (eds.) *The Self-Regulation of Health and Illness Behaviour.* Routledge: London, 2003: 42–65.
45. Klein CTF & Helweg-Larsen M. Perceived control and the optimistic bias: A meta-analytic review. *Psychology and Health.* 2002; **17**: 437–446.
46. Branstrom R & Brandberg Y. Health risk perception, optimistic bias, and personal satisfaction. *American Journal of Health Behavior.* 2010; **34**: 197–205.
47. Helweg-Larsen M & Shepperd J. Do moderators of the optimistic bias affect personal or target risk estimates? A review of the literature. *Personality and Social Psychology Review.* 2001; **5**: 74–95.

48. Slusher MP & Anderson CA. Belief perseverance and self-defeating behavior. In: Curtis R (eds.) *Self-Defeating Behaviors: Experimental Research, Clinical Impressions and Practical Implications*. Plenum Press: New York, 1989.

49. Ekman P, Levenson RW & Friesen WV. Autonomic nervous system activity distinguishes among emotions. *Science*. 1983; **221**: 1208–1210.

50. Adelmann PK & Zajonc RB. Facial efference and the experience of emotion. *Annual Review of Psychology*. 1989; **40**: 249–280.

51. Nisbett RE & Ross L. *Human Inference: Strategies and Shortcomings of Social Judgment*. Prentice-Hall: Englewood Cliffs, NJ, 1980.

52. Kahneman D, Slovic P & Tversky A. *Judgment Under Uncertainty: Heuristic and Biases*. Cambridge University Press: New York, 1982.

53. Kahneman D & Tversky A. Prospect theory: An analysis of decisions under risk. *Econometrica*. 1979; **47**: 263–291.

54. Thaler RH & Sunstein CR. *Nudge: Improving Decisions About Health, Wealth and Happiness*. Yale University Press: New Haven, CT, USA, 2008.

55. Owen N. Sedentary behavior: Understanding and influencing adults' prolonged sitting time. *Preventive Medicine*. 2012; **55**: 535–539.

56. Owen N, Healy GN, Howard B *et al*. Too much sitting: Health risks of sedentary behaviour and opportunities for change. *President's Council on Fitness, Sports & Nutrition: Research Digest*. 2012; **13**: 1–11.

57. Baumeister RF & Vohs KD. *Handbook of Self-Regulation: Research, Theory, and Applications* Baumeister RF & Vohs KD (eds.). Guilford Press: New York, 2004.

58. Hofmann W, Friese M & Strack F. Impulse and self-control from a dual-systems perspective. *Perspective on Psychological Science*. 2009; **4**: 162–176.

59. Baumeister RF & Vohs KD. Self-regulation, ego depletion and motivation. *Social and Personality Psychology Compass*. 2007; **1**: 115–128.

60. Epstein S. Integration of the cognitive and the psychodynamic unconscious. *American Psychologist*. 1994; **49**: 709–724.

61. Reyna VF & Farley F. Risk and rationality in adolescent decision making: Implications for theory, practice, and public policy. *Psychological Science in the Public Interest*. 2006; 7: 1–44.

62. Reyna VF & Ellis SC. Fuzzy-trace theory and framing effects in children's risky decision making. *Psychological Science*. 1994; **5**: 275–279.

63. Inhelder B & Piaget J. *The Growth of Logical Thinking from Childhood to Adolescence. An Essay on the Construction of Formal Operational Structures*. Routledge: London, 1958.

64. Fishbein M & Ajzen I. *Belief, Attitude, Intention, and Behavior: An Introduction to Theory and Research*. Addison-Wesley: Reading, MA, 1975.

65. Deutsch R, Gawronski B & Strack F. At the boundaries of automaticity: Negation as reflective operation. *Journal of Personality and Social Psychology*. 2006; **91**: 385–405.

66. Deutsch R & Strack F. Duality models in social psychology: From dual processes to interacting systems. *Psychological Inquiry*. 2006; **17**: 166–172.

67. Friese M, Hofmann W & Wiers RW. On taming horses and strengthening riders: Recent developments in research on interventions to improve self-control in health behaviors. *Psychology Press*. 2011; **10**: 336–351.

68. Wiers RW, Gladwin TE, Hofmann W *et al*. Cognitive bias modification and cognitive control training in addiction and related psychopathology: Mechanisms, clinical perspectives, and ways forward. *Clinical Psychological Science*. 2013; **1**: 192–212.

69. Gollwitzer PM. Implementation intentions: Strong effects from simple plans. *American Psychologist*. 1999; **54**: 493–503.

70. Wegner DM. Ironic processes of self-control. *Psychological Review*. 1994; **101**: 34–52.

71. Gawronski B, Deutsch R, Mbirkou S *et al.* When "Just Say No" is not enough: Affirmation versus negation training and the reduction of automatic stereotype activation. *Journal of Experimental Social Psychology.* 2008; **44**: 370–377.

72. Deutsch R & Strack F. Duality models in social psychology: Response to commentaries. *Psychological Inquiry.* 2006; **17**: 265–268.

73. Bargh JA & Ferguson MJ. Beyond behaviorism: On the automaticity of higher mental processes. *Psychological Bulletin.* 2000; **126**: 925–945.

74. Bargh JA, Gollwitzer PM, Lee-Chai A *et al.* The automated will: Nonconscious activation and pursuit of behavioral goals. *Journal of Personality and Social Psychology.* 2001; **81**: 1014–1027.

75. Sheeran P, Gollwitzer P & Bargh J. Nonconscious processes and health. *Health Psychology.* 2013; **32**: 802–809.

76. Aarts H. Health and goal-directed behavior: The nonconscious regulation and motivation of goals and their pursuit. *Health Psychology Review.* 2007; **1**: 53–82.

Chapter 4

ENVIRONMENTAL INFLUENCES: THE CONTEXT OF CHANGE

People typically live in environments where OS processes generate undesirable options to HTM behaviours too frequently, and/or does not have capacity to regularly generate or maintain HTM behaviours without continual assistance from the ES (see Figure 2.1). This means environmental change can be an important means of shaping behaviour, although within the limits of OS sensitivities.

Modern society has become pretty good at reducing some of the adverse effects of the natural environment, including mitigating many natural threats. We now live in homes that provide good protection from the environment and can heat or cool them to increase comfort. We no longer have to hunt for food, but merely go to the local shops. Most people in developed countries now live in cities, where even aspects of the physical environment (e.g. parks and gardens) are managed to maximise utility and minimise threats. All of this activity has been good for human health. People in developed countries live on average longer than in just about any other society.

However, the good has come with undesirable side effects: more people are becoming obese as a result of a combination of less need for physical exertion and an excess of food. The huge energy demands required to achieve the increased comfort and convenience may also not be sustainable; so, we should be prepared for a possible need to readjust our lifestyles towards the more demanding ones we have forsaken. The rise in bicycling rather than use of motorised transport is one example of a change that provides benefits for physical well-being as well as reduces societal energy consumption.

The problematic behaviours that emerge in a society at any time will be partly a function of broader social conditions that create excessive cues for these behaviours to occur and/or be sustained. However, the environment is not only central to the generation of HTM behaviours, but it also plays a role in determining what makes behaviour patterns and states of the OS adaptive or maladaptive. Thus, in a situation of famine, cues to eat are adaptive as they do not trigger overconsumption but rather facilitate survival. In periods of feast, the same predispositions drive obesity.

This chapter has two main functions: to discuss ways by which the proximal environment in which people live, their interactional environment, affects their behaviour, particularly their interactions with other people; and to discuss the ways

Understanding hard to maintain behaviour change: A dual process approach, First Edition. Ron Borland.
© 2014 John Wiley & Sons, Ltd. Published 2014 by John Wiley & Sons, Ltd.

by which broader environmental forces affect the nature of proximal, interactional environments and how they can be changed from without. As broader forces impact interactional environments, it is convenient to consider these forces first.

Ecological models of behaviour are the most useful framework for understanding environmental effects, including the effects of cultural factors and social norms [1]. While these theories acknowledge a role for intra-individual effects, most focus on determinants of behaviour that emanate from outside of the individual: forces that originate from interpersonal, neighbourhood, community, organisational, through to society-wide ones, including policy interventions. CEOS is an ecological model, but differs from many other ecological models in that it considers how the environment affects the OS directly, as well as how our interpretations of the environment both influence our reactions and allow for systematic changes in the environment in pursuit of culturally shared goals.

Sallis and colleagues [1] identify four core principles that ecological theories hold about how health behaviour is influenced by environmental factors. First, there are multiple levels of influence on specific health behaviours; and second, these influences interact across these different levels. Third, ecological models need to be behaviour-specific as the environmental influences differ markedly from behaviour to behaviour. Fourth, multi-level interventions should be most effective in changing behaviour because they maximise the likelihood of environmental factors systematically supporting the change. This is all consistent with CEOS.

Influences that operate or which can be changed at the level of entire societies set the agenda around which the interactional environments of individuals and their social networks operate. Some of these societal factors are taken for granted, and only when people experience other societies do they realise that they are not inevitable. Societal-level influences are a result of the laws and customs of the society, institutional forces (including commercial ones), cumulated knowledge, various forms of mass media and increasingly the role of communications technology to allow more interactive communication at a distance. These set the context that individuals and their social circles interact in and provide limits on what is possible and/or desirable.

In considering where to intervene on systems, it is important to work out where the power to enact change lies, and, where possible, to act at the highest level of that power structure. That said, where there is resistance at higher levels of systems, progress can be made by acting with or on lower level processes, but only where they are part of the relevant system of control.

The relatively stable environment

The environment in which people live and behave consists of the physical environment (natural and built) and within it, the social environment, both of people and the ways they communicate.

A range of aspects of the environment need to be considered in analysing the likely ease of behaviour change, for either increasing or decreasing behaviours. These are briefly described in the following paragraphs.

Most critical is the extent to which the micro-environment provides opportunities to act, including accessibility of places to act (e.g. access to places to exercise safely and enjoyably) on the one hand, and places where the behaviour is not normative or is actively prohibited on the other. This also includes any degree of obligation to act (e.g. places where the behaviour is expected or allowed) and any demands of the physical environment (e.g. having to go outside to smoke in freezing weather or during a rainstorm). The greater the range of places where behaviours can readily occur, the more these behaviours are engaged in. Smokers smoke less when subject to bans from smoking at work and other places [2, 3]. For recreational exercise, living near a gym or a pleasant park is associated with higher levels of exercise [4, 5]. Having safe paths for bicycle transport is leading to marked increases in the proportion of people cycling to work and other places, as well as for recreation.

The availability of tools or resources to enable, facilitate or sustain action also needs to be considered, for example, one can't smoke without tobacco. Availability relates to such things as their source (e.g. of drugs), variety of options and variation in quality (e.g. psychoactivity). The density of outlets for particular products influences consumption or use patterns [6, 7], and while it is also true that density is influenced by demand, there appears to be interactive effects, that is, density or availability also drives consumption as well as responding to it. In the early phases of change, sources of information about the need for, and benefits of, change may be more important resources than the physical resources required to act.

The pattern of rewards and costs associated with engaging in behaviours in different contexts provides another set of influences. The costs associated with engaging in the behaviour (either to do it or to pay for what is required) are an important consideration as most people have limited financial resources, and increased cost is known to reduce consumption or use of most things. Even addictive behaviours such as smoking are price sensitive [8]. Costs also include such things as the amount of effort required to obtain the products or get to the place where the behaviour is to take place (e.g. the local gym). Rewards need to be higher than costs. The net reward is a mix of experienced and assumed benefits of the behaviours.

One aspect of value is the extent to which the behaviours of interest occurs among the person's social circle and/or among those they admire. This affects both value and opportunities for behaviour modelling, which can facilitate uptake.

Finally, the number of cues in the environment that stimulate action tendencies towards the behaviour is critical. In addition to the cueing aspects of the above-mentioned sources, cues can also come from the amount and kind of advertising for relevant products and services that occur. In cases such as smoking, where commercial advertising is banned, this has eliminated a whole range of cues that used to be present. There is now a lot of evidence that antismoking advertisements both encourage quitting [9, 10] and can help prevent relapse [11]. Reactions to health warnings on cigarette packs are reliably increased with stronger warnings [12] and these reactions predict subsequent quitting [13], and active use of warnings is associated with reduced rates of relapse [14]. Similarly, point-of-sale warnings also seem to encourage quitting [15]. On the other side of the equation, putting cigarettes out of sight at point of sale reduces spontaneous purchasing [16], and the evidence is generally consistent with all forms of advertising restrictions reducing smoking, although such effects are difficult to demonstrate [17]. The range of environments the person needs to operate in and the extent to which, and predictability with which, the environment changes both determine variability in the distribution and nature of cues to act, and thus the ability of the individual to sustain action across contexts.

Environmental variables have both direct and indirect effects on behaviour. The environment directly affects the OS, and thus behaviour, via innate or conditioned responses. The indirect effects are via how the various aspects of the environment are interpreted by the ES, including what others tell us about it. This leads to expectations on people as to how to behave. Changing HTM behaviours can involve either or both: changing the environment, or changing the way we conceptualise environmental conditions in relation to the behaviour, that is, change the inferences about the desirability/necessity of the behaviour. This includes normative beliefs about the value of the behaviour to the society, either because of its impact on others and/or what it signals about a person behaving in that way.

There are different challenges for optimising the environment (in so far as is possible) for behaviours where excess is the problem (e.g. alcohol and gambling), rather than any level of use (e.g. tobacco smoking), or where the goal is to increase the behaviour (e.g. exercise). It is useful to think of four forces on individuals that affect the balance of desirable and undesirable behaviours. Two focus on desirable behaviours: forces promoting desirable behaviours and forces distracting attention from desirable behaviours, the latter being important as rarely are there forces actively discouraging desirable behaviour. The other two focus on undesirable behaviours: forces discouraging them and forces stimulating them (often incidental to other goals rather than deliberately). The intention of purveyors of unhealthy products is not to make people unhealthy; it is merely to make a profit, and they don't see themselves as being responsible for designing and promoting their products in ways that encourage abuse by some.

Many of these forces on behaviour come from the broader environment, while others are very much a function of people's micro-environments, the things they have around them, their normal routines and the people with whom they interact. For some forms of change, all four sets of forces need to be considered, but for others, especially where no replacement behaviour is required or no other behaviours need to be foregone, the focus can be on only one pair, for example the balance of pro- and anti-environmental forces influencing smoking.

There is increasing evidence that both physical aspects of the environment and people's perceptions of their environment affect the likelihood of engaging in and persisting in behaviour change efforts. This has been demonstrated for physical activity [1, 18] and for smoking cessation, where perceptions of social integration and environmental safety seem to have as much impact if not more than real indicators in predicting capacity to quit smoking successfully [19].

Most people's macro-environments are fairly constant over a period of months or even years. Most people spend the majority of their lives in a small number of fairly predictable micro-environments, such as home, work, and less commonly, recreational venues, friend's places and vacations/work travel. People generally have quite predictable routines for how they deal with most of the variability in these settings, and have varying capacity to deal with unexpected variations and novel situations.

The social environment and social norms

The social environment is arguably the most important influence on behaviour. It can be thought of as a complex, somewhat hierarchical, network, from the society to interpersonal influences. The focus of this section is on the broader or macro-environmental factors that include the society or culture in which the person lives and its laws and customs, the society or culture they identify with (often but not always the same, for example, for migrants and members of minority groups), the organisations or institutions to which they belong and/or to which they come into contact (including religions) and the local communities in which they live or work or otherwise spend time with. The extent to which societies divide into subgroups is a function of things such as size (the bigger the more likely), the homogeneity of the population and their history of past mixing.

The ways that social forces are thought to influence behaviour are partly mediated through seeing others behave (discussed later) and partly through social norms. Norms with respect to behaviours refer to broadly shared beliefs about the desirability of the behaviours and the contexts in which they are more or less desirable, ranging from socially taboo to expected. In essence, norms are what you expect others to think or do. As a result of past experiences and communication, people within any particular culture tend to share common beliefs, or norms, when generalised to the society as a whole. Norms are not physical things, they only exist conceptually, but they are important to understand as they help us predict how others will behave and how they will react to our behaviour.

The normative context can vary depending on such things as who you are (e.g. gender, religion social status) and the subgroup you belong to (e.g. drug use is condoned in some subgroups, particularly user groups). More generally, some behaviours are condoned for some groups but not for others, for example, gender differences in the acceptability of sexual activities.

The desirability of any given behaviour (or behaviour change) is not fixed: something previously seen as either desirable or unproblematic can come to be recognised as a problem needing to be changed (or vice versa). For example, society's position on the desirability of smoking slowly changed after its massive adverse health consequences were discovered. For some, this knowledge was enough to motivate quitting, but for many, knowledge alone was not enough, it also required strategies that made the risks emotionally real, and/or changes in societal norms legitimating change, before effective action was possible (i.e. experienced as worth pursuing). Even with almost complete reversal in norms, only some smokers have been able to quit, leaving many who continue in the face of considerable social pressure to stop. Norms are only one set of influences on behaviour, and for many HTM behaviours, they are unlikely to be the main determinant, at least for maintenance. They play a more central role in influencing the desirability of behaviours.

The normative societal context can often be taken as a given at any point in time in any one place, but it can change massively over years, and in doing so greatly affects the ease/difficulty of engaging in related behaviours. Understanding this requires a credible theory of how the environment sustains behaviour. This is hard to research directly as the processes by which the determinants change typically occur over a number of years, or even decades. These are not time intervals that can be encompassed within individual research studies, and often take place over periods where the necessary data is not collected, or where it is collected in different ways, all of which makes comparisons difficult.

Because normative change is slow, under most circumstances it is unlikely to act as a dynamic predictor for individual behaviour change. One exception is around cusp points in societal acceptance where prevailing assumptions can rapidly change and thus the way the context is perceived also changes (see next subsection). As described in diffusion of innovation theory [20], change begins slowly in the face of normative opposition, but at some point, the norms shift and this is accompanied by a rapid shift in the behaviour, until only a few laggards are left engaging in the old pattern. The rapidity of this shift is a function of the extent to which the change is contested and to which the behaviour is socially determined. For example, there has been quite a rapid uptake of smoke-free homes, but much slower reductions in smoking prevalence. Patterns of smoking prevalence show no clear evidence of increased quitting with increased denormalisation [21]. This suggests that, at least among regular smokers, normative influences are not the major determinant of continued smoking.

At a societal level, changing norms to be less accepting of undesirable behaviours and more supportive of desired behaviours should be a key goal. People often talk of the need to normalise an adaptive behaviour or denormalise an undesirable one – for example smoking – as if this were something that could be done directly. However, norms are an emergent property of the ways a society, or relevant subgroups within it, treat behaviours. Thus, norms cannot be changed directly. Norms emerge out of socially shared interpretations of perceptions of patterns of social reinforcement of behaviour to become beliefs about what is acceptable. These beliefs cumulate across individuals to create the social climate. Changing norms can lead people to discover what they thought to be freely chosen behaviours, are at least in part driven by social forces. Once behaviours become routinised, they become part of the context determining normative beliefs; so, only tend to be a focus of attention when their desirability becomes the focus of executive considerations.

Modelling and vicarious learning

Humans are essentially social, and one key aspect of sociability is the tendency to imitate the behaviour of others. What other people do is an important influence on behaviour and we tend to copy what others do. The tendency to model behaviour appears to be deeply biologically determined, with evidence of learning from observation in birds and other higher animals. One of the first people to focus on the importance of modelling for human behaviour was Bandura [22]. Bandura identifies several functions modelling can play: it can result in observational learning, that is, capacity to perform new tasks; to changes in frequency of behaviours as a result of seeing others rewarded or punished for engaging in them; it can act as an immediate cue to act in a similar way, and it can stimulate similar emotional responses to those in the person behaving, that is, by modelling what someone else does you experience some of the same accompanying affective reactions.

At its base, modelling can operate through OS processes, but it can and often is overlaid by ES activity. An individual has some choice in whom they attend to, and thus who has the potential to influence them as models. Modelling can be of desirable and undesirable behaviour patterns, and to be a positive force there need to be people engaging in the desirable behaviours who are seen as models to emulate. It should be noted that modelling works best for actual behaviour, and its role is less well understood and it may play no role for not doing things, as there are no specific acts to model, unless there are incompatible alternatives (e.g. using an e-cigarette rather than a cigarette). Beyond the person's interpersonal circle, modelling can be used in therapeutic settings, and it is particularly important in mass communications (TV, radio and internet) both because of the capacity to disseminate images to large audiences, and because it can model behaviours that are unlikely to occur in the person's environment. This means that the media can be used to demonstrate potentially effective novel strategies, and/or allow the repetition of events that are likely to be rarely seen. Modelling via high-profile people in popular media can be important in setting norms by helping to define what is new and fashionable in behaviour. Seeing admired figures acting in particular ways attracts those who identify with these people and thus want to be seen to be acting in the same ways.

Changing the broader environment

The goal of environmental change is largely to change social conditions in ways that are more supportive of desired behaviours and less supportive of ones we wish to reduce. It can be useful to think of three kinds of forces acting on individuals: two have been discussed previously, namely, those encouraging and discouraging the desired behaviours, and a third force, comprising governments and other institutions that regulate to affect the balance between the two [23, 24]. Forces can emanate from interpersonal influences through to the transnational policy environment. Social forces that value a form of behaviour act to try to normalise it and give it a privileged position, while forces that oppose the behaviour try to denormalise it, thus reducing the potency of one set of forces supporting it. Work with Young and other colleagues [23–25] provides an analysis of how, in Western societies, the system that is dealing with tobacco has changed from one supporting and encouraging use, to one managing use down gradually, and of the need for systemic change to hasten this process.

Elaborating on the analysis of Young et al. [25], it can be useful to conceive of three broad stages of societal change: acceptance when there is a problem;

arguments over appropriate solutions; and institutionalisation of solutions. Before the need for change is accepted, a case needs to be made both that there is a problem and that it is of sufficient importance for action. Until this point is reached, the to-be-changed behaviour is regarded as normative, and attempts to control it are considered unusual, with anyone making the change likely to be seen as eccentric. Once the point of accepting a problem is reached, the next step is the search for solutions, something that can be seemingly simple, but in most cases of HTM behaviours is particularly difficult to achieve. Deciding what societal actions are required for change tends to go in phases, with the simplest possible solutions tried first, and only when they fail are more intensive solutions countenanced. The exception is where the behaviour is seen as extremely threatening, in which case quite draconian measures might be taken, for example, prohibiting various kinds of drugs with heavy penalties. In the intermediate stage, action by individuals may be seen as optional, in the sense that institutional forces do not yet support it, or other people don't really expect it. The final stage is where a new set of rules are instituted, the new behaviour is now normative and continuing to engage in the old behaviour may require justification. The second and third stages tend to alternate with each other until a set of strategies is found that results in a satisfactory resolution. This may require a series of changes both by individuals and institutions. It should also be recognised that sometimes progress stalls, and there is a need for a reconceptualisation of the nature of the problem, that is, a return to first-stage issues. Thus, these three stages may be better thought of as a process that may occur multiple times as a complex problem is addressed and initial solutions come to be seen as inadequate, or in some cases even counterproductive.

Achieving change in the social acceptability of a behaviour is an important early strategy to change its frequency of occurrence. It is important because it both allows those who are most subject to social influence to change without (much) other external help, and because it hastens the level of commitment of the broader society to act in ways that are consistent with facilitating the change. On the basis of insights from diffusion of innovation theory [20], it is clear that some people are better placed to change than others. Part of this may be explained by a general disposition of some people to enjoy novelty, but part of it is also likely to relate to the relevance of the behaviour to their lives. Supporting and/or encouraging more rapid change among those who are most likely to be able to do so may prove a more effective strategy for facilitating societal change than broadly based strategies that try to motivate change in everybody before the early adopters have shown it has potential worth. One group who it might be important to target early are those who are likely to be most influential in changing the norms around the behaviour. Therefore, it might be productive to focus initial efforts at achieving health-related changes on doctors and other health professionals. Historical analysis suggests that in countries where health professionals (largely doctors) led the move away from smoking, progress has been greater than in those where they ignored the issue and continued to smoke. However, this is not commonly articulated as a key strategy; rather, there is often an implicit (and wrong) notion that change should be equally easy for all at all times.

A rational society should not encourage or facilitate organisational forces that systematically create cues to trigger those behaviours that society wants to discourage. However, social systems have developed which support existing undesirable behaviours [23] and powerful institutional forces often benefit from this situation, either directly or indirectly through the markets they create. It is socially unacceptable to be seen to be directly encouraging unhealthy behaviours, but it is possible to oppose societal change by appealing to other normative beliefs or values, for example, by arguing against restrictions on a behaviour or the promotion of a behaviour based on the importance of individual autonomy and/or of competitive markets and profit-driven activity. Thus, while people might agree that for-profit marketing of tobacco is problematic, they can claim to legitimately oppose constraints on the basis of those other norms or values. What society is prepared to do is not just a function of what might be best for any isolated problem. Change at both institutional and individual levels is a continual battle for the priority of some values over others.

The normativeness of a behaviour is one important factor that influences governments and other institutionalising forces to take action in support of behaviour change. Public support for change, and particularly the lack of strong opposition to change, makes it easier for governments to act. Normativeness both provides a basis for action and increases the likelihood that those values will be shared by those in positions to influence the decisions. Achieving public support for action requires an ongoing public debate about what sort of supports for individual lifestyle optimisation we want from an open society when the needs of individuals and their goals and priorities may legitimately differ. In addressing this issue, we need to realise that the freedom for institutional or collective forces to act may constrain our freedom as individuals. Conversely, constraints on organised activities may be essential for maximising individual freedom.

In the remainder of this section, I consider the main kinds of social forces and give some examples of specific environmental changes that have been shown to facilitate behaviour change or are theorised to do so.

Regulation and legislation

The process of normalisation/denormalisation described in the previous section is largely one of bottom-up societal change, and the regulatory approach by contrast is a top-down process, albeit one designed to produce, or at least influence, normative change. In many countries, government is the main institutionalising force in a society; however, in some countries, where religious practices are institutionalised as laws (e.g. in Islamic societies), religious laws can be at least as important in shaping HTM behaviours that the religion has taken an interest in (e.g. use of some drugs, some forms of food and sexual activities).

Organised society, through government action or other means, can change the nature of the 'playing field' to facilitate the adoption of behaviours it favours and to discourage ones it does not. That said, there tends to be more focus on laws to prohibit or restrict activities than on efforts to promote desired behaviours. Laws often act to institutionalise normative changes rather than being an important force in the changing of norms. However, in all cases laws add extra structure and clear definitions of what is acceptable, and often include penalties for transgressions. That said, penalties only apply when transgressions are detected, and where societal support for a law is sufficiently compromised, enforcement can become virtually impossible. For example, one hears reports that use of marijuana is as high or higher than of tobacco in some parts of the world, where only the latter can be legally sold. Legality is clearly only an influence on behaviour. This may be surprising to some. For many people, laws are taken as things to obey, and where the required actions are found to be acceptable, they can rapidly lead to normative change. However, where the experience of complying is experienced as negative, for instance, when the laws run counter to cultural traditions, or they incur unexpected (to the law-makers) negative effects, there can be resistance, and the desired normative transformation may not occur. CEOS treats laws as a form of incentive, which influence behaviour but does not determine it.

There are different forms of laws and regulations that can be used to shape the environment to facilitate desirable choices. Laws can target behaviour directly or have indirect influences by affecting institutions that influence behaviour. Of laws focussing directly on the target behaviour, the most obvious is prohibition. Making something illegal creates costs (risks of punishment) associated with a behaviour, which should reduce its frequency. However, it also pushes any continued use into private environments, where it can flourish with limited capacity for governments to intervene in discourse on its costs and benefits. For common HTR behaviours, prohibition is rarely a part of the solution, although it can be effective in preventing a problem emerging.

Prohibition need not be of all forms of a product. Only the more harmful forms need to be prohibited, either because they are more inherently dangerous or because they are more likely to be subject to abuse. Thus, alcohol content of drinks can be limited, and the drink absinthe used to be banned in many places because of concerns about it being a particularly harmful form of alcoholic drink. In the area of tobacco use, many countries including most of the European Union and Australia have prohibitions in place on most forms of smokeless tobacco, while some countries also have bans on newly developed alternative nicotine delivery systems such as e-cigarettes. This is even though the current evidence is that these forms of nicotine use are far less harmful than smoking cigarettes [26], which remain legal. Legal anomalies like this can make resolving a problem harder.

Laws can also constrain when and where some forms of behaviour can be undertaken, such as bans on smoking in indoor areas, restrictions on when and where alcohol can be consumed or on places where gambling is allowed. I have done a lot of research on the impact of smoking bans on smoking behaviour. This has shown that restrictions on smoking tend to be highly complied with, and often result in significant reductions in cigarette consumption, but do not appear to have a large effect on smoking prevalence [2, 3]. This implies that compliance with where to smoke is largely under social and volitional control, while stopping smoking altogether is less socially determined. The creation of smoke-free places and the acceptance of these by smokers and non-smokers alike have almost certainly sped up the process of the denormalisation of smoking. For example, where there are more extensive bans on smoking in public places, smokers are more likely to report that smoking is banned in their home [27].

Restrictions on places that one can purchase requisites for behaviour are also important. There is good evidence that the greater the number of alcohol outlets, the higher the consumption [6, 28]. Price is another means of influencing the choice of products, and thus associated behaviours (e.g. alcohol consumption [29]). Price can also affect usage of resources such as gymnasiums. Governments can influence prices in two main ways, through taxes and through setting minimum and/or maximum prices for products and services. Placing larger than normal taxes on products to discourage use and removing taxes from products to encourage use are known to influence consumer choices, including tobacco use [8]. Differential taxation is a potentially powerful means of encouraging shifts in behaviour within a product class. Thus, differential taxing of alcoholic drinks according to the level of alcohol and/or the extent to which the alcohol content is masked by sweet flavours can tilt the consumption away from the less desirable products. From a behavioural perspective, price is just one method of changing the balance of costs and benefits associated with a behaviour; however, where it can be used, it is one of the most powerful.

Laws can also affect behaviour indirectly: these include laws constraining marketing activities; laws about the form of built space and the availability of public space (particularly important for physical activity); laws to require product information and product warnings and to enhance personal choices and sometimes even laws designed to influence other behaviours. A good example of the last law is the reduction in gambling revenues that resulted from the introduction of bans on smoking in poker machine (gambling) venues [30].

Modern marketing is arguably the most powerful set of forces on individual behaviour that modern societies have developed. Marketing has emerged out of the desire to profit from increased commercial activity. HTR behaviours are particularly vulnerable to, and thus attractive to marketers wanting to sell more and thus are part of the problem, while with HTS behaviours, marketing can be a powerful ally.

Marketing is usually divided into the 4 Ps: product, price, place and promotion. Laws can be used to control aspects of marketing, including limits on discounting, rules prohibiting or limiting advertising, bans on give-aways and other special offers, restrictions on the kinds of places products can be sold (e.g. licensed outlets for alcohol and for legal gambling) and on the number of outlets. Advertising is a particularly powerful tool, and attempts to control it have ranged from restrictions on advertising during children's programming through bans on all advertising in some media, to virtually complete bans such as those found in Australia for tobacco products. In Australia, tobacco products now have to be sold under the counter (i.e. no display of products except at certain tobacconists); no advertising except point of sale price boards; and only allowing the name and variant name on the pack with the part of the pack not covered by warnings in a common dark olive brown colour (plain packaging). Many of the restrictions on promotion and advertising have been shown to be effective, but some only indirectly, as it is easier to show positive effects for advertising than it is to show effects of its removal. One recent direct effect colleagues and I were able to show is of a reduction in unplanned purchases of tobacco following the implementation of bans on displays of tobacco products in stores [16].

Laws and, more commonly, governmental policies can also affect the design of the built environment. Thus, requirements for footpaths can encourage walking, the provision of bike lanes, cycling and the presence of amenities in parkland, the extent to which these areas are used for exercise and the kinds of exercise encouraged.

All of these things help create conditions that make some behaviours easier and place constraints on others. As noted earlier, to maximise individual freedom, institutional forces that push behaviour in undesirable directions may need to be constrained. For a liberal society, the aim should be to create, short of prohibition, a set of conditions that maximally encourage what the society desires, and discourage what is undesirable, limited by the freedom of individuals to choose inappropriate options if they really want to. This is partly an issue of freedom, and partly a recognition that some things that are bad for most may actually provide net benefits for a minority. I understand that in all societies there is some form of intoxicant use, if only by a minority, suggesting that for some it is a desirable part of life even if others can live fulfilled lives without it.

It is hard to estimate the relative contribution of the various forms of regulatory interventions that are put in place, especially when they involve removing things that were present (like bans on advertising), as the effects tend not to be sudden, and almost certainly interact with other interventions [31], but in total, they can make a considerable difference.

Public education

An important part of the environment is the knowledge environment. The main vehicle for this is mass media, where people can be exposed to information they are not seeking. However, for those seeking information, the internet is now probably the most important source. Another source of unsolicited information is information on product packaging, such as health warnings on cigarette packs, which as noted earlier in this chapter, can have desirable effects from increased knowledge [32] to supporting quitting [12–14].

There is now a large body of evidence on the effectiveness of mass media for health behaviour change, especially of TV advertisements. There is no doubt that sustained campaigns can lead to behaviour change, although as might be expected the findings indicate that it is harder to change habits than encourage one-off behaviours (such as screening for illness) [33]. In the area of smoking cessation, where the effects of the mass media are most studied, there is now a lot of evidence that anti-smoking advertisements can stimulate increased calls to help services, which result in more quitting activity and when available during the early period of quit attempts reduce relapse [9, 11]. The research also shows that advertisements that graphically portray the adverse health effects of smoking are overall the most effective, consistent with dual-process theories. However, they are inconsistent with other theories such as Prospect theory and theories that they act as punishment and thus only suppress the behaviour [34]. It appears that warning messages act as discriminative stimuli warning of adverse effects, not as punishment. The messages that work best appear to be those that are conceptually simple and evoke OS reactions consistent with their propositional content.

Newspaper stories, news and current affairs programs on radio and TV play important roles in both educating the public and helping to define what is normative. They are an important source of new knowledge for most, and through repetition, help keep the knowledge remembered and salient. The additional graphic capacity of electronic communication channels also means that they will be more effective in linking propositional knowledge to affective OS processes. Media stories are also important for influencing people's perceptions of the importance of an issue (if it is in the news, it must be important, and if it isn't, then perhaps it isn't important). Seeing something as important increases the likelihood that people will engage with it, which is a prerequisite to contemplating action.

Popular culture can also play an important role in both educating about problems and their consequences and in helping to change the normative context [35]. It provides a rich source of potential models for behaviours and scripts as to how to integrate them into one's life (or free oneself from them), and is extremely powerful at engaging OS processes.

The influences of popular culture on norms may be greater than that of more information-based communications, while the reverse is likely the case for dissemination of factual information. However, as the distinction between education and entertainment is increasingly blurred in the mass media, it is important to consider the dual roles of all forms of mass communication. Mass communication can produce changes in beliefs and norms more rapidly than would normally occur. That said, the speed will be more constrained for HTM behaviours as their determinants are only partly social; so, there will be more resistance to social trends to encourage change.

The interactional environment

To have any effect on behaviour, things must impact on the person in some way. Some of those influences, like those discussed earlier, are pretty much externally determined and all that the person can do is change his/her patterns of attention or the ways he/she interprets them. However, other aspects of the environment are interactional. These include the ways resources are used when engaging in behaviours, and the influence of others with whom one interacts.

Requisites for behaviour

Some behaviours such as eating and drug use require the appropriate resources, while others can be made easier with suitable resources (e.g. clothes that are more suitable for exercise). Thus, what is already present in the person's immediate environment will influence his/her behaviour quite directly. For example, if nobody has bought healthy food options, it is not possible to eat at home in a healthy way; or if the person buys cigarettes in cartons, it may lead to them smoking more than if they buy them by the pack. The person's perceptions of the resources also affect his/her influence. Thus, people's perceptions of product quality and appropriateness to the situation interact with availability to influence behaviour.

For some behaviours such as smoking, rituals develop around the use of the cigarette that can come to be valued in their own right (thorough processes of conditioning). Seeing others engage in similar rituals can both act as cues and enhance the strength of other cues to smoke. As noted in Chapter 2, the acceptability of potential substitutes for harmful forms of behaviour is constrained by the extent to which usage rituals are similar. This can occur even with apparently irrelevant aspects of the product. For example, following the introduction of plain packaging in Australia, some smokers called talk-back shows complaining how the taste of their cigarettes had changed. As far as we know, there were no changes to the product; so, smoking from a plain-coloured pack with bigger warnings on it had clearly disrupted the experience of smoking for some. This phenomenon is part of the reason that smokers and regular users of other products are very brand loyal.

Interpersonal influences

The interpersonal environment consists of a person's network of friends, family and, more generally, everyone they interact with. Clearly the influence of those they interact with more regularly are likely to be more influential than chance encounters. The degree of influence will also be affected by their relationship with the persons involved; thus, those seen as authorities may be more influential, as are those that the person wants to please or build or maintain a relationship with.

Interpersonal aspects of the environment can be the strongest influences on behaviour, and they are also the most subject to change. There are three aspects of interpersonal influence. The first is through the ways other people behave, which can create direct effects through processes of modelling (imitation) and vicarious learning. The second is through direct requests or demands on the person to act in various ways. In both cases, the direction of influence is clear although it can be resisted. The third form of influence is indirect, involving inferences from what others are saying and doing, including non-verbal cues. Inferences can be about possible reactions of others to behaving in particular ways.

Emotional expressions are important for communicating to others about possible consequences of behaving in particular ways, but they are also important for providing information to a person about how others are likely to behave. Because emotional expressions are communicative, rather than instrumental, they only affect others who can decode the messages, something that can be done unconsciously via OS processes, regardless of whether it subsequently reaches consciousness or not. Seeing others do something that you have chosen not to do, especially if they seem to enjoy it, can make it more difficult to resist, both through direct exposure triggering the action tendencies, as well as indirectly via a re-evaluation of its desirability.

People are influenced by the way their friends and family react to them and by their professed opinions as to what they do, and this process is reciprocal. Interpersonal factors coalesce to create local social norms that are an emergent property of the ways groups (including dyads) think and act. Interpersonal norms are among the strongest cognitive influences on behaviour, but they do not occur in a vacuum, and thus are harder to sustain when they are inconsistent with either cultural norms and/or laws, especially when the person is interacting with others who do not share the local norms.

It is hard to act in ways that differ markedly from the rest of your social circle, especially if what you do (or resist doing) is not valued and understood by them. When change is not normative, the person may need to justify his/her actions to others, but once change has become normative, if any explanation were necessary, it would be around any decision not to change. Where people need to justify their behaviour, they need a story that is credible to their audiences; else they may feel unable to persist. Stories can also inhibit change; for example, a story justifying not taking action in the past can act to inhibit subsequent attempts to change unless it can be credibly changed.

It is not just what other people do that can affect the kinds of reactions they get, who they are also matters. Influences of other people can range from those due to observable physical characteristics (e.g. gender, age and physical appearance) to the nature and history of your relationship with the person. For example, when acting in an equivalent way, women get different reactions to men in some settings, and similar reactions to a situation by men and women can be interpreted quite differently. These relationships are dynamic and reciprocal, and although initially driven by OS processes, can be modified by ES conceptualisations.

The main form of indirect influence of the micro-environment is through assumptions the person makes using his/her story as to how a particular situation will work out. Take the example of a smoker who has quit, but is offered a cigarette by a friend. The inner dialogue might go like this: 'If I say no to a cigarette, he is likely to bring up all my previous failures to quit, so I'll just have this one now rather than succumbing after his tirade', thus relapsing. On a more positive front, a story about convincing oneself to go for a run with a friend might go like this: 'I have been complaining about not being fit enough, so although I don't really feel like it, I will go for that run, else I will look bad in my friend's eyes and it is not worth the grief I will get from her'. The beliefs we have about the behaviour of others can affect the ways we behave independent of their truth value, when they remain untested. The friend who was assumed to denigrate a quit attempt may have been supportive, and would have helped maintain the quit attempt, but the other friend might have been looking for an excuse not to run themselves. The rule would seem to be only question assumptions when they threaten what you really want to do!

The environment constrains the content of stories that drive our volitional behaviour, not just our OS-generated actions. This is in part because action stories are partly constrained by the cast of characters within them (i.e. other people), and a story has to be consistent with the environment it seeks to describe or in which action is to take place. The situational specificity of stories is one reason why intentions formed in one context can lose their potency/relevance in other contexts, something that is common for HTM behaviours.

To do something new, you need to be capable of dealing with public reactions: these may range from awe, through curiosity, to hostility. Thus, change that may be extremely difficult to engineer when it is non-normative, but can occur spontaneously when the norms change. For example, early research on the effects of behavioural interventions to encourage the introduction of smoke-free homes found that they were remarkably unsuccessful, but sometimes there were large changes in control conditions. In parallel, population monitoring was showing marked increased in prevalence of smoke-free homes [36]. This demonstrates that some forms of change can occur without external help when conditions are right, but even quite intensive interventions may be able to contribute little when social conditions are not conducive to the change. The power of the normative context varies with the nature of the behaviour; as I have noted before, it is only likely to be a dominant influence when the main determinants of the behaviour are social.

Different aspects of the social environment (institutional, cultural or normative and interpersonal), although often positively correlated, can conflict and push individuals in different directions; for example, interpersonal networks might encourage challenging social taboos on a behaviour, or institutions might offer rewards for performing a behaviour that one's friends disapprove of. From the perspective of someone trying to engineer change, it is important to understand where the various forms of influence emanate from as that is usually the level of organisation that needs to be intervened on to produce the desired changes. In the early stages of behaviour change, at a population level, it is the subgroups who value the change that begin the process of advocacy for change or of demonstrating the worth of change, often in the face of considerable societal opposition or resistance. However, once norms change, it tends to be local norms that act to sustain undesirable behaviours within some subgroups. This can be because the subgroup does not value the change or because the behaviour may have come to be so strongly associated with the group that it becomes accepted as both a badge and cost of subgroup membership, making change difficult. In this regard, I am reminded of some work we were doing years ago to develop an intervention to reduce smoking. We were engaged with a group of school students who were seen as *rebels*. Only one member of the group did not smoke, and in a group discussion, several other members expressed their admiration of him not being a smoker, but still being one of their group (this was done in a way that was unambiguously positive). At the same time, they were disdainful of other kinds of non-smokers who were not part of their group. They were even more disdainful of other kids who took up smoking or said they did so to try to become part of their group. Deep down, I suspect most people are admiring of others who take actions based on what is best for them, especially if they do not impose expectations on others to do likewise where they are not ready or able to act in similar ways.

As a society, we can act to change the balance of forces promoting behaviour we want to increase or decrease. However, top-down processes have only limited capacity to influence subgroups, and here it falls on the individual to negotiate their relationship with their friends in ways that maximise their ability to engage in what they decide is in their best interests.

Summary

This chapter has two main functions: to discuss the ways the proximal environment in which people live affects their behaviour, particularly their interactions with other people; and to discuss the ways in which broader environmental forces affect the nature of personal environments and how they can be changed from without. It treats CEOS as one of a group of ecological models and briefly reviews influences on behaviour of places to act, cues to act, norms about behaviour and interpersonal factors.

References

1. Sallis J, Owen N & Fisher E. Ecological models of health behavior. In: Glanz K, Rimer B & Viswanath K (eds.) *Health Behavior and Health Education Theory, Research and Practice*. 4th edn. Jossey-Bass A Wiley Imprint: San Francisco, 2008: 465–485.
2. Borland R, Chapman S, Owen N et al. Effects of workspace smoking bans on cigarette consumption. *American Journal of Public Health*. 1990; 80: 178–180.
3. IARC. *IARC Handbooks of Cancer Prevention, Tobacco Control, Volume 13: Evaluating the Effectiveness of Smoke-Free Policies*. [http://www.iarc.fr/en/publications/pdfs-online/prev/handbook13/index.php]. International Agency for Research on Cancer: Lyon, 2009.
4. Humpel N, Owen N & Leslie E. Environmental factors associated with adults' participation in physical activity: A review. *American Journal of Preventive Medicine*. 2002; 22: 188–199.
5. Saelens B, Sallis J & Frank L. Environmental correlates of walking and cycling: Findings from the transportation, urban design, and planning literatures. *Annals of Behavioral Medicine*. 2003; 25: 80–91.
6. Campbell CA, Hahn RA, Elder R et al. The effectiveness of limiting alcohol outlet density as a means of reducing excessive alcohol consumption and alcohol-related harms. *American Journal of Preventive Medicine*. 2009; 37: 556–569.
7. Gruenewald PJ, Ponicki WR & Holder H. The relationship of outlet densities to alcohol consumption: A time series cross-sectional analysis. *Alcoholism: Clinical and Experimental Research*. 1993; 17: 38–47.
8. Jha P & Chaloupka F. *Curbing the Epidemic: Governments and the Economics of Tobacco Control*. The World Bank: Washington, DC, 1999.
9. Durkin S, Brennan E & Wakefield M. Mass media campaigns to promote smoking cessation among adults: An integrative review. *Tobacco Control*. 2012; 21: 127–138.
10. Wakefield M, Spittal M, Durkin S et al. Effects of mass media campaign exposure intensity and durability on quit attempts in a population-based cohort study. *Health Education Research*. 2011; 26: 988–997.
11. Wakefield M, Bowe S, Durkin S et al. Does tobacco control mass media campaign exposure prevent relapse among recent quitters? *Nicotine and Tobacco Research*. 2013; 15: 385–392.

12. Borland R, Wilson N, Fong G *et al*. Impact of graphic and text warnings on cigarette packs: Findings from four countries over five years. *Tobacco Control*. 2009; **18**: 358–364.
13. Borland R, Yong H, Wilson N *et al*. How reactions to cigarette pack health warnings influence quitting: Findings from the ITC Four Country survey. *Addiction*. 2009; **104**: 669–675.
14. Partos TR, Borland R, Yong HH *et al*. Cigarette packet warning labels can help prevent relapse: Findings from the International Tobacco Control 4-Country policy evaluation cohort study. *Tobacco Control*. 2013; **22**: e43–e50.
15. Li L, Borland R, Yong HH *et al*. The association between exposure to point-of-sale anti-smoking warnings and smokers' interest in quitting and quit attempts: Findings from the International Tobacco Control Four Country Survey. *Addiction*. 2012; **107**: 425–433.
16. Li L, Borland R, Fong GT *et al*. Impact of point-of-sale tobacco display bans: Findings from the International Tobacco Control (ITC) Four Country Survey. *Health Education Research*. 2013. doi: 101093/her/cyt058. Epub May 2.
17. National Cancer Institute. *The Role of the Media in Promoting and Reducing Tobacco Use*. Department of Health and Human Services, National Institutes of Health, National Cancer Institute: Bethesda, MD, USA. NIH Pub. No. 07-6242, 2008.
18. Sugiyama T, Neuhaus M, Cole R *et al*. Destination and route attributes associated with adults' walking: A review. *Medicine and Science in Sports and Exercise*. 2012; **44**(7): 1275–86.
19. Siahpush M, Borland R, Taylor J *et al*. The associated of smoking with perception of income inequality, relative material well-being, and social capital. *Social Science and Medicine*. 2006; **63**(11): 2801–2812.
20. Rogers EM. *Diffusion of Innovations*. 5th edn. Free Press: New York, 2003.
21. Warner KE & Mendez D. Tobacco control policies in developed countries: Today, yesterday and tomorrow. *Nicotine & Tobacco Research*. 2010; **12**: 876–887.
22. Bandura A. *Social Foundations of Thoughts and Action: A Social Cognitive Theory*. Prentice-Hall: Englewood Cliffs, NJ, 1986.
23. Borland R, Young D, Coghill K *et al*. The tobacco use management system: Analyzing tobacco control from a systems perspective. *American Journal of Health Promotion*. 2010; **100**: 1229–1236.
24. Young D, Borland R & Coghill K. Changing the tobacco use management system: Blending systems thinking with actor-network theory. *Review of Policy Research*. 2012; **29**: 251–279.
25. Young D, Borland R & Coghill K. An actor-network theory analysis of policy innovation for smoke-free places: Understanding change in complex systems. *American Journal of Public Health*. 2010; **100**: 1208–1217.
26. Etter JF. *The Electronic Cigarette: An Alternative to Tobacco?*. Version 3, Jan 2013 edn. Jean-Francois Etter: Geneva, Switzerland, 2012.
27. Borland R, Yong HH, Cummings KM *et al*. Determinants and consequences of smoke-free homes: Findings from the International Tobacco Control (ITC) Four Country Survey. *Tobacco Control*. 2006; **15**: iii42–iii50.
28. Livingston M, Chikritzhs T & Room R. Changing the density of alcohol outlets to reduce alcohol-related problems. *Drug and Alcohol Review*. 2007; **26**: 557–566.
29. Wagenaar AC, Salois MJ & Komro KA. 'Effects of beverage alcohol price and tax levels on drinking: A meta analysis of 1003 estimates from 112 studies. *Addiction*. 2009; **104**: 179–190.
30. Lal A & Siahpush M. The effect of smoke-free policies on electronic gaming machine expenditure in Victoria, Australia. *Journal of Epidemiology and Community Health*. 2008; **62**: 11–15.

31. Chapman S. Unravelling gossamer with boxing gloves: Problems in explaining the decline in smoking. *British Medical Journal*. 1993; **14**: 429–432.
32. Hammond D, Fong GT, McNeill A *et al*. Effectiveness of cigarette warning labels in informing smokers about the risks of smoking: Findings from the International Tobacco Control (ITC) Four Country Survey. *Tobacco Control*. 2006; **15**: iii3–iii11.
33. Wakefield M, Liken B & Hornik R. Use of mass media campaigns to change health behaviour. *The Lancet*. 2010; **376**: 1261–1271.
34. Peters G-JY, Ruiter RA & Kok G. Threatening communication: A critical re-analysis and a revised meta-analytic test of fear appeal theory. *Health Psychology Review*. 2013; 7: S8–S31.
35. Browne K. *An Introduction to Sociology*. 4th edn. Wiley, 2011. ISBN: 978-0-7456-5008-1.
36. Borland R. Theories of behavior change in relation to environmental tobacco smoke control to protect children. Background paper to WHO International Consultation on Environmental Tobacco Smoke (ETS) and Child Health 11–14 January 1999.

Chapter 5

CONCEPTUAL INFLUENCES ON CHANGE

The ES operates through a set of interrelated stories that conceptualise problems, contexts, and possible solutions, and how solutions might be implemented. The way we think about a problem affects the kinds of solutions we seek. However, the way our OSs react influences our capacity to act in the ways we think we should. This chapter is concerned with the generic thematic content of stories that are used to help engineer change.

As elaborated in Chapter 3, the ES creates three kinds of stories: descriptions of situations or events, explanations or stories of why we act the way we do and scripts or stories of pathways to action.

Collectively, our stories allow us to create conceptualisations of possible futures, generate goals with respect to those stories, and develop plans for achieving those goals, including seeking out environments more amenable to the achievement of our goals. The distinction between setting and/or refining goals and the subsequent development and refinement of plans or scripts for action is an important one for HTM behaviours, as goals are rarely achieved immediately after they are formed. Several attempts, often over a period of years, may be required and for some, the goal will never be attained.

This chapter focusses on the kinds of beliefs that are relevant to behaviour change and how such goals contribute to the development of goals for action. The ways in which people move from goal development, to behaviour change, to sustained behaviour change, is the topic of the next chapter. This chapter contains an overview of the main conscious determinants of action, with a focus on understanding those aspects that are particularly important for HTM behaviours.

Goals for behaviour change, especially for HTM behaviours, are typically formed in a context where the desirability of change has been known for some time, and may have been either ignored or downplayed over the course of that time period. This means people are likely to have access to plenty of material when they do actively consider change. Following goal setting, there is often an extended period of trying to change and failing.

The thoughts being considered are not just those that support action. The experience of failure is likely to result in people who have not yet been able to make desired changes constructing justifications for their failures, which can themselves then act as barriers to change. Such beliefs may need to be challenged before subsequent attempts to change are likely. As a result, this chapter also considers the nature of beliefs that can constrain behaviour change, as well as those that support it.

The stories of change that we use to guide our behaviour are social constructs. They have no independent identity. As a result, they should be judged on both their capacity to lead us in ways we desire, and to do so in ways that are consistent (or a least not conflicting) with other aspects of our lives. To understand the potential and limitations of stories to guide us, we first need to consider the ways stories are framed.

Framing the problem

The idea of framing comes from the work of Bateson [1], who introduced the idea, based on a picture frame, to help conceptualise what was part of a story from what was not. This idea has been extended to have greater generality within communication theory [2, 3], so that now it relates to what is taken into consideration by a story, and by default what is ignored. It is also about the perspective from which the issue is approached, which is typically from the person's point of view for a script, but even here it can contain elements that take other positions (e.g. what science says, what I think my friends will want). Framing occurs at several levels; first, defining the scope of the problem, second, in the ways the problem is conceived and third, in the way solutions are approached. The framings chosen are likely to be an amalgam of a basic story frame provided by others (e.g. from the person's culture) modified by inputs from internal thought processes, experiences and external sources of information to try to best make sense of the situation, and do so in a way that facilitates the achievement of relevant goals.

The scope of the frame is dependent on the nature of the issue under consideration and how it relates to broader life goals. The scope determines what is relevant to consider, and thus can constrain how the problem is analysed. For example, someone whose basic idea of themselves is that of a fearless person, someone who espouses an indifference to risks, can find it harder to justify adopting behaviours to protect long-term health than someone for whom future health is an acknowledged priority.

Framing a potential task too broadly can result in it becoming too complicated for our limited-capacity ESs to deal with. However, framing too narrowly can result in important features being ignored, which can adversely affect possible outcomes, and/or the assessment of the utility of acting. For example, in the area of outcome expectancies, basing a health decision on the effects that decision has on one disease may actually result in increased health risk, if the net effects on all-causes mortality/morbidity are in the other direction.

There is no *a priori* best frame for a problem or issue. The utility of the chosen frame can ultimately only be evaluated in terms of the outcomes it helps to deliver. Finding a useful frame is something that is often informed by framings that others have used successfully in the past, or that are provided by some external change agent. The person can then use this base frame or modify it as necessary to fit their needs.

One important aspect of the way a problem is framed is the way the person includes himself/herself in the frame. Two critical aspects are whether they see themselves as the agent of change or expect others to produce the changes for them, which then determine whether they are oriented to act; and where they situate themselves. The latter can range from considering either their OS or ES as the *real* them, to seeing themselves as some integration of the two.

HTM behaviour change affects the person in diverse ways, and bringing a simplistic view of self into the task can be problematic. If people frame themselves around thought-through decisions as to what they would like to be (i.e. ES dominant), then they may be ill-equipped to deal with emotional (OS dominant) challenges associated with trying to achieve such a vision. By contrast, if they frame inputs from the OS as reflecting what they want, then they may frame externally sourced arguments (however compelling) as ego-alien, and thus be prone to reject any notion of change. CEOS postulates that the model of the self that is optimal for HTM behaviours requires some integration of both OS and ES processes.

Related to the person's sense of who he/she is the extent to which external influences, such as scientific knowledge, religion, laws, rules and other forces, are seen as legitimate influences on personal executive decisions. If I see myself as a rational actor, then taking these factors into consideration is an important part of 'who I am'. However, if I view myself through what I want (i.e. OS-centric), then many of these external influences can come to be seen as barriers, and thus things to overcome or deny. The potential importance of this implication of framing has been neglected as theorists tend to focus on the way rationality can be used to improve our understanding, and thereby help us to live our lives more effectively. Population-level behaviour change would be well served by gaining a better understanding of the mechanisms by which a person comes to own a compelling argument or injunction as part of his/her own justification for acting, rather than as a case of others (e.g. the 'Nanny State') trying to tell them what to do.

At the next level is the degree of specificity with which the problem, and thus the goal for action, is defined; for example, 'I must do something about my health' as opposed to 'I need to quit smoking'. The more specific the goal, the easier it is to develop a plan for action and the greater the likelihood that action will ensue.

Within the context of the chosen goal, several components of frame comprehensiveness need to be taken into account:

- Whether contemplating taking up a new behaviour includes consideration of what would have to be forgone as a consequence of taking up that behaviour (e.g. considering what you no longer have time for as a result of a new exercise regime), or considering what new behaviours can be adopted instead of just eliminating an unwanted behaviour (do you just quit smoking or take up a range of alternative activities at the same time?).
- The implications of potentially competing priorities. This primarily relates to the period when active self-regulation is required, as it reduces the capacity to allocate this limited resource to deal with other life challenges. The importance of considering these other factors will be a function of how strong other forces are in determining priorities for action.

- The extent to which the goal covers the range of contexts in which the person lives (e.g. both work and home lives). This is particularly an issue in complex modern societies where people often have two or more different roles with quite different kinds of expectations. The values that emerge out of engaging in those roles can result in divergences in beliefs by context. This can be seen when a person behaves differently at work to at home. Core beliefs are ones that transcend societal roles, but what they are may only become clear when a value from one sphere attempts to be asserted in another. Many people keep different aspects of their lives quite separate to prevent conflicts between values becoming overt. This can make it difficult to frame the kinds of challenges that by necessity must transcend social roles (e.g. quitting smoking needs to transcend all roles).

Frames are not necessarily fixed, but they tend to remain stable unless explicitly challenged by inconsistent experiences or by argument. In general, people find it easier to adjust lower level aspects of their frames than to challenge the basic assumptions that partly define the broadest level of framing. The absence of a suitably framed script for action can be a catalyst for relapse, given that it is difficult to come up with new or modified stories in times of high-cognitive load (i.e. when trying to resist temptations to relapse); so, having the right script, or set of scripts, available can be critical to success. The development of strategies to both improve framing and ensure that the appropriate information is considered when needed are among the strategies for facilitating change described in Chapter 7.

Message framing

The way justifications for action and consequences of action are framed is also important. Framing is sometimes analysed in terms of whether statements designed to motivate action are framed in terms of gains or losses. On the basis of Prospect theory [4], Rothman and Salovey [5] argue that because people are more willing to take risks when faced with loss framed messages, the influence of the framing on behaviour should be a function of whether the behaviour change risks an unpleasant outcome (loss superior) or the risk is reduced (gain superior). Thus, they argue that gain frames should be preferable for behaviours designed to prevent disease.

By contrast, CEOS and other dual-process theories [6] argue that what drives the potency of message framing is its capacity to elicit desired affective (OS) reactions. In particular, it is important for communications to avoid negations with evaluative statements. The idea of negation first requires the activation of what is to be negated (the ironic problem [7]). Statements elicit OS reactions to their elements via the rippling activation of associations, rather than via the idea of their absence (i.e. ignoring the negation). The negation of an element is not incorporated in activation of associations until executive processes eventually extract the desired meaning, by which time the opposite valence has come to dominate. This can either weaken the desired affective response to the eventual interpretation, or even lead to a misreading of the message (i.e. one consistent with the OS reactions). The latter is increasingly possible as the complexity of the communication increased, and thus the effort required to decode it accurately increases.

The implications of this analysis become clearer if we consider the statements in Table 5.1. First, some of the statements, especially those involving negations are cognitively complex and would be elaborated more to increase clarity in normal communications. Second, it makes a difference whether the target is to reduce or increase a behaviour. CEOS analysis comes up with some different predictions as to the optimum communication mode to those from Prospect theory [8] for hard-to-reduce behaviours such as smoking. CEOS predicts greater effectiveness of loss framing as this is both simple and evokes congruent associations from operational and executive analyses, while Prospect theory predicts that gain framing will be superior. The evidence from applied studies clearly shows that loss-framed messages (smoking is harmful) are more effective than any other form of message [9].

Table 5.1 Affective reactions to processing by OS and ES of health-related statements varying in valence of outcome (gain vs loss) and presence of absence of the behaviour

Statements	Frame	OS	ES	Comment
Smoking (HTR behaviour)				
Smoking is bad/smoking causes illness	Loss	−ve	−ve	Congruent and easy to understand
Smoking is not good/smoking impairs health	Loss	+ve	−ve	Mismatch
Not smoking is good/not smoking improves health	Gain	+ve	+ve	Mismatch: OS +ve about smoking, ES +ve about not smoking
Not smoking is not bad/not smoking reduces harms	Gain	−ve	−ve	Mismatch, but congruent: OS −ve about smoking, ES positive about not smoking. Very hard to understand
Exercise (HTS behaviour)				
Exercise improves health	Gain	+ve	+ve	Congruent and easy to understand
Exercise reduces harms	Gain	−ve	+ve	Mismatch
No exercise reduces health	Loss	+ve	−ve	Mismatch, but congruence: OS +ve about exercise, ES −ve about no exercise
No exercise increases illness	Loss	−ve	−ve	Mismatch: OS −ve about exercise, ES −ve about no exercise

Graphic health messages that realistically depict the harms of smoking (i.e. loss framed messages) are an effective means of encouraging smokers to try to quit [10, 11] and there is increasing evidence that such warnings can also help prevent relapse [12], although perhaps only if this information is used actively [13]. A recent review of experimental studies of such messages [14] concluded that they may only work when the audience has adequate self-efficacy for change. While this may be true for isolated instances of communication, over multiple exposures it is likely that fluctuations in self-efficacy mean most will end up getting the message at times when they feel capable of making an attempt to change.

Undertaking a similar exercise for an HTS behaviour (like exercise) makes it clear that the comparisons do not work in the same way. If exercise is good, engaging in it is good too; so, gains are easy to understand all the way. Here, gain framing would seem to be likely to be preferable, consistent with Prospect theory. For HTR behaviours such as smoking, at some point the proposition 'quitting is desirable (not smoking is good)', needs to occur, but perhaps it is best if the person generates this in a context where he/she has a firm sense that smoking is bad, rather than it being a primary communication from others.

All the thinking and research mentioned earlier is about making decisions and acting and so may not apply to messages designed to resist relapse (i.e. those occurring after behaviour change), a situation that is critical for HTM behaviours. Once a person has stopped engaging in an undesirable habit, not acting is their current experience, and associative processes might facilitate making the desired affective links (my current situation – not smoking – is good). That said, these thoughts are most important in the context of a temptation to relapse, a time when positive associations with the old behaviour (smoking) have been generated. Here, self-talk needs to both counter this existing positive link and create positive associations for the alternative of resisting. How this is best done requires research. These problems do not seem to arise for encouraging desirable behaviours as gains continue to be a reasonable focus.

As noted in Chapter 3, negative affect motivates action of some sort, while feeling good can be demotivating for immediate action. CEOS theorises that unless there is some affectively charged sense of a deficit, the positive framing of messages will be less effective in stimulating action, particularly action repeated or sustained over time. Thus, for a positive outcome to motivate change, it has to relate to an existing need or generate a need for that outcome [15]. This explains why sated animals don't act for food rewards. By contrast, for HTR behaviours, negative framing helps to create motivation for action. It is then necessary to ensure that the desirable action is what is carried out, rather than an action that reduces the negative emotion, without solving the problem (e.g. psychological avoidance).

Mechanisms of persuasion

Coming to a decision to change, and maintaining that goal in the face of difficulties, are the two central cognitive challenges of behaviour change. Such decisions need to be grounded in OS experiences, so that the person not only thinks that change is a good idea, but feels a need to make it, and is able to resist competing urges. Unfortunately, the most influential theories of persuasion tend to neglect the role of OS processes, especially affective reactions. CEOS postulates a three, rather than two-path model of persuasion. CEOS adds the experiential path [16] to Petty and Cacioppo's [17] peripheral and elaborated paths (or the heuristic and systematic paths [18]). That is, the experiential path produces change through direct or vicarious experiences which, in turn, elicit emotional responses from the OS that provide drive to the analytically generated plans of the ES. The central, or *elaborated*, route to persuasion is through an analysis of the evidence, and it can lead to firmly held beliefs. The peripheral route is still an executive-led activity, but it relies on shortcuts, such as accepting views of influential others and relying on the number of arguments, all of which act to influence intuitions with minimal executive processing. Attention to peripheral cues tends to result in unstable attitudes in the absence of concurrent elaborated processing, or strong affective reactions, but where strong enough, can threaten the certainty of our beliefs (e.g. noticing others we admire holding a contrary view may imply that they know something we don't).

Of the three paths, the experiential is the strongest, and beliefs that are formed via this route can only be fully changed by direct experience, although the consequences of past experience can be reinterpreted, thereby increasing or decreasing the impetus to act [16]. For example, a person reinterpreting strong cravings for cigarettes as necessary signs of their body cleaning itself out, rather than evidence of the need to smoke, and thus the cravings no-longer constituting a reason for relapse.

Experience shapes beliefs by demonstrating ways to achieve outcomes and by affecting emotions. Conditioned associations are often imputed as causal links, and one mode of challenging behaviours that are supported by conditioned links is to demonstrate that the link is a learnt one and that the valued outcome is achievable in other ways. When direct experience is not possible, vicarious experience can play a similar role. Knowing or seeing someone tackle a problem, or failing that, viewing realistic mass communication about what is involved, can have some of the same emotion-inducing effects as direct experience.

Where the causal links between experiences and behaviour are contingent, attitude change is almost automatic. However, this does not happen when the consequences are not contingently linked to the behaviour. This is common for HTM behaviours, but not for their alternates. Consequences of HTM behaviours are often delayed and/or involve avoidance of adverse outcomes, and unless the thing to be avoided is present in some way (either in reality or as an envisaged possibility) there is no direct OS engagement, and where the object is present, the OS reactions will, unfortunately, be towards the unwanted behaviour. This is a key reason why HTM behaviour change is dependent on elaborated processing, and why negations should be avoided where possible.

Attitudes have to have an element of OS engagement if they are to result in action. This engagement is not necessarily related to the intrinsic value of the behaviour: engagement can be through a desire to be right, to be socially accepted, an expectation of benefit, or concern over possible adverse consequences. The emotional reactions are the input of the OS, and for the most part conceptualisations need to be consistent with felt experiences if they are to be credible (to the person). Experience ultimately leads to change in behaviour patterns via processes of rewards for new behaviours, extinction for eliminating old ones and/or counter-conditioning for replacing the old ones with the new.

Emotions are signals to the ES of operational readiness to act in various ways, with emotional expressions signalling similar things to others. Thus, where the ES does not need to be engaged, there is no need for conscious experience of emotions, and action tendencies and needs are only experienced when the ES acts to monitor or interrupt ongoing behaviour. NB: This is not a problem, as in these cases no important decisions need to be made because action is adequately managed by the OS.

The experiential path is neglected in theories of persuasion because it is not readily modifiable in experimental contexts, and is therefore difficult to study outside of real-world issues. The neglect is especially curious in the case of Petty & Cacioppo as in other aspects of their work they have focussed on the potency of emotional reactions [19]. One theory that does consider the role of emotions is Witte's Elaborated Parallel Processing model [20, 21]. Witte argues that high levels of negative affect (fear), especially in the context of low self-efficacy, leads to avoidance behaviours, which are generally maladaptive, while with high self-efficacy, the perceived threat can be directly confronted and resolved. There is a lot of empirical evidence from analogue studies in support of this model. However, it cannot explain why nearly all smokers make quit attempts after having a heart attack, something that certainly generates fear of mortality. What seems to be missing in Witte's analysis is a consideration of the ease of avoiding the threat. A real heart attack precludes most forms of avoidance, and thus makes confronting one's smoking and quitting the most likely solution. Avoidance is only a viable option where direct action is difficult and avoidance is relatively easy and likely to reduce concern sufficiently to be a satisfactory short-term solution.

One other problem with most existing models of persuasion is that they are rather mechanistic, implicitly assuming that it is simply one agent trying to convince another. The reality is that it is usually a dynamic process; people who are the target of persuasion are active participants in the process. Change in attitudes tends to occur over an extended period, rather than suddenly, as a person reflects on information he/she is given and relates it to his/her own experiences, and on whether change is both desirable and achievable. People who stand to lose something of value if they change are (quite reasonably) likely to require a higher level of proof and/or a larger anticipated gain to be convinced of the need for action.

Being persuaded to act is not enough; for action to occur, there must be a confluence of events that produces cues to act that stimulate the necessary affective engagement. These cues can come from environmental stimuli or from thoughts, either self-generated, or indirectly, via the implications of what others say or do. Such cues are what stimulate a decision to try to change now, rather than at some other time. The strength and experienced immediacy of the need to act make a difference. For example, smokers typically try to quit before there is a major manifest health problem. However, in the absence of symptoms, quitting is always easy to put off. Work by Wang [22] suggests that the strength of the desire to act now mediates the effects of more stable beliefs on quitting such as outcome expectancies, and value placed in long-term outcomes.

The above-mentioned analysis does not imply that action can only occur in the presence of strong affective force. In areas where there are no competing action tendencies, it requires little affective force to lead to action. However, where there are competing forces, as there are by definition with HTM behaviours, then ways of increasing affective force are required to counter the affective force of competing alternatives, either by adding affective links, or strengthening the evidence to reduce the power of doubt.

The processes of persuasion are not just involved in the decision to change, they are also important in understanding, and thus coming to resist, pressures to reverse or undermine decisions once made, whether this be due to experienced or anticipated adverse effects, or a simple nostalgia for the old behaviour. We may need to regularly re-convince ourselves that our choices are for the best until situational factors no-longer cue alternatives sufficiently to require self-control to resist.

Organisation of concepts about change

The process of change is organised around two key summary concepts, namely, beliefs about the desirability of change and beliefs about the achievability of change. However, the beliefs are organised in different ways when focussing on the development of goals compared to the development of scripts to achieve the goals. CEOS also theorises that the determinants of these two summary beliefs vary as a function of the nature of the problem and of the behaviour change required, making it quite different to existing theories that posit fixed pathways of influence. This changed perspective suggests that the Theory of Reasoned Action [23], which posits attitudes and subjective norms as the two main determinants of desirability, may be most useful when considering behaviours with a strong interpersonal component, for example, negotiating condom use or negotiating for a smoke-free home. On the other hand, behaviours with less social facets may be influenced in somewhat different ways, for example, using the considerations of susceptibility and severity of the problem [24]. This approach is very similar to the COM-B model of West [25].

Goals are based on relatively stable preferences. They emerge out of ES processes evaluating more stable aspects of desire based on the assessed utility of change and any associated costs. This is done (implicitly or explicitly) in terms of broader life goals and values, complemented by some general assessment of the viability (achievability) of the change (Figure 5.1). Operational factors may act to help drive the activity of goal setting, but are not central to the process. By contrast, they play a central role in both the development and implementation of action scripts because affective charge is needed to generate appropriate action tendencies.

It is worth noting here that cognitive theories such as the Theory of Planned Action and the Health Beliefs Model claim to be theories of behaviour change, but, in reality are only theories of trying [26]. That is, they are theories of the

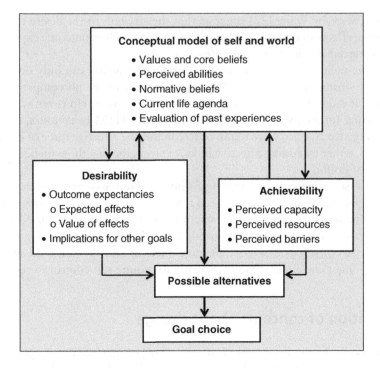

Figure 5.1 Determinants of goal choice.

determinants of decisions to act, or in some cases that action is worthwhile. Thus, they are only useful for predicting behaviours that follow quasi-automatically from a decision that they are desirable and feasible.

In analysing the role of various conceptual determinants of change, I make a distinction between analytical concepts that describe aspects of what is, of possible plans for action, and evaluative concepts such as attitudes, which include elements of value. Further, among attitudes, it is important to try to differentiate the affective elements that come from the person's values and long-term goals, and those which are generated by the contingencies of any given moment.

Core beliefs and values

The organisation of a person's thinking on any issue is framed by his/her concep- tualisation of himself/herself and of the world in which they live and act. Critical to the conception of self are the core beliefs the person holds and the consistency of those beliefs across contexts. A person's core beliefs can be about values (what I should or should not do), overarching life goals (what I want to achieve materially, for self and well-being, and for my social groups) and general capacities (what I believe I am capable of). Life goals include a mix of material, self-maintenance, and social goals, and how they interrelate may vary over the person's life, thus resulting in changes in their relative priorities for action.

Conceptualisation of the world concerns beliefs about what actions are possible in any given environment, what is socially acceptable (normative beliefs) and what kinds of resources are around to facilitate action. Knowledge about the world is not only based on memories of past experiences, but also includes propositional information, including scientific knowledge. Normative beliefs include beliefs about how others might react, and an understanding of relevant societal rules (secular or religious) together with associated sanctions and rewards. It should not be assumed that the analytic framework that leads to goal formation is always, or even mostly, a logical analysis based on empirical evidence. It may be based on social or religious edicts or on what the person wants to believe.

For any particular task, parts of the above complex of beliefs, along with knowledge, and ideas about possible solutions, can be thought of as the raw materials for the analysis of the desirability and attainability of possible goals and of the constituents of scripts required to achieve them.

The desirability of change

The most critical determinant of both goal choice and the subsequent development and implementation of action scripts is the person's assessment of the desirability of changing their behaviour. Because goals need to persist independent of context, affective factors in goal formation tend to be those that are driven by values and attitudes towards long-term consequences. By contrast, because behaviour is contextually determined, momentary affective factors play a much greater role in influencing the desirability of acting now and, especially, of persisting. Analysis of the desirability of change is not completely independent of achievability, but the links are generally small and the nature of the considerations involved so different, that it is useful to treat them as separate. Further, consideration of achievability usually only occurs once a decision has been made that change is, or could be, desirable.

Influences on goal desirability

A person's assessment of the desirability of a behavioural goal is a function of the effects expected, and the value placed on them, which combine to form outcome expectancies (Figure 5.1). This can be complemented by comparable evaluations of alternatives to arrive at an assessment of the relative desirability of the available options.

Outcome expectancies describe the person's synthesis of the likely consequences (positive and/or negative) of the target goal in relation to the current, problematic behaviour pattern. This consideration needs to be from the perspective of longer term or persisting effects if it is to remain stable. Net outcome expectancies are negative for HTR behaviours, while they are positive for HTS behaviours.

The way a person thinks about the desirability of change (i.e. the way they frame it or have it framed for them) is a major factor in determining if he/she sees a problem in the first place, then in determining its magnitude, the solutions he/she might seek and the desirability of action. Subsequent action is strongly influenced by the degree of affective force associated with the analysis. Abstract analysis does not drive action unless it gains affective clout.

For a health-related behaviour, the kinds of issues that one might encourage a person to take into account in forming outcome expectancies include the likely impact on his/her personal health and well-being, including both risks avoided/reduced and benefits gained; the urgency of making changes to get all or some of the expected benefits; the implications of action on their relationships with others (via normative beliefs); the impacts on their day-to-day life (other priorities) and to what extent the work involved in achieving stable behaviour change is likely to take up limited self-regulatory capacity and/or involves patterns of behaviour that might interfere with the pursuit of other life goals.

Considerations about what is desirable can be based on varying mixes of existing beliefs, propositional knowledge, vicarious experiences and actual experiences. The conceptualisation of long-term benefits is likely to involve some analysis of the relationships between personal values, relevant past experiences, independent empirical evidence, reference to authority (e.g. secular or religious laws and known societal opinions) and/or logical analysis as to the various implications of action or inaction. If the goal that results from this analysis is to be sustained, then the analysis needs to be relatively independent of moment-to-moment OS influences. More stable OS influences operate through the affective aspects of values and attitudes. What is included will depend on the frame the person chooses (or finds themselves using) to address the problem, which will in turn be influenced by what they know, what their thoughts trigger during conscious analysis and what is emotionally salient at the time they do the thinking. People also vary in whether they focus on maximising likely outcomes, minimising effort or some balance between the two. They also vary in the extent to which they discount outcomes that are more distant [27, 28], or in CEOS terms, in their ability to develop and sustain as strong affective links with ideas about future outcomes as compared with more immediate consequences.

It should be stressed that a person's analysis of outcome expectancies will have the greatest impact on future behaviour when it is strongly linked to the person's values, whether positively or negatively. The value attributed to each possible outcome has two main components: the ES elaboration of why it is important and OS reactions to it. The elaborated part is what people believe to be in their best interests, while the operational aspect is what they feel to be desirable. The two need not point in the same direction. Affective reactions to possible outcomes are likely to be relatively stable, but can be enhanced by personal and vicarious experiences. It is the sum of OS-generated components that turn abstract desirability into something that is enough to motivate action. Health-related outcomes from HTM behaviours are inevitably overwhelmingly longer term and probabilistic in nature. The level of discounting that occurs is theorised to be a function of any change in affective response either due to delay or the probabilistic nature of the expected outcome. Decisions made on the basis of probabilities, and avoidance of undesirable future outcomes, are particularly vulnerable to competing arguments.

It is both harder to form affective links with abstract possibilities and easier to find rationalisations as to why these events might not occur, than it is to rationalise away experienced effects. One of the challenges for HTM behaviours is to encourage the development of affective links with the most likely outcomes (i.e. the benefits of the change), while discouraging the development or maintenance of affective links with less probable and potentially self-defeating beliefs (e.g. I will be one of the lucky ones who aren't adversely affected). HTM behaviour change represents a triumph of rational appraisal over the competing contingencies of immediate value.

Another key factor influencing decisions is how the various component influences are organised. One aspect of the structuring of ideas is the need for simplicity, given the limited capacity of working memory. There is value in organising ideas quasi-hierarchically to cope with this limited capacity. The final determinants of our choices (i.e. at the highest level of the hierarchy of ideas) are typically summaries of more complex analyses, with reference back to the supporting detail only when the potency of the summary is brought into question. The nature of the summaries can make a difference, particularly when implementing an action script. One of the challenges of behaviour change is that the non-contingent benefits of acting tend not to spontaneously occur to the person at times when their OS is pushing them towards relapse. Not being able to think of the appropriate reasons when pressed can result in failure to resist and thus relapse.

Which of the possible influences on outcome expectancies outlined earlier are most likely to be important can vary from goal to goal, and also vary as a function of the task; that is, different emphasis might be required for goal setting than for having affectively charged thoughts available to resist pressures to relapse. Part of the analysis of each kind of goal should include which of these factors are likely to be primary and which subsidiary, in terms of how they feed into the main summary conclusions that direct and/or sustain action. In Chapter 7, the use of a strategy called *implementation intentions* [29] is elaborated as a method for maximising the likelihood that appropriate thoughts and actions will be triggered when they are needed. For the appropriate intentions to be formed, the key determinants of success for achieving the task need to be identified, and thinking organised to place these factors at the top of the hierarchy of ideas.

The scope of the frame determines which motivational factors are taken into consideration; missing negative (for change) motivational factors (e.g. ignoring the enjoyment you get out of smoking) can lead to more rapid action, but can cause problems later if these become manifest, while missing positive factors can reduce the likelihood of taking action, as there is less apparent reason for acting (at the time). Taking into account the different needs/goals of the OS and ES can also be critical, as they both help to determine what is desirable and affect the ease with which change is likely to be negotiated.

When relatively stable factors (e.g. that there are no substitutes for cigarettes) are assumed to be fixed, they are excluded from the frame (i.e. not considered), but where they have changed or need to, there will need to be ways to broaden thinking to encompass them. From time to time, especially after failures, it is useful to question whether the past framing was sufficiently comprehensive or too complicated.

In Chapter 6, the way the role of outcome expectancies varies as a function of the stage of the behaviour change process is discussed. Outcome expectancies are critical for setting goals and for the initiation of change, but their role post-change is more complicated.

Priority

There are many possible options that each of us could pursue in life. Priority refers to the ranking of those possibilities. It is a function of the perceived importance of the task and the urgency of action, assessed in relation to the same judgements about other needs for executive action, either emerging from other life goals, or through OS processes. Thus, priority can change if a re-evaluation of the goal concludes that there is less value for effort, or if other priorities demand more self-regulatory capacity. The importance of priority for action is neglected in most behaviour change theories, perhaps because most studies of behaviour change start with the target behaviour; so, the choice of behaviour is outside the frame of thinking. However, in the real world, choices are usually compromises between competing priorities; so, for any comprehensive theory, priority needs to be considered.

The importance of an action stems from its outcome expectancies in relation to those for other life goals. Because change makes demands on self-regulatory capacity, a new goal may disrupt other activities that are dependent on working memory. Priority is not a major issue for goal setting; it only becomes an issue when the effort of implementing change threatens the pursuit of other life goals. The goal with the highest priority is usually the one pursued most strongly. For example, a quitting smoker who experiences negative affect and is grumpy and short-tempered as a result (or sees themselves in this light) may justify relapsing so as not to further strain his/her relationship with his/her partner because this relates to a more highly valued, and hence important, goal. Importance also influences the amount of time and effort the person is prepared to commit, for example, a person might decide not to exercise regularly because she convinces herself that she cannot spare the time from competing life priorities. (She is too busy at work.)

The second element of priority relates to timing. This has two elements, namely, urgency, the relative benefits of acting now as compared to some time in the future, and opportunity, the possible existence of contextual factors that might affect the chances of success: 'Now seems a good time' or 'Hearing that my friend has started to run regularly and will let me run with him makes getting into a regular exercise routine now easier than it would have been'.

There are two main task-related factors that affect timing. First, where the core benefits are in the future, it is easy to put off action because there is often no compelling reason for acting now as compared with some other time. Analysis of the costs of delay determines the urgency of acting; it is easy to justify small delays, although if repeated they can result in large, consequential delays. Secondly, the further in the future or the more probabilistic the expected benefit (or loss avoided), the harder it may be to generate strong affective links to the desired outcomes and the easier it is to discount them. Discounting occurs because outcomes are less certain and thus may not occur, and/or because they are of less worth than they would be if received immediately. This latter form is the way discounting is understood in economics and in Temporal Self-regulation Theory [27].

Two aspects of delay influence affective reactions, and thus the salience of the outcome: first, anything that takes the consequences out of the range of OS processes; that is, no immediate effects, and thus no automatic OS reactions; and second, any additional discounting that occurs as a result of ES analysis of the implications of the delay and/or the ability to imagine the outcome and its consequences. The ability to take more distant possible futures into account may be a relatively stable characteristic of people [27]. Much of the research on temporal discounting and of probabilistic outcomes uses money as the basis, and is often interested in finding out where biases lie. This is useful for those interested in maximising wealth, but for non-monetary outcomes, it is not clear whether rational actuarial decisions are always the best. Kahneman [30], in his excellent book *Thinking Fast and Slow*, summarises several such studies. One finding is that people will tolerate greater harms from inaction than from action. This appears to be a deeply held human value, and one that may be adaptive in the general sense, even if it leads to some sub-optimal decisions; the sort that researchers in this area love to create. Seen from the perspective of CEOS, we should exercise some caution in concluding that the rational solution is the right one when the rational choice occurs within an artificially constrained framing of the problem.

The existence of strong OS forces opposing action, and the sense of ambivalence that this often creates about initiating change, has the effect of making postponement of efforts to change often seem like a reasonable strategy. Establishing a belief that action is required now, and countering arguments about putting it off (where these arguments are not well-grounded), is an important part of decision making, and one that requires finding ways to override OS reluctance.

Decisional balance

Decisional balance refers to the net value the person sees in continuing to pursue his/her identified goal, and is experienced as what the person wants to do (experienced desire). What the decisional balance is at any one moment is determined by the extent to which the person is able to evoke the full range of outcome expectancies at points where the behaviour change is challenged by immediate desires to do otherwise. The affective (OS) forces which the ES must compete against will automatically be generated by the context, although their strength can be affected by the ways in which the ES thinks about them.

In CEOS, decisional balance represents the balance between moment-to-moment OS-generated action tendencies and outcome expectancies (longer term perceived net consequences), rather than the net balance between costs and benefits as it is used in other theories (Figure 5.2). In situations where the best long-term choice is unclear, there is a need for a more executive-driven analysis, and when this suggests no important differences, it doesn't matter if the final choice is the one that feels best. This is not an issue for HTM behaviours because what is desirable is always clear.

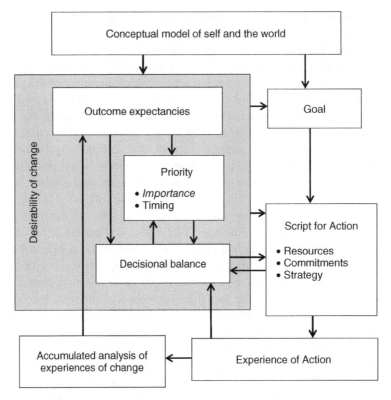

Figure 5.2   Interrelationships between key determinants of the desirability of change and how they relate to goals and scripts.

In situations of conflicting desires, each time a decision is made or an action taken, it is immediately followed by feedback that will sometimes lead to the generation of inhibitory tendencies resulting in the action being put on hold (inhibited) awaiting further consideration of competing alternatives. This can result in a new decision being made, which can then feedback to a re-triggering of other alternatives, and so on, until one set of forces comes to dominate and action occurs. This period of indecision is experienced as ambivalence as to which path to take. Such situations are experienced as stressful and thus requiring resolution. Stress typically triggers associations that favour the behavioural option most likely to reduce stress in the short term, and this is most likely not the desired behaviour.

Once behaviour change has been initiated, experiences associated with the change have a major influence on overall decisional balance. These experiences can override past experiences and/or replace or modify relevant expectations with experience-based interpretations. These influences operate in a similar way to how competing options create ambivalence in decision making. The contingencies of the moment compete with the longer term goals to determine the path of action. Also, as for goals, ES expectations and assumptions can affect the interpretation of experiences and thus their potency. For example, if getting strong cravings after giving up a drug is interpreted as evidence of the futility of trying, it will facilitate relapse, but if used simply as a cue for the need to act decisively, it can be used to reduce the risk of relapse.

Goal achievability

The second main influence on goal setting is believing that there is some possibility of achieving the goal (Figure 5.3). This can include an analysis of the following:

1. Perceived capacity to act. For goal setting, the focus tends to be on the abstract possibility of acting, something usually relatively easy for HTM behaviours. However, once failure has been experienced, it can also take into account issues associated with the challenges of persisting, which is where most of the problems lie.
2. Resources for action. These are relatively stable resources, not situational factors, that can assist change. They can be physical resources such as evidence-based aids such as pharmacotherapies and cognitive behavioural therapies, and non-evidence based ones that the person nevertheless thinks can help. Potential resources can also include support from others in the person's social environment, independent of whatever effects social factors have on the desirability of the behaviour.
3. The nature and magnitude barriers to change, which determine perceived task difficulty. These can be social or physical, and represent the challenges to be overcome.
4. Finally, these are combined to provide an analysis of the person's sense of self-efficacy or capacity to succeed on the current task in the current context.

We tend not to set goals that we believe are unachievable, but at least initially we often don't think too hard about the nature of the challenges as most HTM behaviours appear easy to adopt until the person has tried and failed on a number of attempts to sustain the change. Indeed, once a behaviour change is seen as desirable, it can become a goal unless there is a spontaneous reaction that leads to the questioning of achievability. Detailed consideration of achievability is more likely after experiences of failure to maintain change.

Analysis of the challenge (task difficulty)

An analysis of the challenge or the difficulty of the task being attempted involves consideration of both transaction costs (i.e. costs of making the change) and any ongoing challenges in persisting. This involves an evaluation of the task and of the viability of change in the current environment, and includes an evaluation of influences of environmental factors, OS influences and the interaction between the two. It has both stable and time-varying components. Time-varying components include opportunity (e.g. a friend invites you to join in a new exercise regime) and

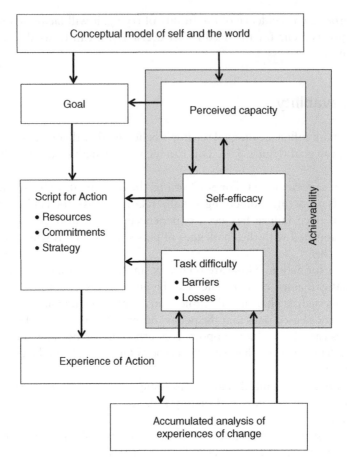

Figure 5.3 The main determinants of achievability and how they relate to goals and scripts.

a consideration of competing demands. The varying aspect is critical for answering the question: How feasible is behaviour change now?

Task analysis need not be cognitively elaborated, especially for future needs, but some deliberative analysis is likely to be beneficial to prepare for the challenges of maintaining HTM behaviour change.

Task analysis involves consideration of the following:

1. The habit strength of the old behaviour, including an assessment of how much effort is likely to be required to resist urges to continue it (e.g. give in and smoke, overcome inertia to exercise).
2. The extent to which the desired behaviours are cue driven (including the time taken for cues to become triggers). This includes the extent to which there are common antecedents associated with the times when the desired behaviour is needed, and thus the capacity for it to become cue-driven, and the extent and nature of anticipatory responses.

3. The extent to which the behaviour pattern is self-sustaining, that is, generates intrinsic rewards from its performance (becomes governed by the OS), and the possible effects that re-engaging in the old behaviour has on subsequent capacity to maintain the new one. A key element of giving up a habit, particularly an addictive habit, involves maintaining vigilance to be able to implement resistance strategies whenever urges to re-engage in the old behaviour occur.
4. The extent to which new skills and/or aids need to be acquired and how easy they will be to get.
5. What alternatives exist, both in terms of potential replacements for the intrinsic value of the old behaviour, and for the instrumental functions it serves. For behaviours to increase, it includes an analysis of whether any other valued activities are going to be reduced because of lack of time. This involves consideration of whether the new behaviours can co-occur with existing behaviours or whether they are incompatible (e.g. running and sitting are incompatible). HTM behaviour change usually involves situations where substitutes are at best only partial (at least initially), such that some intrinsic value of the old behaviour is lost.

Making behaviour-specific decisions needs to occur in the context of a contextual analysis; analysis that involves using the model created by the ES of the environment, and how the OS relates to it, ideally including how relevant non-cognitive variables can have direct impacts on behaviour change (independent of any effect they may have via cognitions). These include the following:

*   The contexts and actors that are likely to trigger impulses that are either supportive of change or not, and an assessment of what is required to utilise/defuse them.
*   The extent of competing demands. Opportunity (space to do it), both to initiate change and to engage in any additional activity (including help seeking) required to facilitate maintenance of the change.

These two sets of factors combine to provide the basis for working out an action plan for coping, designed to maximise the chance of success. They should culminate in an assessment of difficulty, and degree of persistence, required to extinguish the old behaviour pattern to the point where it can be easily resisted. The summary assessment of task difficulty, along with general perceived capacity, combines with contextual factors to determine self-efficacy.

Self-efficacy

Self-efficacy is the person's perception of his/her capacity to achieve his/her goal under the conditions in which the individual's script for action is to be or is being implemented. It is only once some form of decision to act has been made that the person can take into consideration the amount of effort he/she is prepared to put in, resources available, and the specific challenges he/she is likely to face. These considerations influence self-efficacy, but not overall perceived capacity. Further, unlike some other theories (e.g. the TTM), task difficulty and self-efficacy are treated as related, but independent constructs, with task difficulty being the expected or experienced challenge and self-efficacy the perceived capacity to overcome it in the context of the supports and commitments made.

Self-efficacy is an extremely useful summary concept, and thus predictor of a person's readiness to act and/or persist. It can be based on anything from some intuitive sense of what can be achieved through to a comprehensive analysis of OS, ES and environmental factors, including the availability of assistance (advice, skills training or drugs). Re-evaluation of self-efficacy on the basis of feedback or evaluation is also the main means by which more abstract beliefs about capacity can be modified.

The specificity of self-efficacy means that the focus of efficacy changes as the process of change progresses; thus, self-efficacy for the initiation of an action script can be differently determined to that for maintenance of change, and can be different again to that for recovery from any setbacks. These distinctions follow those of Schwarzer's [31, 32] HAPA theory. In addition, CEOS posits two forms of maintenance self-efficacy. The first is concerned with the ability to withstand the negatives and losses associated with cessation of a behaviour and to persist with this for as long as is required. The second is concerned with ability to create change such that the losses are replaced, the period of loss is shortened and/or an acceptable long-term balance has been achieved (i.e. where the gains consistently outweigh the losses). Overconfidence due to misconstruing the task as nearing completion, when only the first of these tasks is in hand can result in increased risk of relapse [33, 34].

Internal factors (excluding the motivational ones covered earlier) that can influence self-efficacy include the following:

- People's assessment of the implications of past experiences of this or similar behaviour changes, including an assessment of how their OSs will react and of their capacity to deal with these reactions.
- Their assessment of their capacity to let go of valued aspects of the old behaviour and accept the loss.
- Their ability to accept some degree of uncertainty, including the possibility of failure.
- Whether they have the skills, both generic self-regulatory capacity and any task-specific skills, required to successfully achieve the behaviour change.
- An analysis of competing demands and level of self-control capacity, including the level of exhaustion.
- Their assessment (evaluation) of progress to date, where relevant.

The predictive capacity of self-efficacy is likely to vary as a function of how much of the above-mentioned people includes in their assessments, that is, how accurate they are. However, as self-efficacy feeds back into motivational factors such as degree of commitment, an optimistic bias for self-efficacy can be adaptive. Indeed, requiring too high a level of certainty for self-efficacy can result in self-fulfilling failure because it can result in never trying. For any given individual, his/her goal should be having a level of self-efficacy that maximises the likelihood of success.

NB: When sought outcomes (goals) are behaviours (or the experienced conse-quences of behaving), then self-efficacy for achieving those outcomes equates to outcome expectancies. For example, the extent to which an ex-smoker feels com-fortable as a non-smoker (the outcome) is the evidence as to how successful he/she has been so far (their self-efficacy) for achieving a non-smoker lifestyle. In HTM behaviours, the ultimate goal extends beyond the behaviour (e.g. quitting smoking to improve health); so, the capacity of the behaviour to achieve the goal is an issue that can emerge after change is initiated if the expected benefits are not realised, or are not observable. In this way, feedback on progress towards the ultimate goal can influence outcome expectancies, and through this other motivational factors independent of self-efficacy. In addition, the capacity to enjoy life with the new behaviour pattern, at least enough to make the change bearable, needs to be seen as part of the behavioural challenge. Anybody not seeing a possibility of coming to value the new behaviour will be likely to react to perceived or experienced losses by relapsing.

Beliefs that can interfere with behaviour change

Changing HTM behaviours involves costs, that is, whatever was valued about the behaviours to be forgone as a result of adopting new behaviours. Some of the losses may be replaceable in other ways, but there may be real losses. These need to be dealt with, either by seeking replacements, or by coming to accept the loss as a price worth paying for the benefits of the change. The extent that this can be achieved before change, or be left to after change, when the implications become more real, is unclear. Beyond real costs, many people develop additional beliefs that justify not changing, which can disrupt attempts to pursue identified goals, lead to the pursuit of less desirable goals and/or be used as excuses for abandoning efforts altogether.

These beliefs include the following:

- Rationalising beliefs such as that the problem is overstated [35], and thus action is not as important.
- Self-exempting beliefs, that is, that the person is less vulnerable to the potential harms than average.
- Compensatory health beliefs [36], that is, that engaging in some healthy options compensates for not engaging in others. This can include strategies such as switching to low tar cigarettes instead of quitting, and exercising instead of quit-ting smoking. At best, these strategies only provide a fraction of the benefits and in some cases none (e.g. switching to low-tar cigarettes).
- Reframing the problem so that behaviour change is not appropriate at that point. For example, deciding that you don't need to quit smoking before you are 30 because if you quit then you will avoid most of the harm.
- Choosing an easier option. The tendency to choose a simple easy to achieve goal over a more complex one that rationally should deliver greater probability of

benefit is a significant form of human weakness. We have a clearer conceptualisation of the task than of the consequences; so, false claims about the benefits
of change can sway thinking much more than false claims about ease of implementation.

- Exaggerating the adverse effects of change. A story I have heard several times
  from smokers goes something like this: 'Whenever I try to quit, I am such a
  terrible person to be around that once the wife handed me a cigarette and said
  either you smoke or I leave. So I gave up trying to quit. What else could I do'?
  Clearly this justifies relapse if it is true; if the only thing that could be done about
  the anger is to smoke. By not considering the possibility of otherwise managing
  anger, the excuse seems credible.

- Believing that you really have to want to before there is any point in trying to
  change. In one study a few years ago, we asked people about the importance
  of aspects of will power and found that most smokers believed that will power
  was a necessary and sufficient condition for successful change: that is, if you
  really want to, you just will [37]. CEOS sheds new light on this, in that while it
  acknowledges that first coming to want to change might represent one path to
  change, the alternative of using self-control until adaptation takes place is also
  a viable alternative. For some, that there is value in an undesirable behaviour
  they continue to pursue is self-evidently true; so, challenging this belief can
  be difficult.

Related to beliefs about the appropriateness of acting are beliefs that you should be
able to do it alone and without help. Indeed a stronger version of this is that help,
particularly from an advisor who clearly wants you to change, might interfere with
what you want to do and in some sense fool you into giving up something you value.
When made explicit, this belief tends to disappear as it doesn't stand up to close
scrutiny, but unless confronted, it may inhibit seeking assistance that could help.

All these beliefs have potential potency because they engage with OS reactions
against change, and thus have inherent motivational force, which unless confronted
can drive action away from the desired goal. Many of these *questioning* beliefs
are sustained by the inevitable doubt that accompanies any predictions about the
future. Unless this doubt is dealt with appropriately, it can cripple attempts to
change. In moments of stress, when there is neither time nor capacity to think rationally about an issue, an argument with affective force can easily dominate a more
rational argument that has less affective force.

The challenge that CEOS helps make clearer is that resisting these beliefs either
requires building countering beliefs supporting the change that will, concomitantly
generate strong action tendencies themselves, and/or using strategies to try to reduce
the affective strength of these maladaptive beliefs. Two important aspects of this are
framing the analysis to minimise the doubts about goals and ensuring that beliefs in
the desirability of acting are elicited at moments when there are strong OS-generated
action tendencies that are opposed to the desired behaviour pattern. Some of the
potential strategies for doing so are discussed in Chapter 7.

Summary

This chapter focusses on the kinds of personal beliefs that are relevant to behaviour change and spells out how such beliefs contribute to the development of people's goals for action. The framing of the problem, expressed in terms of what is considered, and how it is thought about, influences both the conclusions reached and the affective reactions generated. Choices of goals for action are grounded in basic beliefs and the eventual choice invariably represents a balance between what is perceived to be desirable and what is believed to be attainable. It also explains how feedback from experiences, both immediate experiences as well as those that arise as a consequence of longer term reflection, provide ongoing influences on the course of behaviour change. Desirability, moment to moment, is shaped by experiences (both tangible and envisaged) and the priority of the behaviour, while achievability is influenced by the perceived difficulty of, and self-efficacy for, the various tasks required to achieve a given goal.

References

1. Bateson G. *Steps to an Ecology of Mind*. Paladin: Frogmore, St. Albans, 1973.
2. Penman R. *Communication Processes and Relationships*. Academic: London, 1980.
3. Wilden A. *System and Structure*. 2nd edn. Tavistock: London, 1980.
4. Kahneman D & Tversky A. Prospect theory: An analysis of decisions under risk. *Econometrica*. 1979; **47**: 263–291.
5. Rothman AJ & Salovey P. Shaping perceptions to motivate healthy behavior: The role of message framing. *Psychological Bulletin*. 1997; **121**: 3–19.
6. Strack F & Deutsch R. Reflective and impulsive determinants of social behaviour. *Personality and Social Psychology Bulletin*. 2004; **8**: 220–247.
7. Wegner DM. Ironic processes of self-control. *Psychological Review*. 1994; **101**: 34–52.
8. Rothman AJ, Bartels RB, Wlaschin J *et al*. The strategic use of gain- and loss-framed messages to promote healthy behavior: How theory can inform practice. *Journal of Communication*. 2006; **56**: S202–S220.
9. Durkin S, Brennan E & Wakefield M. Mass media campaigns to promote smoking cessation among adults: An integrative review. *Tobacco Control*. 2012; **21**: 127–138.
10. Borland R, Yong H, Wilson N *et al*. How reactions to cigarette pack health warnings influence quitting: Findings from the ITC Four Country survey. *Addiction*. 2009; **104**: 669–675.
11. Wakefield M, Spittal M, Durkin S *et al*. Effects of mass media campaign exposure intensity and durability on quit attempts in a population-based cohort study. *Health Education Research*. 2011; **26**: 988–997.
12. Wakefield M, Bowe S, Durkin S *et al*. Does tobacco control mass media campaign exposure prevent relapse among recent quitters? *Nicotine and Tobacco Research*. 2013 **15**: 385–392.
13. Partos TR, Borland R, Yong HH *et al*. Cigarette packet warning labels can help prevent relapse: Findings from the International Tobacco Control 4-Country policy evaluation cohort study. *Tobacco Control*. 2013: **22**: e43–e50.

14. Peters G-JY, Ruiter RA & Kok G. Threatening communication: A critical re-analysis and a revised meta-analytic test of fear appeal theory. *Health Psychology Review*. 2013; 7: S8–S31.
15. Rescorla RA. Pavlovian conditioning: It's not what you thing it is. *American Psychologist*. 1988; 43: 151–160.
16. Leventhal H, Brissette I & Leventhal EA. The common-sense model of self-regulation of health and illness. In: Cameron LD & Leventhal H (eds.) *The Self-Regulation of Health and Illness Behaviour*. Routledge: London, 2003: 42–65.
17. Petty RE & Cacioppo JT. *Communication and Persuasion: Central and Peripheral Routes to Attitude Change*. Springer-Verlag: New York, 1986.
18. Chaiken S. Heuristic versus systematic information processing and the use of source versus message cues in persuasion. *Journal of Personality & Social Psychology*. 1980; 39: 752–766.
19. Petty RE & Cacioppo JT. The role of bodily responses in attitude measurement and change. In: Cacioppo J & Petty R (eds.) *Social Psychophysiology: A Source Book*. The Guilford Press: New York, 1983: 51–101.
20. Witte K. Putting the fear back into fear appeals: The extended parallel process model. *Communication Monographs*. 1992; 59: 329–349.
21. Witte K. Fear control and danger control: A test of the extended parallel process model. *Communication Monographs*. 1994; 61: 113–134.
22. Wang S, Borland R & Whelan A. Determinants of intention to quit: Confirmation and extension of Western theories in male Chinese smokers. *Psychology and Health*. 2005; 20: 35–51.
23. Fishbein M & Ajzen I. *Belief, Attitude, Intention, and Behavior: An Introduction to Theory and Research*. Addison-Wesley: Reading, MA, 1975.
24. Rosenstock IM, Strecher VJ & Becker MH. Social learning theory and the health belief model. *Health Education & Behavior*. 1988; 15: 175–183.
25. West R & Brown J. *Theory of Addiction*. 2nd ed. Wiley: Chichester, UK, 2013.
26. Bagozzi R & Warshaw P. Trying to consume. *Journal of Consumer Research*. 1990; 17: 127–140.
27. Hall PA & Fong GT. Temporal self-regulation theory: A model for individual health behaviour. *Health Psychology Review*. 2007; 1: 6–52.
28. Hall PA & Fong GT. Temporal self-regulation theory: Integrating biological, psychological, and ecological determinants of health behavior performance. In: Hall PA (eds.) *Social Neuroscience and Public Health*. Springer Science + Business Media: New York, 2013: 1–19.
29. Gollwitzer PM. Implementation intentions: Strong effects from simple plans. *American Psychologist* 1999; 54: 493–503.
30. Kahneman D. *Thinking, Fast and Slow* 1st edn. Farrar, Straus and Giroux: New York, 2011.
31. Schwarzer R. HAPA theory. [http://userpage.fu-berlin.de/health/hapa.htm] [updated 10th December 2011, 4 July 2013].
32. Schwarzer R. HAPA website. [http://userpage.fu-berlin.de/health/hapa.htm] [updated 10 December 2011].
33. Borland R & Balmford J. Perspectives on relapse: An exploratory study. *Psychology and Health*. 2005; 20: 661–671.
34. Segan CJ, Borland R, Hannan A *et al*. The challenge of embracing a smoke-free lifestyle: A neglected area in smoking cessation programs. *Health Education & Behavior*. 2008; 23: 1–9.

35. Borland R, Yong H, Balmford J *et al*. Do risk-minimizing beliefs about smoking inhibit quitting? Findings from the International Tobacco Control (ITC) Policy Evaluation Survey. *Preventive Medicine*. 2009; **49**: 219–223.
36. Rabiau M, Knauper B & Miquelon P. The eternal quest for optimal balance between maximizing pleasure and minimizing harm: The compensatory health beliefs model. *British Journal of Health Psychology*. 2006; **11**: 139–153.
37. Balmford J & Borland R. What does it mean to want to quit? *Drug and Alcohol Review*. 2008; **27**: 21–27.

Chapter 6

THE STRUCTURE OF THE CHANGE PROCESS

This chapter focusses on the process of change. It explores the different factors and forces involved in setting a goal for change, and for any given attempt, on the decision to change, the initiation of attempts to change, in the maintenance of change and on challenges of recovering from setbacks. It is clear that there are a number of discrete tasks in each of these steps. The acceptance of a problem, the formation of a goal for change, the decision to change and the initiation of change are all primarily driven by ES processes, with OS engagement only really important in generating sufficient emotional engagement to make the change seem worthwhile, and for initiation, to overcome any initial resistance. By contrast, contingent OS reactions are critical for maintenance, with negative experiences linked to the change particularly important in triggering relapse, thus requiring active resistance by ES-led processes, of self-control and/or of strategies to retune OS processes, if relapse is to be prevented.

CEOS theory conceptualises the process of behaviour change as one that may be cycled through a number of times with varying degrees of success before finally achieving stable change; indeed it accepts that some will never get there without more effective strategies to help them. For this reason, CEOS reconceptualises many of the determinants of change to separate out their stable and dynamic aspects and to help differentiate the long-term goals for change from specific attempts to achieve them.

In this chapter, I begin by discussing the establishment of goals for behaviour change, before focussing on the long-term process of achieving the goal. The factors that determine action include those involved in goal setting, as well as more dynamic elements. The determinants of goal choice tend to remain relatively stable, and thus exert less apparent influence on goal attainment unless they change.

I also consider the implications of repeated failures to sustain change. Most theories of behaviour change seem to assume that the person is approaching change for the first time, yet most attempts at behaviour change are repeated efforts. Thus, the paradigm case for a HTM behaviour is not the initial attempt to change the behaviour, but a subsequent one. Finally, there is an analysis of the implications of repeated attempts, both in terms of the feedback from past experiences and in terms of changing characteristics of the population that have been unable (so far) to change.

Tasks involved in behaviour change

There is more than one way to approach behaviour change. Different paths have different waypoints, that is, points when either decisions need to be made or when the context of, or nature of, the tasks involved changes. Different paths may require the same set of tasks, but in a different order; perhaps as a result of some not being significant challenges or others requiring considerable effort. Some paths also require extra steps, for example, when a person seeks some form of help and/or needs to develop extra skills. Furthermore, some tasks may be implemented in an instant because the preparatory work has been done, while others can require significant extra dedicated effort that can delay implementation of the full script.

A comprehensive theory of change needs to consider whether there are waypoints common to all pathways, the range of pathways and whether some waypoints are discontinuity points where fundamentally different processes are required to progress to them to those required to progress beyond them. Theories that include discontinuities are typically referred to as *stage-based theories*. In some senses, CEOS can be thought of as a stage-based theory of behaviour change, but it treats stages differently to other theories.

Stage-based approaches to behaviour change owe their popularity to the Transtheoretical Model of Change (TTM) [1, 2] The idea is that there are distinct periods of change with quite different determinants, and in the strong version of stage theory, that progress follows sequentially through the stages, only allowing for relapse to previous stages. Stage-based theories have been questioned in part because the TTM stages are fundamentally flawed [3, 4]; for example, the boundaries between the pre-quit stages have been shown to be arbitrary and lacking in any predictive utility [5−7] and the stages of Action and Maintenance also do not map any identified discontinuities in the period post cessation.

There is increasing evidence that change is not a continuous process. In particular, the determinants of the initiation of behaviour change differ from those influencing the maintenance of change. For smoking cessation at least, the evidence is compelling [8−10] and would seem to support a return to an active consideration of stage-based models. These studies found that measures of outcome expectancies and overall attitudes that were strong predictors of making quit attempts were often not positively associated with maintenance of change. Indeed, some of these studies have found negative relationships, most clearly one of ours [8]. We asked smokers about a range of beliefs and behaviours that can loosely be described as indices of motivation to quit, including outcome expectancies and expressed reporting of the extent of wanting to quit. As expected, all these measures were positively associated with making quit attempts in the following year, with wanting to quit the strongest predictor. However, among those who tried to quit, the measures most strongly predictive of trying were most predictive of failure. That is, the more you want to quit, the less likely you are to succeed, given that you have tried. Clearly, what motivates trying is different to what motivates maintenance. We think the negative association is because smokers who really want to quit and are still smoking are in some way more addicted, and thus less able to change.

There is also increasing evidence from smoking that the determinants of relapse vary systematically with time quit, perhaps related to some underlying mechanism, such as the period of withdrawal, or the period when self-control starts to be exhausted [11, 12]. This possibility is taken up later in this chapter.

CEOS accepts that the determinants of the initiation of behaviour change (a waypoint) differ from those of maintenance (the ultimate outcome), and is concerned with specifying the determinants of each (including spelling out common determinants). In this respect, it divides the change process up into two fundamental stages. All stage-oriented theories of which I am aware accept this, or something close to it, as a stage boundary. The initiation of behaviour change is the distinction made by the TTM [1, 2], Rothman's dual theory [13], the theory of trying of Bagozzi and associates [14], the ASE model of De Vries [15] and Weinstein's PAP model [16]. HAPA theory [17] makes a slightly different distinction focussing on the decision to act as the boundary point. If there is discontinuity, then the point should be able to be quite accurately specified, although discontinuities need not be instantaneous; so, absolute precision may not be achievable.

The focus of CEOS is on the specific tasks involved in behaviour change, to better understand how these tasks interrelate, when and how their determinants might differ and how they impact on progress to the eventual goal of sustained behaviour change. In particular, I am interested in waypoints that are both necessary and ordered within the change process. The ordering of some of the tasks is not completely fixed. For example, planning for maintenance can occur both before and after changing the behaviour, but planning for how to make the change must occur before, but not necessarily before a decision to change has been made.

The core tasks involved in behaviour change are listed in Table 6.1. These relate to any single attempt to change. This table also lists some tasks that can occur, but not inevitably. These include the acquisition and use of aids, and development of strategies to cope with major challenges, such as strong negative reactions to

Table 6.1 Key tasks involved in behaviour change

Necessary tasks	Possible additional tasks
Setting a goal	Seeking assistance
Deciding to act	Developing new skills
Initiating action	Seeking support
Dealing with failures to cue the new behaviour	Making commitments
Dealing with urges to relapse,	Dealing with withdrawal, pain associated with engaging in new behaviour, for example, pain from too much exercise too quickly
Institutionalising/sustaining change	Coping with setbacks

change. The person's script for change can specify if and when such tasks will be undertaken. It should be noted that the script does not need to be developed in advance beyond decisions to take particular actions. This means that elements of scripts can be developed after the decision to change or even after the initiation of change. Scripts can also be conditional, for example, 'This is what I will do when I decide to change'.

Getting behaviour change on the agenda

The first major task of behaviour change is going from simply knowing about a potential problem to deciding that change is desirable and is something that should be pursued, that is, setting a goal. Goal setting is an executive activity, although OS factors can influence it.

Before anyone is likely to contemplate change, they need to have reasons for change. For HTM behaviours, accepting that their behaviour is harming them typically comes in the face of experience of little or no adverse effects, and is thus an intellectual decision with causation inferred, not grounded in direct experience. Once the person accepts that his/her current behaviour is putting his/her future health at risk, the next task is to come to identify behaviour change as a reasonable solution. As noted in the previous chapter, this involves not only thinking of it as a possibility, but seeing it as potentially achievable. Once the person has a goal, he/she is in a position to act when suitably cued.

Propositional knowledge that a behaviour is causing harm and that the solution is behaviour change is not generally sufficient to engender change in HTM behaviours. Take the example of smoking. Smoking rates did decline [18] following the publicity given to major reports demonstrating the health harms and recommending quitting in the first half of the 1960s [19, 20]. However, smoking is still common in these countries and millions who have grown up with this information have still ended up smoking. While more than half of ever-smokers eventually quit successfully, many do not, even though virtually all have tried and failed multiple times, at least in countries where the population are acutely aware of the adverse consequences [21].

While it might have been different in the past, when nobody knew that the behaviour of interest was potentially harmful or of sufficient benefit to take up even if it doesn't inherently appeal, HTM behaviours are now ones that we as a society have known about for some time, in many cases, all our lives. All adolescents know smoking is harmful; we all know that some level of physical activity is good, and that some patterns of eating and drinking are healthier than others. Most of us aspire to do better, and our unhealthy patterns tend not to be actively chosen. It is notable that very few people actively take up smoking as a result of setting themselves the goal of being a smoker. Indeed, the best indicator of vulnerability to uptake of smoking is anything other than a firm commitment not to [22]. Most younger smokers hold vague goals about quitting, such as 'I'll quit before I am 30', or deny that they are a long-term smoker: 'I'm really just a social smoker,

I can quit whenever I decide to'. Thus, we take as our starting point people who are aware that they and/or society consider their current behaviour pattern deficient in some way, regardless of whether they are engaging in undesirable behaviours or not engaging in enough desirable ones.

Before volitional change is possible, the person needs to identify a behavioural goal. Until the person has contemplated the possibility of change, they are not in a position to think through the possible implications. Goal choice can involve a comparative analysis of the costs and benefits of possible goals and of ways of achieving them. The choice of options is often what is presented to them by others, augmented sometimes by creative discovery of others. The cost–benefit analysis can include consideration of what is socially acceptable, and what the person thinks he/she can tolerate, and not just abstract utility. Such an analysis may not appear to be an issue for smoking, where cessation is an established behavioural goal, but it is for exercise or diet, where means of improvement are many. However, if we consider the possibility of choosing sub-optimal goals, then goal choice also applies to smokers who too often decide on alternative goals such as cutting down or define cessation to allow an occasional cigarette. Choices are important, because the nature of the choice both determines the potential net benefits to be obtained and the likelihood that the behaviour change will be successfully adopted. As we have seen, there is internal pressure on people to adopt smaller, less beneficial changes because they require less effort.

Goals

Goals refer to any conceptualisation of future possibilities that guide behaviour systematically towards their realisation, in whole or part. Forming a goal can be thought of as being the equivalent of putting something on a 'To Do List'. Scripts, on the other hand, are specifications for implementing the goal when the conditions are right. This separation of goals and scripts is useful for helping us to understand the sporadic nature of attempts to change behaviour and the changing nature of the specific efforts as past (failed) attempts accumulate; issues which past efforts at conceptualising behaviour change have largely ignored.

Goals can vary in degree of specificity, including the extent to which they specify the means by which they are to be achieved; for example, 'I want to live a healthier life', compared with 'I am going to quit smoking'. Goals can also vary in the extent to which they are based on executive decisions (e.g. increase my exercise to four 30-min sessions per week), rather than to meet primarily OS needs (e.g. to do whatever it takes to be happy).

Goals around HTM behaviours are invariably those where the goal is some consequence of the behaviour change, not the change itself. This is because things worth doing for themselves are typically easy to do, or don't require constant reminders. The choice of a goal for behaviour change should take into account the extent to which it can deliver on the ultimate goal, and how this compares with alternative goals. An analysis of this, coupled with the analysis of what is achievable, will determine the eventual goal that is pursued.

A separate focus on goals is important for CEOS because goals, once formed, can persist until modified or abandoned; so, they can act as a guide to behaviour over an extended period. This means a goal can continue to exist without any specific plan to achieve it. As a result, a goal can re-emerge fully formed when conditions activate thoughts about the possibility of achieving it.

A person is usually pursuing a range of goals at any point in time, and also has a range of established habits. When the pursuit of one goal threatens the stability of any of the other goals or behaviours, there is a potential problem. Where the new goal is identified as more important than ones it challenges, the person will at least try to adapt, but where the other goal(s) is of equivalent or greater importance, problems are bound to ensue. Often such problems will not be identified immediately, but will emerge over time as it is seen that pursuit of the new goal is disrupting progress on achieving others, or that a valued behaviour is being lost. Such re-evaluations can have consequences for persisting, the means used to attain the goal or for reviewing the nature of the goal. For example, if disturbed mood as a result of quitting smoking leads to marital discord, the quitting smoker might decide that the goal of quitting is less important than his/her marriage and thus abandon (at least temporarily) the goal of becoming a non-smoker. The more adaptive alternative would be to find alternative ways of managing emotions while quitting, but to form such an alternative goal would involve reframing the problem, something that typically requires a suggestion and/or assistance from an external agent to happen.

At some point, a specific goal needs to be chosen, although what it is can shift throughout the change process if feedback from progress (analysis and/or experience) results in changes in what is seen to be either or both desirable and achievable. This fluidity of goals is more likely in areas such as dietary change and exercise where the options are huge, but can still occur for something such as smoking, where options to complete cessation exist, such as switching to a less harmful form of nicotine. Early on in the change process, a goal does not need to be precisely specified; indeed it might only be implied by the strategy used to achieve it. However, after failed attempts to change, the person may need to refine his/her goal to fit with the reality of what can be achieved and/or to be more consistent with other life priorities. One place where refinement is likely is when progress to the ultimate goal stalls, and the potential for further change or benefit from change is assessed as being marginal. This can be adaptive where it results in a stable and acceptable outcome, but maladaptive where the compromise errs too much on ease of attainment over potential benefits.

Changes to goals can involve an analysis of the implications of past efforts to change, including the experiences of change (evaluative feedback), along with new information that may come along about desirability (e.g. new information on the health consequences of the current behaviour) or of achievability (e.g. new aids for change such as new drugs or a new gym opening up nearby). The process of choosing or refining a goal can also provide feedback and lead to changes in framing: conceptualisation is rarely a linear process.

Making an attempt to change

Once there is a goal, the next major task is making an attempt to change, or for those who have tried and failed, to make another attempt. It may be useful to distinguish three key tasks: deciding to act, initiating the attempt and getting to a point where the attempt can be said to have really started. Deciding is primarily an ES process, while the other two also involve engaging the OS.

Understanding initiation requires consideration of three sets of factors: the mechanisms of change or the nature of the script, motivational factors (the desirability of change) and the person's ability to successfully enact the change. Moving to action requires an assessment that the challenges involved in undertaking it (task difficulty) can be overcome (self-efficacy); deciding that the effort is worth any pain (decisional balance), that now is a good time (priority) and that the necessary effort can be put in (commitment). The links between these influences are depicted in Figure 6.1, also showing how feedback from the experiences of beginning to implement an action script influences the dynamic determinants that influence initiation and persistence.

The initiation of a decision to act can come from an idea or an event in the environment that generates a behavioural schemata or set of action tendencies towards the goal. These can either trigger an immediate decision or some period of contemplation, depending on how compelling the situation is in triggering action and how well prepared the person feels to act. Thinking about change requires it to be high enough on the person's agenda to justify spending time on, while the criterion for action is higher. Thus, if the person is to decide to act, contemplation of change either needs to lead to or be accompanied by a strengthening of beliefs about the desirability of change or a reduction in concerns about achievability. Once a decision is made, other forms of commitment can also be made, which creates another force for change. Commitments can be made conditional on a decision to act (e.g. If/when I decide to act, I will …). Commitments can only be brought to bear once a decision change has been made. Once made, their existence can provide feedback to influence other determinants.

In principle, one can decide to act and initiate action independent of any consideration of task difficulty or self-efficacy, but this probably only occurs for an initial attempt to change. For HTM behaviours, an unthinking decision to change is unlikely to be successful, and if it were, it would not be a cause for concern for the theory, merely suggesting that person was one of the group for whom is the behaviour was not problematic.

For HTM behaviours, the benefits of change lie in the future; so, deciding to change is a victory of the foresight of the ES over the contingencies of the moment. Because the potential harms are largely in the future, there is also a challenge in getting change onto the present agenda and keeping it there in the face of other life priorities. The value of changing now needs to be made concrete, which may involve creating a story as to why *Now* is the time to act, and of how the change can enhance the person's sense of self and/or worth, especially where the short-term signs of benefit are less salient or absent.

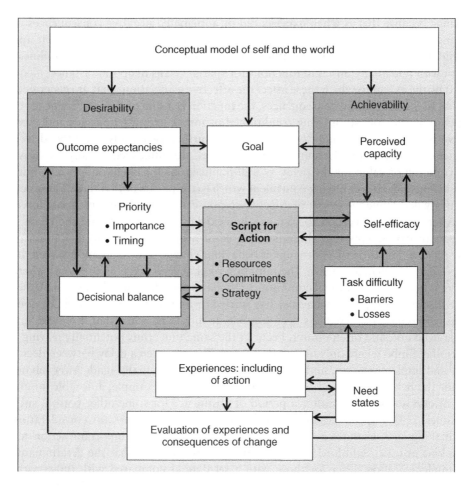

Figure 6.1 The main influences on the development of the action script. This shows feedback loops from the experiences of action to influence both the decisional balance and the perceptions of task difficulty and self-efficacy. This represents a synthesis of Figures 5.2 and 5.3.

Once persuaded, maintaining the appropriate decision is not straightforward. Work is involved. Motivational gradients for positive and negative outcomes have different slopes, with the slope for avoidance (negatives) steeper [23]. One consequence of this is that the balance between costs and benefits will be constantly shifting, except in situations where there is no psychological change in proximity of outcomes. In particular, the influence of costs will increase relative to benefits, the closer the outcome comes to being realised. As the immediate benefits of behaviours generated by the OS are always salient (as they are immediate), and never more so than when suddenly deprived of this value or where there is a threat of them being withdrawn, motivation to change is likely to come under its strongest challenge at exactly the time that the task is most difficult. This is the period around enacting change because that is when experienced or anticipated negative consequences of change are at their strongest. This analysis does not assume that approach and avoidance gradients are linear, rather they are more likely to follow a curvilinear path with potentially different functions for spatial versus temporal distance, mediated by the extent to which these affect the affective associations that are generated. Close to the anticipated consequences, the function is a sum of the joint influence of operational factors stimulating conditioned or innate action tendencies and executive processes adding additional ones, while further away only executive-driven factors are important. Executive considerations are influenced by any cognitive discounting of value for the delay as well implications for likelihood of outcomes occurring and of them having equivalent worth to the person at that time. These collectively determine the extent of affective response and thus the motivational force.

After making a decision to change, the next key task is to initiate the change. CEOS theory accepts that there is a degree of arbitrariness in any definition of the point of initiation of an attempt at behaviour change (the waypoint between the pre- and post-change stages). The initiation of change is taken as the point where there is both some volitional commitment to make the behaviour change; and either one instance of the new behaviour has started or an instance of the old behaviour that would have occurred has been forgone. It should be noted that these two criteria need not, and often do not, occur at the same time, thus potentially leaving a period of limbo where only one has been met. There is often a delay between deciding and implementation, and for some the decision is actually made after having made the behaviour change for some other reason. For example, a notable minority of quit attempts start after a period of abstinence for some other reason, such as illness [24], and changes in other behaviours can occur before any consideration of making such changes permanent. Pre-commitment is an important action for smoking at least. Balmford *et al.* [7] provide some evidence that the determinants of implementation differ for those with a set date as compared with those without, and thus may need to be treated separately. Indeed Schwarzer [17] treats the decision point as the critical distinction. We know little about attempts that started with action for some other reason and were then translated into attempts to sustain the change.

The initiation of a new behaviour pattern may not be the best point to define the implementation of an attempt to change. It may be better defined as having completed one cycle of the new behaviour because what is changing is a pattern of behaviour. Changes in a pattern can only be recognised externally when at least one cycle of the change has occurred; for example, for an activity that is assessed in terms of times per day, a day of activity (or for abstinence, of abstaining) would constitute one cycle. Until there has been one cycle of change, abandoning the attempt may be best defined as a failure to fully implement the change, and only beyond this point defined as relapse. Related to this are situations where the target behaviour pattern is approached gradually; for example, cutting down to quit, or gradually increasing the amount of exercise. Naturally this will extend the period of the uncertain status between initiation and full implementation. In some cases, particularly for more continuously varying behaviours, it is not uncommon to halt attempts to change at some intermediate point and change the target to some lower level, and thus have achieved implementation of the reduced target at the point it is set. The above distinctions may be of more importance to an outside observer than the person making the change, so capacity to be observed and or for the person to report reliably on them may be as important as what they are. The positioning of these various points varies by behaviour and by such things as the use of structured help which may introduce necessary delays.

Where the decision to quit is not implemented immediately, both the reasons for delaying and activities engaged in during this period can affect both the likelihood of the quit attempt being implemented and of it succeeding. Delay can relate to use of resources; for example, enrolling in a course, getting in to see a doctor for a prescription for stop-smoking medications and using medications that require a period of use before quitting. It can also relate to planning and strategy, for example, cutting down to quit, rather than stopping abruptly, spending time planning and/or identifying some date in the future as a target date to start. The path to implementation might affect outcomes independent of the advantages of any resources (e.g. medications) used. For example, smokers who retrospectively report cutting down on their last quit attempt are less likely to succeed in the medium term [25], although some forms of cutting down protocols have been shown to be effective [26].

Moving from making a decision, to initiation and then to implementation brings in more immediate OS factors as reactions to the decision and to the impending change. Experiences related to the change are fed back into ongoing management of the change, initially primarily affecting decisional balance, but as implementation begins, increasingly also affecting perceptions of task difficulty. The cognitive task thus changes to one of resisting pressures to change the decision, including resisting questioning of perceived desirability, not just questioning of self-efficacy.

There is no set pattern for getting a goal onto or back on the change agenda. For some people, attempts at goal attainment appears to occur in bursts, while for others they occur as isolated events with a lot of time in between. Little is known about the implication of these antecedents for outcomes. Recently [27], we found some evidence that repeated attempts to quit smoking were associated with reduced success (in the last attempt), but do not know if this is because there is a need for a rest period between attempts or it reflects the continuing efforts of a group who are otherwise less able to effect the change.

Persuasion is not just needed in goal setting, it is also important in the decision to act, and may need to be renewed after failure if the failure tests the person's views on desirability and/or achievability, for example, undermining self-efficacy.

In the remaining part of this section, the role and contents of scripts for action are discussed. I then focus on one important but neglected aspect of scripts; the nature and kinds of commitments people make with respect to their attempts to change.

Scripts

Scripts refer to the strategies developed to try to achieve goals and relate to specific attempts to change. The term *script* is used rather than plan as it is designed to be broader than plans and includes the implications of resources used and commitments made as well as the implications of strategic choices made. Schwarzer [17, 28] also makes a useful distinction between action plans and coping plans, with action plans that part of the script focussing on the adoption of the new behaviour pattern and coping plans related to strategies to deal with barriers to change. While scripts can be similar from attempt to attempt, they need not be, and as the focus is on a specific attempt to change, consistency is not relevant in the same way as it is for goals.

Building a script involves working out an action plan to answer the following questions: 'What do I want to do'?; 'What are the tasks involved in getting from where I am to where I want to go'?; 'What resources do I need'? and 'How can I maintain my commitment to getting there'? The script does not need to be completed in advance of action, but can evolve as the person progresses. However, as for framing, redrafting the script at times of high emotional arousal can lead to OS factors overwhelming decision making, and a tendency for the script to be *rewritten* towards relapse. In script formation, consideration need to be given to the possible influences of OS processes as they are part of the reality of enacting change.

A person's script needs to be congruent with his/her goals and values and should also be congruent with his/her abilities. Scripts can range from being heavily detailed with attempts to cover all possible contingencies, through to very simple scripts than may say no more than: 'Act now and go with the flow'. A script without a meaningful commitment to act, such as a starting date, is not a real script, rather it is better thought of as a potential plan that could be used when the time is right. A script can begin with a decision to act, or can (but need not) be preceded by a range of activities such as consideration as to whether to act, of resources and/or skills that might be needed and even of plans for dealing with specific situations after the change is initiated.

After a decision to act is made, the next essential element of an action script is to initiate action. This can follow directly from the decision, but where there is a delay, there is a possibility of rethinking and/or of some intervening event occurring that blocks action. Planning and preparation can also occur in any delay between the decision and initiation, but need not. That said, unless the script has some mechanism for triggering its reactivation (i.e. to begin the change attempt), it cannot really be thought of as a script for action.

The decision as to how to make the change can be for abrupt change to the target goal or some gradual process of adjustment. The path chosen can influence both the likelihood of implementing the script and potentially its chances of success. For example, self-managed attempts to cut down to quit appear to be less successful than quitting abruptly [25], but on the other hand, an unfit person trying to abruptly initiate a rigorous exercise regime is likely to result in immediate failure. What is best for one behaviour is not necessarily best for all.

Once action is initiated, there are no specific script items that are invariably essential. However, there are a range of elements that may improve a person's chance of success if they are included. The timing of the various elements that can be included in a script vary as to when they need to occur. As noted above, many can occur at any time from before a decision to act is made (conditional planning) through to after initiation of the change. both before and/or after initiation.

For many HTM behaviours there is compelling evidence that a range of interventions from pharmacotherapies to cognitive-behavioural interventions of various kinds enhance the chances of successful change. Thus including a decision to use evidence-based help, and the subsidiary script of obtaining it and undertaking the prescribed regime of activities, are desirable script elements.

A script is likely to be more useful if it is the outcome of a strategic analysis of the challenge. The main strategic concepts that are important for scripts can also be organised around the content of the script and the desirability and achievability of the actions required to pursue the goal (Figure 6.1). Strategic planning involves consideration of the factors outlined in Figure 6.1. It includes a specification of the nature of the task required to achieve the goal; an analysis of the current value of the goal, something that is a balance between expected positive outcome expectancies that are available to consciousness at the time and affective reactions to the effort being required and/or losses feared; the priority of the task over competing alternatives and degree of integration of the script with other priorities and a consideration of any constraints on what is appropriate action from values or normative beliefs. Achievability involves an analysis of task difficulty or of the challenges being faced, in conjunction with an assessment of capacity and resources available; these combine to determine self-efficacy beliefs. All of the above-mentioned influence the broad strategy the person adopts for change, the resources they choose to use and inform the nature of commitments to change that the person is prepared to make. Commitments include the decision to act, possible timing and the extent of resources and effort to be put in. Together, this set of factors, complemented by any modification of the goal, constitute the script the person tries to enact. It should be stressed that one does not need to elaborate many of these elements. Generally, only the commitment to change is necessary, although if the person temporarily ceases a behaviour for some reason (e.g. not smoking because ill), then the decision might be to continue not to smoke, rather than to resume smoking when recovered.

As the person begins to implement the action script, feedback from the OS on the experiences of behaving influences subsequent action. This can feedback directly to result in fine tuning of action and also impact self-efficacy and aspects of commitment. Challenges, unexpected consequences and changed circumstances can all feedback to lead to change in determinants and thus the form of action. These can, over a longer timescale, also influence other more stable processes, including the form of the behavioural goal. The implementation of an action script, and the subsequent feedback, will also be affected by the state of the OS as indexed by prevailing mood states and degree of exhaustion.

Scripts are built up by linking elements of the environment to a series of actions with potentially some consideration of the ways others will react. This should be done in ways that gain sufficient OS engagement for the scripted actions to occur. The capacity of any particular script to deliver on its outcomes cannot be known with any certainty in advance. Past experiences, including those of others, are a major source of information about likely script effectiveness, along with the internal coherence of the script. People can and often do adopt or modify basic scripts others have used successfully. To adopt a script from others, the person needs to believe that it can lead to the desired outcome and that they can potentially implement it. If they are to be an active participant, they also need to understand how it is going to help.

Having a potentially effective script is not enough of itself to support behaviour change. It also needs capacity to be both able to call on additional resources at times of crisis. It also requires some mechanism for providing the goal with some degree of enduring priority over competing alternatives and to have its elements implemented at appropriate times. Activation and reactivation of scripts is important because action for behaviour change does not occur continuously, but is interspersed with actions to deal with other issues; so, scripts need to include mechanisms to trigger resumption after periods of inaction. All of this flexibility is important for HTM behaviours because typically there is an extended period of potential crises where executive input is required from time to time to maintain the desired behaviour pattern, sometimes in the face of very strong impulses to relapse or to attend to other competing priorities.

Commitments to change

The key mechanism for maintaining behaviour over time is the commitments the person makes. Commitments refer to any act of self-statement that is designed to constrain future action. They include intentions, decisions and promises. The importance of commitments to change and the effects of specific commitments on outcomes are neglected areas in behaviour change. This may change with the focus that is now taking place around implementation intentions [29, 30], which is one important form of commitment. There is very little systematic consideration of the nature of the basic commitment to change. Some theories focus on intention, often defined as the person's subjective assessment of the likelihood of change (within some time frame) and skip consideration of the actual decision completely. Others focus on the decision to change, but without any real consideration of the nature of that decision. For simple easy-to-implement behaviours, this may be enough, but for HTM behaviours this is not sufficient.

Commitments are ES strategies to maintain stable efforts towards the attainment of goals in the face of fluctuating experienced value. CEOS theory postulates that the nature of the decision to change can be a critical determinant of outcome; for example, there is a large difference between committing to trying and to succeeding. Commitment only becomes a factor from the point where a decision to act is made, a form of commitment in itself. Commitments also include the priority given in relation to other tasks, how much effort will be put in and over what period and any specification of consequences for failure. While commitments cannot be made before the point of deciding to change, ideas about making them can, and such consideration can be important in decision making.

Linking commitments to relevant environmental cues such that they are remembered at appropriate times is important. Implementation intentions are one way of doing this [29, 31]. Implementation intentions are the specification: 'when a particular situation arises, a specific behavioural response will occur'. Gollwitzer and colleagues have shown that implementation intentions increase the likelihood of action. They are typically related to specific acts, but analogous processes can be applied to the initiation of routines. The making of a commitment in the form of setting a quit date both increases the likelihood of action and changes some of the predictors of following through [7, 32].

There are several other factors that may plausibly affect the impact of commitments on subsequent behaviour: whether it is public or private, whether it comes with sanctions (e.g. if I fail I will donate money to some organisation I detest) or rewards for achieving various levels of progress, whether it includes a commitment of resources or effort (e.g. it will remain my number one priority for at least the next 2 weeks) and whether it is specific enough so there is no wriggle room for compromise.

There is a need for research on the relationship between various forms of commitment and success. Plausibly the stronger the commitment, the greater the likelihood of success, but there may be fewer prepared to make such a commitment, and if a lot more act on a weaker commitment, it may overall result in better outcomes (at a population level). Commitments need not be absolute, but where they are vague or conditional, unless there is some clear specification of what constitutes failure, they may be less likely to be sustained in the face of pressure to relapse as it will be easy to find some way of having 'just one', or not bothering today, or accepting that a small amount of progress as enough.

With HTM behaviours, commitments that relate to success are typically violated. Most change attempts fail. Little thought has been given to the implications of people being unable to follow through on sometimes quite explicit commitments. Should commitments include conditions under which they can be modified or abandoned? Is the psychological pain of breaking a commitment an important component of its ability to sustain behaviour in the face of immediate urges to give up? What are the best forms of commitment for working towards something where you only have limited volitional control over the outcome? The answers to these questions need to take into account the implications of failure on subsequent attempts. The reality is that people who need to make the strongest commitments (i.e. the ones with most likely adverse effects if they are violated) are those for whom the task of changing is most difficult, and are thus most likely to fail and face these consequences. Research is needed to address this dilemma.

Maintaining change: perseverance

The final major task of behaviour change is to persevere. Most attempts to change HTM behaviours end rapidly. Once someone has changed, the new behaviour and its consequences are no longer an abstraction; they have become the reality with which the OS has to deal. The immediate effects of behaviour are inherently more salient than long-term ones; so, it is remarkable that behaviour change in the interests of the future ever occurs where it is challenged by the experiences of the moment. Maintaining change is a triumph of rationality over the impulses of the moment.

Relapse rates are initially high, but decline overall on a log-timescale, but do not reach zero, at least for smoking cessation [33]. This means that the theory of maintenance must explain both the predominance of relapse early and why relapse curves do not asymptote to zero chance of relapse. One important need for a behaviour change theory is to identify ways to help self-regulatory processes operate effectively, not just in the early days of an attempt to change, but episodically over extended periods to ward off risks of relapse and allow the stabilisation of the change.

CEOS postulates two key tasks post-implementation: dealing with temptations to relapse where the emphasis needs to be on enhancing self-control and coming to integrate the new behaviour as a valued part of the person's lifestyle, that is, reorienting operational processes towards supporting the new behaviour. Self-control is an executive function and thus takes up limited working memory. Exercising self-control is effortful and subject to exhaustion [34, 35], perhaps more so than for other executive activities. Thus, self-control needs to be thought of as a temporary solution that can sustain activities while operational processes are being reoriented. For example, reorienting to reduce expected value of smoking will result in temptations to smoke being weaker and easier to resist. The process of reorienting occurs to some extent through the experiences of behaving in new ways, but for HTM behaviours this may not be sufficient, active executive facilitation also appears to be required.

The need for self-control will be greatest in the period immediately after the behaviour is changed, as at this point habit strength of the new behaviour is low, while it is high for the old one. Piasecki *et al.* [12] postulates two main demands on self-control: withdrawal effects that dissipate over the early days post-change, and stressors and temptations that tend to show a pattern of slow oscillation towards an eventual decline, overlaid by sudden spikes indicating high-relapse propensity. The end result is that fatigue tends to peak several weeks after the initiation of change. CEOS sees withdrawal as just another potential source of negative affect, albeit one that peaks in the early days of behaviour change, especially for HTR behaviours. Withdrawal is theorised to either lead to undifferentiated desire for remedial action, or to increase cue sensitivity to trigger old behaviours that have stress modulating effects. That is, there is no need to postulate any direct effects (see Chapter 3). Regardless of how the contribution of withdrawal and related phenomena is treated, the early days are typically associated with the highest level of potential relapse crises due to some combination of poor cueing of replacement behaviours, lack of time or opportunity for extinction of conditioned relationships between cues and the old behaviour and a greater likelihood of negative mood states.

The second task of reorienting the OS may proceed more slowly. The challenge is to speed it up so that both the magnitude of the task is kept within the limits of an ES with less and less resources to commit to this task and eventually to have the new behaviour stably under OS control, or only requiring non-conflicted executive choices. Clearly those who successfully change are able to make this shift. For some, it occurs as a sudden shifts towards a realisation of benefits, triggering a cascade of re-evaluation and an unambivalent desire to pursue and maintain the change; for others it is more gradual and may be incomplete, with residual beliefs in the value of the old behaviour (e.g. smoking [36]) remaining long term. How common the various forms of adjustment are is not known.

This analysis of forces and tasks suggests that there are at least two discrete periods post-change before a stable new behaviour pattern is achieved. First, there is a variable-length period of consolidation characterised by self-control being a priority, but a high risk of relapse due to high levels of high risk situations. Relapse is most likely early in this period as any withdrawal from the old behaviour or pain associated with the new behaviour will add to other pressures to relapse. A comparable period for HTS behaviours would be where there is residual muscle pain associated with doing more exercise than you were used to.

The second maintenance period starts somewhere within a month post-change but timing may vary both by behaviour, the experienced difficulty of the task and needs to deal with other life priorities. It is conceptualised to begin when self-regulatory activity, including self-control, begins to decline, either through exhaustion of this limited resource or because of its reallocation to other life tasks, either fully or that they now take priority. During this period there is a gradual synthesis of the new behaviour pattern in the person's lifestyle and an increased marginalisation of the old behaviour pattern. The speed with which this happens may be a function of active attempts to reorient the OS, although to date there is no good evidence that interventions can speed this up, at least for smoking cessation [37]. Because self-regulatory processes are no longer so available, relapse can occur at lower levels of stressors/temptations; so, in theory, relapse should become somewhat more likely at this time. The risk of relapse is theorised to persist until temptations are so rare and weak that they can be resisted without any real executive effort. Even when this has become the norm, heightened risk of relapse can recur from time to time. There are a number of possible reasons for this. The most general is spontaneous recovery, where after periods where a previously extinguished cue recurs, the accompanying response tends to recur, in executive terms, a nostalgia effect. On top of this, from time to time, people can find themselves in situations where the response has not been extinguished. For example, it is quite common for ex-smokers to relapse when seeing old friends they used to smoke with. Also, for stress-related behaviours, where the level of stress is greater than normal, the urge can recur. The likelihood of relapse in such situations may be heightened if residual beliefs about the value of the old behaviour remain. For example, if an ex-smoker still believes that a cigarette is a great way of managing acute stress, it will be more difficult to muster resistance to stress-induced urges to smoke, particularly as the stress results in perceptual narrowing (i.e. reduced effective working memory). As a consequence, temptations to engage in old patterns will re-emerge from time to time and unless the person is prepared to resist, they may precipitate relapse.

The main challenge over the maintenance period is to continue to integrate the new behaviour into the person's lifestyle, but also requires maintaining commitment to persevere, and is helped by framing the conceptualisation of what has been achieved in a way that is consistent with, or ideally enhancing of, the person's sense of self. This involves having strategies in place to trigger self-control mechanisms when needed and to ensure that the appropriate arguments are also triggered; so, the internal argument is readily resolved and thus resisting temptations is relatively easy. That is, maintenance is essentially a vigilance task.

If this model of relapse proneness is correct, we would expect to find differences in relapse as a function of levels of self-regulatory oversight. Such a shift has not been observed, but this could be because it is masked as a result of the timing of the shift varies considerably between individuals and the spikes in temptations that are the immediate triggers for relapse are irregular. Overall, the chances of relapse decline on a log-timescale [33]. However, there is evidence of discontinuities in the determinants of relapse over time. Herd et al. [11] found that some theorised determinants of relapse change over the early weeks of an attempt to quit smoking, with factors normally thought to be risk factors (e.g. frequency of strong urges to smoke, number of smokers as friends) actually associated with abstinence in the early days and with the expected relationship only clear from around 1 month quit. Other studies have found similar patterns [9]. The exhaustion model of self-control [35] predicts faster drop-off of self-control among those for whom the task was hardest (i.e. the most addicted), which should translate into a relatively greater probability of relapse among the more addicted once self-regulatory processes are exhausted. However, what evidence there is suggests that some measures of task difficulty, for example, the Heaviness of Smoking Index for smoking, the strongest measure of relapse proneness [38, 39], while being more strongly predictive in the first weeks of a quit attempt, are not significantly predictive beyond around 1 month [11, 40]. O'Connell et al. [41] explicitly tried to test the exhaustion model in relation to temptations to smoke following quitting smoking. They found that frequency of temptations actually predicted resistance, not relapse as was predicted. This is consistent with our work showing that temptations do not predict relapse in the early days of an attempt, but come to do so later on [11], a period when the activity has no longer become the focal one for self-control.

These findings explain why CEOS argues that the main factors influencing the allocation of self-regulatory effort are both the priority of the task in relation to need, with the degree of exhaustion only being an influence on what capacity is available. In the early days of a quit attempt, quitting can be given high priority, and as it is used frequently, it is easy to self-justify maintaining self-control. However, as the task becomes more episodic, the likelihood of effort being reallocated to other activities increases, and if it is required when being used for another activity, it can be hard to reallocate it back, as doing so guarantees disruption of the other activity. Thus, in a period of no other challenge, it should be easy to reactivate self-control; however, when it is being used elsewhere, something has to give. Reallocation of self-control resources can occur because of exhaustion (I have done enough of that) or the perceived lack of need. This reallocation need not be deliberative and if it is not, may not be represented in consciousness when it occurs.

The maintenance period ends when there are virtually no temptations to revert to the old behaviour pattern and no serious residual beliefs about the value of that pattern; that is, the behaviour change has become the unthinking norm. This means that the preferred outcome of behaviour change is having come to value the new lifestyle and what it brings (e.g. reduced risk of premature health problems), in such a way that it is integrated with and becomes an element of the person's sense of who they are. Without this, there will continue to be potential to generate arguments to justify relapse. When and how such a realisation comes about is not well understood. Some people never get to this point and they require some ongoing capacity to continue to trigger ES involvement whenever sufficiently strong urges to relapse occur.

Determinants of maintenance/relapse

The analysis of relapse that emerges from CEOS is essentially the same as the revised version of Marlatt's relapse prevention theory [42–44]. Both take a systems approach and view relapse as a setback in a process of striving towards a goal, and that it is useful to make a distinction between more stable and momentary or phasic determinants. Unlike theories of behaviour change that tend to focus on expectancies, theories that focus on maintenance/relapse focus on experiences as the primary set of determinants [12, 13, 42, 45]. Relapse is a joint function of environmental conditions, which produces both conditions and cues to behave, and influences within the individual, including need states, unmet goals and interpretations of experiences. The roles of environmental factors in maintaining a desired new behaviour are likely to be very different from those involved in resisting relapse to an unwanted behaviour. Maintaining a new behaviour is threatened by a lack of cues, and/or an excess of cues towards competing behaviours, while for an HTR behaviour, the threat is from a surfeit of cues for the unwanted behaviour and perhaps a lack of cues to activate self-control. Where there is an alternative behaviour that competes with an unwanted one, all these factors will be important. Having the right cues present and ensuring they trigger appropriate executive responses is important. Beyond the role of cues, the cognitive and evaluative processes involve the same set of factors for all HTM behaviours, although their relative importance varies.

A schematic diagram of the main internal determinants of maintenance for HTM behaviour change is displayed in Figure 6.1. This figure shows how the likelihood of maintenance is determined by the outcome of a complex of inputs modulated by several feedback loops. The experiences of action are constantly feeding back to influence moment-to-moment decisional balance and perceived task difficulty, and more slowly outcome expectancies and perceptions of capacity, which in turn affect moment-to-moment self-efficacy to persist. The influence of affective factors beyond the experience of change is through their effects on need states; thus, negative mood creates motivation for action which in turn can affect mood. The feedback cycles make analysing maintenance in terms of simple linear model difficult and necessarily simplistic.

Relapses, or at least lapses, are theorised to occur when the strength of action tendencies towards the old behaviour is greater than the sum of the action tendencies towards any incompatible alternative behaviour, plus whatever commitment to self-control that can be brought to bear. There are four broad sets of factors that affect the likelihood of relapse/maintenance (Figure 6.1): moment-to-moment factors that increase the risks of relapse, more stable factors that influence the stability of beliefs; those that affect self-control; and those that modify the OS to be reoriented to be less responsive to cues to engage in the old behaviour and more responsive to cues for the new ones.

Drivers of relapse

High-risk situations for relapse are those where the unwanted behaviour is strongly cued to occur. Relapse, or more correctly a lapse, can occur in one of two ways. First, as a result of a failure to cue the desired behaviour at appropriate times. This is particularly a problem for HTS behaviours which are under-cued (e.g. I forgot to go for my run until it was too late), and may also be one for HTR behaviours, where resistance is not cued by urges to resume the unwanted behaviour (e.g. lighting up a cigarette without thinking). Second, relapse can occur because of a failure to successfully resist temptations even though self-control mechanisms have been activated. Cues can be either external or internal. External cues gain their potency by triggering the internal states that drive the action.

Negative affect plays an important role in some forms of relapse. Negative affect is a sign of unmet needs, of which the conflict created by resisting urges to engage in unwanted behaviours or to overcome inertia to engage in desirable ones are exemplars. The negative affect motivates a search for appropriate actions. Where the unwanted behaviour is a possible means of dealing with the negative affect, it will be strongly triggered. The stronger the underlying negative affect, the stronger the urge to act will be, unless comparable alternatives can be generated.

Avoidance-coping strategies, a function HTR behaviours play, are particularly effective strategies for removing negative affect in the short term, but because they do not affect the underlying causes, they do not have long-term benefits unless the source of negative affect disappears of its own accord. Thus, ensuring effective management skills for managing affect are likely to be critical for behaviour changes that threaten pre-existing negative affect or stress management strategies.

Increases in negative affect, whether consequent on quitting (e.g. withdrawal effects) or unrelated, are known to increase the likelihood of lapses and other temptation episodes [45]. However, only a proportion of lapses are associated with negative affect or stress, and negative mood seems to be unrelated to these. Less is known about why temptations in these situations lead to relapse. One possibility is that periods of positive affect associated with completion of tasks or satiation of needs are associated with having a break. Thus, it may be harder to generate competing thoughts when unwanted behaviours are triggered, especially where they have strong past associations with pleasure, or finding the energy to engage in desired behaviours that are treated as work rather than pleasure. In one small retrospective study years ago, I found that either positive or negative affect was associated with increased relapse risk compared with affectively neutral situations [46]. Unfortunately, the work of Shiffman and colleagues who have studied the micro-determinants of relapse, has measures affect on a bipolar scale, effectively precluding a separation of possible effects of positive affect from those of negative affect. Thus, at present, we know little of the situational determinants of non-stress-related relapse or lapse.

Some consequences of HTM behaviours do not act as drivers of behaviour. Part of the problem with HTM behaviours is that non-contiguous consequences of behaviour do not affect subsequent behaviour directly, and any effects need to be mediated by executive processes. Thus, the harms associated with behaviours such as smoking only motivate quitting when the executive analyses results in a decision that smoking is problematic. Similarly, even though there are non-contiguous positive effects of quitting smoking on such things as mood states [47, 48], perceived financial stress [49, 50] or even depression [51], these consequences do not directly protect against relapse. Recently, we have found evidence if health warnings on cigarette packs are actively used by ex-smokers to resist relapse, it is protective [52], suggesting that executive use of non-contingent reasons for change is required at the time of relapse risk for them to affect subsequent behaviour.

Maintaining appropriate beliefs

Decisional balance for action and subsequently for the maintenance of action is influenced by both the momentary experiences associated with behaving (including actively resisting behaving), and more stable influences such as outcome expectancies and priorities (Figure 6.1). Outcome expectancies for HTM behaviours are largely about long-term consequences; so, they are not typically affected by the immediate experiences of change. However, temptations to relapse can trigger a re-evaluation of reasons for changing. Unfortunately, the arguments most likely to be salient at times of crisis are those triggered by the immediate experiences, so will tend to be supportive of relapse. This cognitive elaboration of the OS 'need' can crowd out elements of rational arguments from the limited-capacity volitional system (ES), and thus result in a decision to persist in the undesirable behaviour

Continuing to believe expected outcomes will occur remains an act of faith over most of the period when relapse is most likely. This is not just because benefits have not yet been realised, it is also because some benefits cannot be directly experienced: changes in risk cannot be experienced as such, and problems prevented are never experienced. This means that there will be no direct OS engagement with these benefits.

Time perspective is another factor that can change the balance of outcome expectancies [53]. For the most part, ES-grounded decisions to try-to-adopt HTM behaviours are made when the person has a long event horizon; that is, they are thinking about their long-term well-being. If conditions change to reduce their event horizon, as happens when pressing immediate issues arise, or when things are generally bad and the priority is to feel better now, long-term effects can seem far less relevant (i.e. the event horizon has been reduced), and thus priorities for action can change commensurate with this. It is thus important to counteract such tendencies.

Now turning to the set of influences on the right-hand side of Figure 6.1, task difficulty is the primary means by which other aspects of achievability are influenced, although self-efficacy can be affected by more general evaluations of outcomes. The assessment of task difficulty is strongly influenced by experiences, tempered by the way experiences are interpreted. Interpreting cravings as part of the expected challenge is unlikely to affect task difficulty, while interpreting them as evidence that change is fraught with difficulty can be self-fulfilling. Also, similarly to outcome expectancies, predictions about how the difficulty of the task will change (e.g. get easier) will be partly constrained by the experienced trajectory and how this corresponds to expectations. Changes in experienced task difficulty and how this relates to expectations are both major potential influences on self-efficacy, along with the person's assessment of his/her relevant capacities. Self-efficacy is also influenced by evaluations of elements of the action script, including the nature of the commitments to change and any resources that are used.

It is desirable if temptations to review conclusions about expected outcomes or capacity can be restricted to times when temptations are at a minimum, and avoided if possible when confronting challenges to the behaviour change. This can be done through a commitment to only review expected outcomes and their importance at times when there are no strong urges to relapse, thus ensuring that executive processes are best placed to consider factual information, rather than being driven by experienced needs and momentary challenges. Also perceived capacity should not be reviewed in times of crisis. Complementary with this, beliefs that adverse effects are only temporary are important for maintaining high overall outcome expectancies, for if the adverse effects were sustained, they would become part of the outcomes and thus lessen their net benefits. A belief in the transience of adverse effects may prove difficult in situations where they are not declining as anticipated; so there may be costs post-change of being too optimistic about the speed that change takes to be institutionalized.

Maintaining strong beliefs about the value of action is important, but unless these are accessed when needed, they will have little influence. This means they need to be actively brought into consideration by executive processes when they are needed. This is most critical at times of crisis where attempts to resist reviewing the value of action are failing, but will be important for any re-evaluation.

Framing thoughts or messages in ways that generate appropriate OS engagement is important. First, to provide affective force for the desired behaviour; and secondly, the wrong focus can lead to the generation of inappropriate reactions. For example, a focus on one's continued heightened risk of a problem that has not been fully resolved (e.g. residual risk of getting cancer after quitting smoking) can generate just the same level of anxiety as for the original risk (few people can quantify risk beyond a few descriptive categories) [54, 55]. This is a problem for people who changed their behaviour to reduce their worries about future disease because they are still worrying as much, that is, from an emotional viewpoint they have not gained anything. This suggests that it may be important to encourage people to focus on more certain consequences or to frame uncertain ones in ways that do not strongly evoke uncertainty. Unfortunately, there is very little research on message framing and how it related to relapse prevention; either for communications of external agents or the way self-talk is framed. It certainly would seem to be important to place emphasis on the benefit of the change, rather than allowing a focus on the harm that remains unchanged by the behaviour change.

One other way that outcome expectancies can be altered is if the person can come to accept that the experienced benefits of the old behaviour are no longer desirable, thus tilting outcome expectances further towards change and at the same time potentially removing important reasons for relapse. This is easier said than done.

Influences on self-control

Self-control is required to span the gap between the strength of forces activating the undesirable option and the strength of forces for the appropriate action. As this gap will often be larger earlier in an attempt to change, this is the time self-control will be most needed. As noted earlier, people attempting to change typically commit to putting in the necessary effort, but this commitment is effectively time-limited. The demand for action on competing priorities typically builds over time; so, it may become increasingly difficult to maintain a priority for extended periods, even if the effort is not producing self-regulatory exhaustion. Little is known about how people ration their self-regulatory capacity; that is, how they allocate resources across competing priorities. This should involve having strategies to ensure that the appropriate capacity is allocated when needed, and is not wasted at other times. The challenge of prioritising self-regulatory resources is compounded at times of crisis, because here there are competing priorities that need urgent attention. The executive has limited control over what crowds into working memory as operational forces can push immediate concerns into consciousness, and they will not go away unless dealt with, or the context changes sufficiently for new immediate demands to swamp them. Dealing with conflicting demands is particularly fraught when giving in to a temptation would likely facilitate the performance of other urgent tasks, if only by freeing up executive capacity from dealing with the impulse to lapse.

Self-control involves more than just saying NO. It also requires capacity to resist stories that justify a return to undesirable behaviours. Such stories can be stimulated by OS activation patterns when pursuit of these behaviours is inhibited by executive processes. Dealing with justifications requires either capacity to generate competing stories and/or to undermine their elaboration. Justifications thrive on doubt about long-term consequences, in part because they are grounded in the experienced certainly of immediate benefits that are being threatened. There is a need to find ways of reducing doubt about the consequences of HTM behaviours. To the extent that justifications can be neutralised, it is likely to make resisting temptations easier, and thus in principle should mean that self-control could be successfully exercised in a wider range of situations and over a longer period of time.

Self-control can only be exercised when activated. OS processes can activate it when higher order decisions are required. Beyond this, the ES can set conditions for its activation. Unless the ES is activated in such a way as to cue resistance, virtually any strength of action tendency will be enough to generate an undesired behaviour. Chapter 7 covers some strategies for maximising the likelihood of executive engagement.

Influences on reorienting the OS

Reorienting the OS is necessary if behaviour change is to become stable. Reorienting involves some combination of experience leading to the extinction of links between the behaviour and desired outcomes, and executive re-evaluation of the meaning of the experiences associated with use, such that they no longer feedback to further justify the behaviour. Unless the second of these processes comes to dominate, the process of extinction of relevant links is likely to proceed slowly and unevenly driven only by the frequency of successfully resisting temptations across the range of cues previously linked to the behaviour.

The natural adjustment of the OS to a new pattern of behaviour involves several processes:

- Weakening the links between cues and the old behaviour
- Strengthening the associations between cues and the new behaviour
- Increasing the net positive experiences involved in performing the new behaviours (where possible)
- Engineering a decline in the expected value of the old behaviour. This is only likely to occur where the behaviour can occur without the desired consequences. For smoking, this might involve the use of denicotinised cigarettes (i.e. ones with the active drug removed).

All of the above-mentioned can occur (slowly) as a result of the cumulation of experience, but they are likely to be facilitated by appropriate executive interpretations and especially of executive actions to generate appropriate contiguous experiences and to counter self-defeating cognitions. The former involves thinking of positive consequences when engaging in the new behaviour, and the latter involves avoiding regret and having thoughts that make the experience of the new behaviour worse than it would otherwise have been.

A key factor is the capacity to generate positive thoughts about change, and to avoid negative ones is the extent to which the person has psychologically adapted to their new lifestyle. Where the old behaviour is still valued, the cues are likely to trigger positive expectancies for relapse and associated action tendencies, which when resisted will result in cravings and other negative experiences associated with the opportunity to engage in the behaviour being blocked, and this feedback can act to heighten other negative feelings, increasing the pressure to give in. If instead of exacerbating the problem, executive processes could act to effectively diminish the initial tendency towards action, then resistance should be easier. This is an approach recommended by some behaviour change practitioners, particularly for smoking cessation [56]. Unfortunately, there has been little systematic research on this approach; so, we do not know if it works, but given that it is popular, it suggests that it is meeting some need. There is evidence that residual beliefs about the value of smoking are associated with long-term relapse [11, 36]; so, tackling these beliefs is likely to be beneficial if it can be done successfully. An important empirical question is whether it is easier to facilitate adjustment in values after change when the generally positive experiences of the change can be used as supportive evidence, or try to achieve the task before trying to change, which might be harder, but if successful, should make the task easier. A study I did with colleagues a few years ago, which tried to speed up adaptation to valuing a smoke-free lifestyle after the person was no longer getting frequent strong cravings, failed to find any additional reduction in relapse rates [57, 58]. I now think one reason for the failure might have been because we were asking for more work at around the time self-regulatory fatigue was setting in. Trying to achieve this kind of reorientation might be easier in the early days of an attempt when there is more focal executive attention, especially where there are positive outcomes to point to.

One way of at least temporarily reducing the strength of competing OS tendencies is through the use of aids (e.g. quit-smoking medication or attendance at a program to support change). Aids can work in a number of ways. Medications can reduce the strength of the link between an unwanted behaviour and its desirable effects, thus both making resistance easier and potentially reducing the strength of conditioned associations supporting the behaviour, aids can provide an extra layer of commitments and social supports to enhance self-control and they can potentially provide strategies to facilitate the development of alternative skills (e.g. to cope with stress or to make the new behaviour easier). For smoking at least, the capacity of interventions to speed reorienting processes would appear to be limited at present, as no interventions have been shown to be associated with reduced relapse beyond the period where they are actively being implemented [37]. It would appear that the benefit of aids lies in allowing more to get through the difficult early times presumably by reducing self-control demands and/or through providing more support to self-control efforts.

Recovering from setbacks

For many if not all HTR behaviours, a single instance of the behaviour (a slip-up or lapse) often leads to a complete relapse back to the old pattern. Marlatt [43, 44] theorises that this is due to what he calls the Abstinence Violation Effect, where a recurrence leads to negative thoughts and a reduction in perceived ability to persist. There is not a lot of empirical support for this interpretation, feeling bad about a lapse may indeed be a factor supporting recovery. Feeling bad as a result of slipping, as distinct from feeling bad as a result of failing to stay quit, is not predictive of full relapse [45, 46, 59]. CEOS postulates that the low likelihood of recovery from a lapse is more likely due to a commitment violation effect, as a lapse violates the commitment not to behave (e.g. not smoke again), and it is that violation that makes the person feel bad. To renew the attempt, a new commitment has to be made, but it is difficult to commit again to something when the last failure is highly salient, as it invites the question 'What is going to be different next time'?

An important aspect of a lapse is that it is a perspective-changing action, and as such requires new ways of thinking, and is accompanied by quite a different set of experiences to those beforehand. If the experience of the slip is bad, then it will act as a trigger for recovery, but if the experience is positive overall, then it can act to reactivate the strength of desires to resume the old behaviour pattern at the very time when a new set of strategies are needed; that is, to recover, rather than persist. Not enough attention has been paid to the development of strategies to facilitate recovery from lapses. For HTS behaviours, a lapse is more of an opportunity to engage in the behaviour forgone, and here there are potential issues with breaking a routine that is still being established, thus weakening it and, if recovery is to be maximised, a need to resist any tendency to treat the lapse as giving oneself a break. Further, if as we have suggested, commitments add to the threshold of action tendencies to result in the reversion to the old behaviour, if the renewed commitment cannot be made with at least the same strength as the previous one, relapse will be more likely, even if there is a temporary recovery.

Lapses, especially those that cannot be attributed to external causes, represent a challenge to self-efficacy beliefs. Shiffman's [45] work has shown that following lapses, reductions in self-efficacy are predictive of full relapse. These findings are consistent with the above interpretation.

Feedback and evaluation

The ways in which feedback from behaviour is interpreted can have a huge impact as has already been noted in several places. It is useful to think about two kinds of feedback influencing the progress of behaviour change. There is the immediate feedback from behaving, which is driven by OS reactions to attempts to change and their consequences, and second, a more reflective ES-led process where the person attempts to learn from his/her experiences and to adjust his/her future behaviour on the basis of that understanding. The second form of feedback can directly influence the progression of an attempt via an influence on decisional balance, and/or more indirectly through influences on outcome expectancies and, more rarely more fundamental beliefs and values. These evaluations can also influence decisions about subsequent attempts.

Ongoing evaluation of progress of an attempt to permanently change behaviour patterns is important as the nature of the challenges changes, either as a result of environmental changes (e.g. stressors) and/or with adaptation of the OS. The evaluation can include assessments of the ease with which challenges are being overcome and reflections on progress towards the achievement of the expected outcomes.

Particularly important in this regard is the identification of any positive outcomes to date, especially those which are not contiguous with the behaviour as these effects will not directly influence operational processes. For example, if a smoker has generally been feeling better after quitting, then this experience needs to be actively represented in consciousness when operational considerations are pointing to a crisis, as it can help bolster self-control efforts. Where possible, it is important to seek out evidence to challenge inaccurate (but sometimes compelling) beliefs about the value of the unwanted behaviour by helping the smoker understand that smoking actually contributes to the stress and negative feelings that the act of smoking temporarily masks [47]. Success in such re-evaluations would be expected to have longer term effects by preventing destructive positive feedback from the experience of perceived discomfort in resisting temptations reinforcing beliefs that quitting comes with real longer term costs. Indeed, if the person can re-evaluate temptations as merely signs of the need for remedial action, it might even allow him/her to assist in managing the challenge as they will no-longer be seen as bad and thus needing to be got rid of as soon as possible.

The process of change is complex and information feeds back through experiences and evaluations in numerous ways over varying timescales. The person's commitment to the task, and more generally the script they have for action, is perhaps the most important factor in maintenance of change. Major elements of the change script can remain unspecified until after change is initiated. Scripts can be strengthened post-action by adding elements that enhance coping, but they can also be weakened by compromise. If outcome expectancies decline and/or priority declines, some of the justification for the level of commitment can be lost. If task difficulty is seen to increase, then there may be a need to strengthen commitment, but the extent to which this is possible will be affected by the person's self-efficacy. The goal of the script should be to eventually develop action routines that can be automated (brought under OS control), even if this involves the OS calling the ES for occasional conscious intervention. Scripts need not be highly specific, indeed one possible script is to just do what feels right as the situation arises. However, such scripts are unlikely to be as effective as more prescriptive ones. That said, overly detailed scripts that require lots of activity of dubious benefit can also be counterproductive as they are hard to follow and may result in important tasks being neglected, perhaps via the all-too-common tendency to pick the easiest parts of a long list of potential action items. Regular feedback on progress is needed to ensure that the script is resulting in the desired behaviours and that it is having the desired effects, otherwise it provides an opportunity to revise the script, or in extreme cases, abandon it, and perhaps try another way.

Repeated attempts are the norm

HTM behaviours are characterised by repeated failed attempts to make permanent changes to behaviour patterns. There has been remarkably little research on what implications, if any, making a failed attempt makes to subsequent change attempts. In this section, I will focus on some of what we know from smoking cessation.

In western countries such as the United States, United Kingdom and Australia, smokers have been encouraged to quit for decades. Our research indicates that in any 1 year, over 40% of smokers will make quit attempts (defined as deliberately stopping for at least a day), with those trying reporting on an average a little over two attempts each. Furthermore, at least 20% of attempts are forgotten within the year, mainly shorter ones made several months previously. On top of all this quit activity, there are at least as many aborted attempts, that is, decisions to quit which do not result in at least a day of abstinence [21]. Indeed in one recent study, following a group of smokers interested in quitting (when recruited) on a daily basis for a month, Hughes and colleagues [60] found that nearly all days of abstinence were followed by intentions not to smoke, but that only around 10% of those intentions resulted in no smoking the next day. This study also found some smokers making lots of attempts and lots of aborted attempts, others making only one and others doing nothing. This micro-level data is consistent with the reports from large population samples, with some smokers reporting many quit attempts and others one or none over any given period. For smoking cessation, there appear to be at least two main patterns: isolated attempts with often months or even years in between and periods of repeated activity with a mix of failed and aborted attempts over a period of weeks, probably interspersed with periods of inactivity. However, we don't know to what extent smokers swap between the two patterns, although we can infer that smokers making rare attempts don't typically have periods of concerted activity.

Learning-based models would predict that the chances of success should increase by learning about the challenges involved in the change: practice makes perfect. However, at least in countries with long histories of encouraging smoking cessation, we are finding that recent quitting predicts subsequent failure [27]; indeed those reporting having never previously tried to quit have success rates (albeit on low rates of trying) higher than just about every subgroup of those who report previous attempts. This is particularly so for those reporting multiple attempts in the previous year, suggesting that making multiple failed attempts over a short period may have a negative effect on the likelihood of success of subsequent attempts. Does this mean that there is no benefit to be gained from the experiences of past attempts? Anyone who has quit for at least a day will have experienced at least some successful attempts to withstand temptations to smoke, and this should help in future. However, we don't know what the impacts of these experiences are. Could it be that among those prone to eventually fail, the experiences result in increased sensitisation to the negative aspects? We need a better understanding of the implications would-be quitters draw from their experiences of past efforts. We also need to know how and to what extent these effects decay with time, with the length of the attempt and/or effort put in; and/or the nature of the evaluations made at the time of failure, and whether these evaluations are changed over time.

The ways people think about past attempts can influence subsequent behaviour. Relevant beliefs include whether past efforts were considered to be successes or failures; attributions of reasons for the relapses (internal or external); the perceived controllability of these factors and the memorability of the attempts. The attributions about the last failed attempt are likely to be most influential, unless its importance is discounted. From the perspective of CEOS, both the logical implications of the beliefs and the degree of emotional (OS) engagement with them can influence their impact on future behaviour.

Past attempts to change can only influence future attempts to the extent that they have affected ongoing OS processes, especially action tendencies; evaluations made at the time that persist, and/or memories that can inform future evaluations. With evaluations, what is remembered is more important than what actually happened. Memory of how many previous attempts have been made is also likely to be important, but as an indicator of capacity to change. The extent of past success is thought to have two potential predictive relationships with future success: one through its implications for executive evaluations, and the other as an indicator of capacity to change, that is, as an index of degree of addiction, or underlying habit strength.

Perseverance and vigilance are required in continuing to try to change HTM behaviour, and we need a better understanding of the determinants of continuing to try and how this might influence future attempts. For behaviours such as smoking where the average smoker may have failed to quit around 20 times [21], we clearly need to focus more on the implications of failure and on strategies for using failure as a guide to improve the chances of eventual success.

Hardening: the changing nature of the population who have not changed

When change is a part of a social movement to reduce some unhealthy behaviour or increase a healthy pattern, those left with the undesirable behaviour pattern are likely to differ in important ways from those who have already made the change. First of all, for HTR behaviours at least, the person may be more biologically prone to the behaviour pattern or for other reasons find the new behaviour pattern hard to achieve. For example, they may get more benefit than average from the undesirable behaviour. This could be because they live in a local environment where the undesirable behaviour is more normative, which increases the number and strength of cues to engage in it, and/or a lack of cues and opportunities to readily engage in alternative desirable activities. Alternatively, they could differ in underlying biology making change more difficult, or have reduced capacity for self-control making contested change more difficult. For HTS behaviours, a similar process is likely the case. For example, anyone who is grossly obese or physically frail will confront many more barriers to engage in a regular exercise than a physically fit, normal weight person. As more people exercise, the proportion of those not doing so having higher levels of barriers to action is likewise likely to increase, which is likely to have implications for the kinds of interventions that are going to work.

The prevalence of smoking has been declining in many countries, most notably those that have instituted strong tobacco control policies that have encouraged quitting. As the success of quit attempts is not random, the characteristics of the population of smokers is bound to have changed to include an increased proportion with many failed quit attempts.

Under these conditions, it can no longer be assumed that the interventions that have been shown to help smokers quit in the past, will be as effective in future.

The implications of a potentially hardened population can be masked during the period of population change when normative beliefs and social institutions supporting the undesirable behaviours are changing. Ecological models predict that as environmental conditions become more conducive to change, all other things being equal, the rate of change should accelerate, before perhaps tailing off again in the classical diffusion of innovation curve first described by Rogers [61]. Thus, changed social acceptability should lead to changes in the amount of time spent engaging in the activity as well as the numbers engaging. Thus, for smoking, the reduction in places where it is acceptable to smoke should result in reduced consumption, something we are seeing [62]. However, indices of habit strength such as cigarettes smoked per day and time to first cigarette of the day are used as the main prospective measure of addiction. These are useful measures, the best prospective measures we have of success in quitting, so if consumption is declining, then surely levels of addiction are too, and thus we should be seeing an increase in the rate of successful quitting. However, the evidence from population monitoring suggests the opposite; rates of successful quitting appear to be stalling [63] in the United States, and probably also Australia. Rates are certainly not increasing.

The implications of these observations are profound and widely ignored. Manifest behaviour is due to a mix of forces. As the social determinants are reduced, the aspects of the behaviour that are generated by social forces will likewise decline. Those who only smoke for social reasons will likely quit, changing the nature of the smoker population as well as leading to less smoking by at least some continuing smokers. Unless interactions between social and bio-psychological factors predominate, then the bio-psychological factors will remain as the main drivers of behaviour. To the extent that interventions have worked by selectively helping those more socially addicted, their effectiveness is likely to decline as increasingly they are being applied to populations who are more bio-psychologically dependent. This means that findings from past trials of interventions (i.e. those undertaken before hardening) may increasingly overestimate effect sizes as the population hardens, which will favour the continuation of old interventions (mainly trialled in the past) over new ones when making indirect comparisons of effect size.

When we are dealing with changing the way whole populations behave, we can no longer continue to assume that the population hasn't changed when we are at the same time taking credit for the magnitude of those changes.

There is a need to take seriously the possibility that with current technology (including psychological techniques) there exist subgroups of smokers for whom the challenges of permanently quitting smoking are greater than either their capacity or their perceptions of the worth of the effort (and likely similar groups for other HTM behaviours). For those where capacity is the problem, new strategies are required, but for those where the worth is open to question, there may need to be a more broadly based consideration of the challenges they face. The majority of members of some highly disadvantaged groups may not be able to quit successfully. For example, a recent analysis of smoking rates among people with psychotic illness in Australia [64] found that the rates of smoking were around 66% and had not changed in the previous decade or more, a period when community rates had dropped significantly. Similarly prevalence rates of smoking in other highly disadvantaged groups are also up to several times above the national average. Do these people need nicotine more, are they just more addicted, and/or to what extent do the competing priorities in their lives push efforts to quit smoking into the background? We know they are at least as interested in quitting; so, failure to quit is not for lack of interest. The existence of such groups throws up challenges to our theories and our perceptions of our collective capacity to help these people, something we have an ethical obligation to confront.

Summary

This chapter focusses on the process of change. It explores the different factors and forces involved in setting a goal for change, and for any given attempt, on the decision to change, the initiation of attempts to change, in the maintenance of change and on challenges of recovering from setbacks. There are a number of discrete tasks: acceptance of a problem, the formation of a goal for change, the decision to change and the initiation of change are all primarily driven by ES processes, with OS engagement is only really important in generating sufficient emotional engagement to make the change seem worthwhile, and for initiation, to overcome any initial resistance. By contrast, contingent OS reactions are critical to maintenance, with negative experiences linked to the change particularly important in triggering relapse, thus requiring active resistance by ES-led processes of self-control and/or of strategies to retune OS processes if relapse is to be prevented.

References

1. Prochaska J, DiClemente C & Norcross J. In search of how people change. Applications to addictive behaviors. *American Psychologist*. 1992; **47**: 1102–1114.
2. Prochaska J & Velicer W. The transtheoretical model of health behavior change. *American Journal of Health Promotion*. 1997; **12**: 38–48.
3. Sutton S. Stage theories of health behaviour. In: Conner M & Norman P (eds.) *Predicting Health Behaviour: Research and Practice with Social Cognition Models*. 2nd edn. Open University Press: Maidenhead, 2005: 223–275.

4. Sutton S. Transtheoretical model of behaviour change. In: Ayers S, Baum A, McManus C et al. (eds.) *Cambridge Handbook of Psychology, Health and Medicine*. 2nd edn. Cambridge University: Leiden, 2007: 228–232.

5. Balmford J, Borland R & Burney S. Is contemplation a separate stage of change to precontemplation? *International Journal of Behavioral Medicine*. 2008; **15**: 141–148.

6. Balmford J, Borland R & Burney S. Exploring discontinuity in prediction of smoking cessation within the precontemplation stage of change. *International Journal of Behavioral Medicine*. 2008; **15**: 133–140.

7. Balmford J, Borland R & Burney S. The influence of having a quit date on predictors of smoking cessation outcome. *Health Education Research*. 2010; **25**: 698–706.

8. Borland R, Yong HH, Balmford J et al. Motivational factors predict quit attempts but not maintenance of smoking cessation: Findings from the International Tobacco Control Four country project. *Nicotine & Tobacco Research*. 2010; **12**(Supplement 1): S4–S11.

9. Vangeli E, Stapeleton J, Smit ES et al. Predictors of attempts to stop smoking and their success in adult general population samples: A systematic review. *Addiction*. 2011; **106**: 2110–2121.

10. Hyland A, Borland R, Li Q et al. Individual-level predictors of cessation behaviours among participants in the International Tobacco Control (ITC) Four Country Survey. *Tobacco Control*. 2006; **15**: iii83–iii94.

11. Herd N, Borland R & Hyland A. Predictors of smoking relapse by duration of abstinence: Findings from the International Tobacco Control (ITC) Four Country Survey. *Addiction*. 2009; **104**: 2088–2099.

12. Piasecki T, Fiore M, McCarthy D et al. Have we lost our way? The need for dynamic formulations of smoking relapse proneness. *Addiction*. 2002; **97**: 1093–1108.

13. Rothman AJ. Toward a theory-based analysis of behavioural maintenance. *Health Psychology*. 2000; **19**: 64–69.

14. Bagozzi R & Warshaw P. Trying to consume. *Journal of Consumer Research*. 1990; **17**: 127–140.

15. De Vries H, Mudde A, Leijs I et al. The European Smoking Prevention Framework Approach (ESFA): An example of Integral Prevention. *Health Education Research*. 2003; **18**: 611–626.

16. Weinstein ND. The precaution adoption process. *Health Psychology*. 1988; **7**: 355–386.

17. Schwarzer R. HAPA theory. [http://userpage.fu-berlin.de/health/hapa.htm] [updated 10th December 2011, 4 July 2013].

18. Office on Smoking and Health CDC. Achievements in public health, 1900-1999: Tobacco use – United States, 1900–1999. *Morbidity and Mortality Weekly Report (MMWR)*. 1999; **48**: 986–993.

19. Royal College of Physicians of London. *Smoking and Health*. Pitman Medical Publishing: London, 1962.

20. General S. *Smoking and Health. Report of the Advisory Committee to the Surgeon General of the Public Health Service*. US Department of Health, Education and Welfare, Public Health Services, US Government Printing Office: Washington, DC, 1964.

21. Borland R, Partos T, Yong H et al. How much unsuccessful quitting activity is going on among adult smokers? Data from the International Tobacco Control Four Country cohort survey. *Addiction*. 2012; **107**: 673–682.

22. Pierce JP, Choi WS, Gilpin EA et al. Validation of susceptibility as a predictor of which adolescents take up smoking in the United States. *Health Psychology*. 1996; **15**: 355–361.

23. Kimble G. *Hilgard and Marquis' Conditioning and Learning*. 2nd edn. Appleton Century Crofts: New York, 1961.

24. Cooper J, Borland R, Yong H *et al*. To what extent do smokers make spontaneous quit attempts and what are the implications for smoking cessation maintenance? Findings from the international tobacco control four-country survey. *Nicotine and Tobacco Research*. 2010; **12**: S51–S57.

25. Cheong YS, Yong HH & Borland R. Does how you quit affect success? A comparison between abrupt and gradual methods using data from the International Tobacco Control Policy Evaluation Study (ITC). *Nicotine and Tobacco Research*. 2007; **9**: 801–810.

26. Cinciripini PM, Wetter DW & McClure JB. Scheduled reduced smoking: Effects on smoking abstinence and potential mechanisms of action. *Addictive Behaviors*. 1997; **22**: 759–767.

27. Partos TR, Borland R, Yong HH *et al*. The quitting rollercoaster: How recent quitting history affects future cessation outcomes (data from the International Tobacco Control 4-country cohort study). *Nicotine and Tobacco Research*. 2013; **15**(9):1578–87. Epub March 2013.

28. Schwarzer R. Modeling health behavior change; how to predict and modify the adoption and maintenance of health behaviors. *Applied Psychology*. 2008; **57**: 1–29.

29. Gollwitzer PM. Implementation intentions: Strong effects from simple plans. *American Psychologist*. 1999; **54**: 493–503.

30. Gollwitzer PM & Sheeran P. Implementation intentions and goal achievement: A meta-analysis of effects and processes. Advances in Experimental. *Social Psychology*. 2006; **38**: 69–119.

31. Sheeran P, Gollwitzer P & Bargh J. Nonconscious processes and health. *Health Psychology*. 2013; **32**: 460–473.

32. Segan CJ, Borland R & Greenwood K. Do transtheoretical model measures predict the transition from preparation to action in smoking cessation? *Psychology and Health*. 2002; **17**: 417–435.

33. Herd N & Borland R. The natural history of quitting smoking: Findings from the International Tobacco Control (ITC) Four Country Survey. *Addiction*. 2009; **104**: 2075–2087.

34. Baumeister RF & Tierney J. *Willpower: Rediscovering the Greatest Human Strength*. Penguin Press: New York, 2011.

35. Baumeister RF & Vohs KD. Self-regulation, ego depletion and motivation. *Social and Personality Psychology Compass*. 2007; **1**: 115–128.

36. Dijkstra A, Borland R & Buunk B. The motivation to stay abstinent in ex-smokers: Comparing the present with the past. *Addictive Behaviors*. 2007; **32**: 2372–2376.

37. Hajek P, Stead LF, West R, Jarvis M, Hartmann-Boyce J, Lancaster T. Do any interventions help smokers who have successfully quit for a short time to avoid relapsing? The Cochrane Library Published online 20 Aug, 2013. DOI: 10.1002/14651858 .CD003999.pub4 http://onlinelibrary.wiley.com/doi/10.1002/14651858.CD003999 .pub4/abstract;jsessionid=C2C273DF0129F8862144B9FB29045EE5.f03t03

38. Baker TB, Piper ME, McCarthy DE *et al*. Time to first cigarette in the morning as an index of ability to quit smoking: Implications for nicotine dependence. *Nicotine and Tobacco Research*. 2007; **9**: S555–S570.

39. Borland R, Yong H, O'Connor R *et al*. The reliability and predictive validity of the Heaviness of Smoking Index and its two components: Findings from the International Tobacco Control Four-Country study. *Nicotine & Tobacco Research*. 2010; **12**: S45–S50.

40. Yong HH, Borland R, Balmford J *et al.* Heaviness of Smoking Index only predicts smoking abstinence in the first month of a quit attempt: Findings from the International Tobacco Control Four-Country Survey. 2013.
41. O'Connell KA, Schwartz JE & Shiffman S. Do resisted temptations during smoking cessation deplete or augment self-control resources? *Psychology of Addictive Behaviors.* 2008; **22**: 486–495.
42. Hendershot CS, Witkiewitz K, George WH *et al.* Relapse prevention for addictive behaviors. *Substance Abuse Treatment, Prevention and Policy.* 2011; **6**: 1–17. Epub 2011 Open Access.
43. Marlatt GA & Witkiewitz K. Relapse prevention for alcohol and drug problems. In: Marlatt GA & Donovan DM (eds.) *Relapse Prevention: Maintenance Strategies in the Treatment of Addictive Behaviors.* 2nd edn. Guilford Press: New York, 2005.
44. Witkiewitz K & Marlatt G. Relapse prevention for alcohol and drug problems: That was Zen. This is Tao, *American Psychologist.* 2004; **59**: 224–235.
45. Shiffman S. Dynamic influences on smoking relapse process. *Journal of Personality.* 2005; **73**: 1715–1748.
46. Borland R. Relationships between mood around slip-up and recovery of abstinence in smoking cessation attempts. *International Journal of Public Health.* 1992; **27**: 1079–1086.
47. Parrott AC. Does cigarette smoking cause stress? *American Psychological Association.* 1999; **54**: 817–820.
48. Parrott AC. Nicotine psychobiology: How chronic-dose prospective studies can illuminate some of the theoretical issues from acute-dose research. *Psychopharmacology (Berl).* 2006; **184**: 567–576. doi: 10.1007/s00213-005-0294-y. Epub Feb 7 2006.
49. Siahpush M, Spittal M & Singh G. Association of smoking cessation with financial stress and material well-being: Results from a prospective study of a population-based national survey. *American Journal of Public Health.* 2007; **97**: 2281–2287.
50. Siahpush M, Yong H, Borland R *et al.* Smokers with financial stress are more likely to want to quit but less likely to try or succeed: Findings from the International Tobacco Control (ITC) Four Country Survey. *Addiction.* 2009; **104**: 1382–1390.
51. Piper M, Kenford S, Fiore M *et al.* Smoking cessation and quality of life: Changes in life satisfaction over 3 years following a quit attempt. *Annals of Behavioral.* 2012; **43**: 262–270.
52. Partos TR, Borland R, Yong HH *et al.* Cigarette packet warning labels can help prevent relapse: Findings from the International Tobacco Control 4-Country policy evaluation cohort study. *Tobacco Control.* 2013: **22**:e43–e50.
53. Hall PA & Fong GT. Temporal self-regulation theory: A model for individual health behaviour. *Health Psychology Review.* 2007; **1**: 6–52.
54. Borland R. What do people's estimates of smoking risk mean? *Psychology and Health.* 1997; **12**: 513–531.
55. Slovic P. *The Perception of Risk.* Earthscan: London, UK, 2000.
56. Carr A. *The Easy Way to Stop Smoking: Be a Happy Non-Smoker for the Rest of Your Life.* Penguin: Harmondsworth, 1985.
57. Segan CJ & Borland R. Does extended telephone callback counselling prevent smoking relapse? *Health Education Research.* 2011; **26**: 336–347.
58. Segan CJ, Borland R, Hannan A *et al.* The challenge of embracing a smoke-free lifestyle: A neglected area in smoking cessation programs. *Health Education & Behavior.* 2008; **23**: 1–9.
59. Shiffman S, Balabanis M, Gwaltney C *et al.* Prediction of lapse from associations between smoking and situational antecedents assessed by ecological momentary assessment. *Drug and Alcohol Dependence.* 2007; **91**: 159–168.

60. Hughes J, Solomon L, Fingar J et al. The natural history of efforts to stop smoking: A prospective cohort study. *Drug and Alcohol Dependence*. 2013; **128**: 171–174.
61. Rogers RW. Cognitive and physiological processes in fear appeals and attitude change: A revised theory of protection motivation. In: Cacioppo J & Petty R (eds.) *Social Psychophysiology: A Source Book*. The Guilford Press: New York, 1983: 153–176.
62. IARC. *IARC Handbooks of Cancer Prevention, Tobacco Control, Volume 13: Evaluating the Effectiveness of Smoke-Free Policies*. [http://www.iarc.fr/en/publications/pdfs-online/prev/handbook13/index.php]. International Agency for Research on Cancer: Lyon, 2009.
63. Warner KE & Mendez D. Tobacco control policies in developed countries: Today, yesterday and tomorrow. *Nicotine & Tobacco Research*. 2010; **12**: 876–887.
64. Cooper J, Serafina GM, Borland R et al. Tobacco smoking among people living with a psychotic illness. The second Australian survey of psychosis. *Australian and New Zealand Journal of Psychiatry*. 2012; **46**: 851–863.

Chapter 7

INTERVENTIONS FOR BEHAVIOUR CHANGE

There is a wide variety of potential interventions to change behaviour. Michie *et al.* [1] recently identified 93 different discrete interventions, and more are being developed. In principle, a comprehensive theory would be able to accomodate all of these interventions within the same framework and provide hypotheses about what forms of intervention or combinations thereof would be most likely to be effective in what kinds of situations. However, those that owe nothing to dual-process theories, either in genesis or ease of understanding their mechanisms, are not covered here. Interventions can be divided into tools, things used as part of the process of change: resources, sources of information and assistance from an outside change agent; and strategies, ways of approaching the task. Generally, I use the term *strategies* when focussing on what the person needs to do, and *interventions* in other cases.

Most of the interventions discussed in this chapter, and all those for which there is empirical support, have been developed independently of CEOS. Some interventions were explicitly derived from dual-process theorising, while others were not, but are, in my opinion, more explicable from within a dual-process framework. Most of the suggestions are more in the form of arguments as to why interventions in this area should work, with reviews of evidence that they might where it is available.

The interventions are organised into four basic kinds: (i) increasing the understanding and the use of knowledge; (ii) bolstering self-control mechanisms; (iii) reorienting the OS to be more aligned with desired behaviours; and (iv) changing the environment or context, particularly the social environment. Each of these is considered in terms of strategies the person might use in the course of trying to change, and interventions that are, or may be more effectively provided, by some outside change agent (e.g. a therapist, life coach or broader social forces) (Table 7.1).

A central question for behaviour change is which elements from the matrix of intervention options, alone or in combination, need to be included in a package to most readily facilitate the desired behaviour change, and under what conditions does this differ? That behaviours are amenable to change at all means that for at least some people, change is possible without recourse to biological interventions, for example, long-term use of medication or surgery. However, given the diversity

Understanding hard to maintain behaviour change: A dual process approach, First Edition. Ron Borland.
© 2014 John Wiley & Sons, Ltd. Published 2014 by John Wiley & Sons, Ltd.

Table 7.1 A matrix of potential interventions to increase the likelihood of sustained behaviour change

Focus of the intervention		Major agent of action	
		Interactive/external	Self-driven
Strengthening the Executive System	1	Increasing knowledge	Organising knowledge
	2	Tools to enhance executive function	Exercising self-control more effectively
Reorienting the Operational System	3	Tools to change OS functioning	ES strategies to reorient the OS
Changing the context	4	Policy and institutional change	Restructuring personal environments
Integrative		N/A	Optimising scripts

of biological mechanisms underpinning the maintenance of behaviours, and consequences for the individual's well-being, we cannot assume that volitional change is possible for all – it will certainly vary in difficulty, and perhaps in the nature of the strategies that will best facilitate the change.

It should be noted that this chapter is designed more to orient readers to potential interventions, rather than provide detail on specific methods. Most of those interventions canvassed are not theorised to be necessary for successful change, they are only theorised to increase the likelihood of success. Moreover, it should be noted that some may only be needed when the task is difficult; so may paradoxically be positively correlated with failure, even though when implemented they do actually help.

Internal and external perspectives on change

Critical to any analysis of behaviour change is a consideration of whose goal is being pursued: the individual's, some societal ideal, that of a change agent, or some combination of the above. In an individualistic society, the most ethically defensible position is that the choice should be the individual's, with other forces only facilitating by providing information and/or support for the person to choose the path that best meets his/her needs. By contrast, from a more collectivist position, the ethical imperatives are different. Change is, or should be, a negotiated process by which societal agents interact with the individual to jointly determine a goal that comes to be the espoused goal of the person; one that is consistent with societal values, be that of the society as a whole of from some subgroup (e.g. their family).

Regardless of who decides on change, the reality of most HTM behaviours is that the initial impetus to change comes with new knowledge from outside the individual. This can be seen by the individual as pressure to change if his/her sense of self is focussed on what he/she wants to do (OS-focussed) rather than on what he/she sees as in his/her long-term best interests (ES focussed).

A strategic question for change agents helping a person make a behaviour change is whether they should start with the person's current thinking and work on the problem from there, or attempt to get the person to frame the issue in the way that the change agent believes to be optimal. There are different considerations for where the person seeks help, compared to where the forces on the person are part of societal debates. Given that in most cases where a person seeks help, it is because his/her conceptualisation of how to approach this behaviour change is part of his/her problem, some form of cognitive restructuring is likely to be important in clinical contexts. However, if this can be done by modifying the person's existing framework, it is likely to be easier than getting him/her to adopt a completely new and different one. Sometimes the necessary cognitive restructuring involves challenging incompatible values the person might hold; but people can be very resistant to this if it is seen to threaten their core sense of who they are.

In population contexts, where there is less capacity to directly influence a person's framing of his/her situation, it may be more practical to try to work with the existing conceptualisation, unless it is critically flawed. Over a longer timescale, public debate over how we should think about a problem and the implications of various alternatives will have the effect of guiding most people towards either one or a small number of alternate framings of a problem. Having a shared frame aids commonality of understanding. Furthermore, where competing framings continue to exist, it can create challenges. The current social context tends to throw up two major framings. One is of the independent freely choosing individual, a frame that ignores the powerful social forces at work, and usually the challenges of individual differences in capacity. The second is of social determinants; that it is social change not personal change where the focus of action should be, and that with the appropriate social change, individual change will follow. Both disempower the individual, but it is in quite different ways: one by expecting too much of them and the other too little.

Differences between HTR and HTS behaviours

Although CEOS theory sees the underlying mechanisms supporting Hard-to-Sustain (HTS) and Hard-to-Reduce (HTR) behaviours as essentially the same, the implications for interventions are quite different.

First, take the challenges of inhibiting an undesirable behaviour. The sources of input important at the time of the initiation of an attempt to change or of a relapse crisis need to include sufficient affective force to inhibit the undesirable behaviour, the generation of action tendencies for an acceptable alternative and the capacity to produce arguments and affective force in favour of the preferred option. At the time when action is required, the OS will have generated strong action tendencies for the undesired behaviour. Thus, the first need is for an inhibitory response to be generated to allow time for higher level processing. The stimulus for an inhibitory response can come from either concern about the appropriateness of the behaviour and/or from action tendencies for an alternative incompatible behaviour. Where an alternative that has strong enough affective links to dominate exists, the crisis will quickly pass as the person will engage in the alternative behaviour. However, where there is no clear preference, a period of indecision will result, that is, no initiation of a behavioural schemata. This is experienced as anxiety, and is accompanied by a freeze on competing actions and increased priority for finding a solution. There are four possible paths to a short-term resolution, two of which are avoidance strategies: escaping the situation and delaying, both in the hope that contextual supports for the conflict effectively disappear. The second two involve confronting the conflict, either by reviewing the value and priority of the options; or second, by shifting the extent of self-control being exercised: raising it to pursue behaviours currently committed to, or reducing it, to allow a lapse. Reviewing the value of a choice in the context of strongly cued competing arguments is a dangerous activity as it is difficult to achieve a balance. By contrast for HTR behaviours, the escape/delay alternatives are actually likely to result in the desired outcome, as when the situation changes, the forces supporting the unwanted behaviour typically decline, making the decision to resist much easier. Delay can be an effective strategy.

The challenges associated with initiating a desired HTS behaviour at appropriate times are different. First, action tendencies for the behaviour cannot be assumed to occur at the appropriate times, they may need to be triggered using ES-generated strategies. Second, even when appropriate action tendencies are generated, there is a strong likelihood of competing alternatives. Here, a period of inaction associated with indecision favours alternative behaviours, as delay can reduce the timeliness of the desired action. For example, delay can mean there is no longer time to fit in a new exercise regime without getting to work late. Preventing prevarication is important here. The general principle is that delay reduces the likelihood of behaviours that are most strongly cued at any given time because typically the changing context will lead to a realignment of contextual factors, reducing the strength of those cues, and thus effectively favouring alternative courses of action. With HTS behaviours, strategies are required, which strengthen the action tendencies for the desired behaviour to the extent that it can compete with alternatives across a range of contexts. A potentially complementary strategy is to act in ways that reduce the strength of forces supporting the alternatives, including using arguments as to why the alternative is not desirable or as desirable. This can be difficult where the reasons for the alternative are quite different. For example, when waking early to exercise, it is common to feel sleepy; so, the argument that you need more sleep has compelling aspects. Resolving an internal debate over the relative merits of extra sleep versus exercise will be difficult unless those arguments have been previously resolved and the arguments used seem relevant in this new context. Delay usually favours the alternative, but this may be reversed if some action is taken towards the desired activity before making the decision on whether to persist or not. (E.g. Decide after getting into your gear whether to pull out of a run because you are too tired).

This analysis highlights the importance of alternative behaviours. For HTR behaviours, having an identified alternative can greatly simplify the process of change, as it allows a positive focus and a direction for action beyond resistance. Where there is not a pre-identified alternative, one needs to be generated for each situation and this can create challenges when there is nothing immediately cued (naturally or as a result of pre-planning). For HTS behaviours, the alternatives are problematic because they are likely strongly cued and thus need to be resisted in the same way as HTR behaviours.

Enhancing executive function: optimising understanding

This section focusses on ways of increasing understanding, with a focus on new knowledge and the organisation of ideas in ways that facilitate change. It is possible to target the Executive System directly by providing it with information that allows for a clearer sense of purpose and rationale for action, and provide advice as to how to organise that information into stronger stories supporting change or its maintenance. Ill-formed or weak goals are likely to be forsaken in the face of resistance, no matter what skills the person has to achieve them. I begin with the fundamental importance of the basic frame, that is, what is considered relevant and what not.

Framing: defining the problem and options for change

As discussed in Chapter 5, the way an issue is framed is critical to the way it is approached, and thus can have major effects on outcomes. This section focusses on the external frame, while the way information is organised within that frame is a topic for the next section.

The framing that is used in analysing a problem is initially determined by executive assumptions as to what is relevant, but may be subsequently reshaped, particularly by thoughts stimulated by operational processes that force their way into awareness. Relevant information includes things believed (assumed) to be true, but not necessarily the arguments as to why these things are true. The most useful frame is likely to be the one that does not need to change as a result of experiences; so it needs to allow for external factors that might get in the way of successful change, for example, environmental challenges that result in increased cues to engage in the old behaviour and the demands of other life priorities. It is important to anticipate problems; if the frame has to change, it is usually because unanticipated problems have arisen and necessary arguments and/or strategies for countering these are not available within the existing frame. This increases the risk of relapse. The chosen frame also needs to be consistent with the person's values (life story); incomplete, inaccurate or internally inconsistent stories can create problems that lead to inappropriate choices or failure to prepare the person for counterarguments.

Frames typically need to differ by task. Thus, the framing needed to set a behavioural goal is likely to be different from that for an action script to try to attain the goal. The framing of a goal for smoking cessation occurs in the context of the ways smoking has been framed in the society. The current predominant framing is that all tobacco products are harmful and addictive, and we should do all we can to get existing users to quit. Over the last 20 years, an alternative framing has gradually emerged: that while nicotine is addictive, it is the delivery system that is doing most of the harm. Thus, we should be splitting the tobacco problem into two separate problems: reducing the harmfulness of products people use, on top of discouraging use and facilitating complete cessation [2]. This thinking was stimulated by emerging knowledge that some forms of smokeless tobacco are very low in harm [3], and that in Sweden, where males often use smokeless tobacco instead of smoking, disease rates are consistent with smoking rates but seemingly unrelated to the rate of smokeless tobacco use. However, smokeless tobacco does not have quite the same effects as smoked, and smokers in societies where it is not already normative tend not to see it as a substitute. More recently, the development of electronic cigarettes that mimic smoking but deliver far fewer toxins has ignited community interest in alternatives to smoking. This is driving increased focus on the potential for dividing the tobacco problem in two, especially on the first task which would be getting rid of cigarette smoking using less harmful possible substitutes. Writing this in late-2013, I can foresee a future where the focus of tobacco control efforts will be on getting smokers to switch to low-harm forms of nicotine if they are unable to quit altogether. Whether this will be a HTM behaviour change remains to be seen, but it is most unlikely to be as hard as getting smokers to quit nicotine altogether in one step.

For the time being, the preferred framing for smoking is to see it as an addictive (and thus undesirable) habit that threatens long-term health and does not provide the benefits that it at first seems to, and is thus a net burden. This framing attempts to open up the potential for self-reorienting the OS as well as providing reasons to the ES to pursue change. The framing of what is required to bring about change should encompass the range of strategies that are evidence based. In the case of smoking, a combination of pharmacotherapy and a cognitive behavioural coaching program has been shown to provide the best outcomes [4]; so, this provides the best framework for a self-changer.

For the most part, people find it difficult to change the way they frame a problem without some external stimulus triggering a rethink. This stimulus can come from being confronted by evidence that cannot be ignored; for example, the risk of losing one's job for excessive drinking can help redefine a belief that one's drinking is under control very effectively! A crisis can trigger a reframing or at least result in seeking the help of a therapist who can facilitate a rethink.

The focus earlier has been on aspects of framing important for setting goals for action. The framing required for an action script differs. The reasons for the desirability of the goal should be included within the action frame to protect against situationally induced counterarguments. The framing for action also requires more detail on the mechanisms of change; while for goal setting, it may be enough to simply assume that change is possible.

Feedback and evaluation

Relevant experiences are a potentially important part of the frame from which change is considered. Experiences of behaving feedback to directly influence subsequent behaviour, and they can also form the basis of executive evaluations. There are two levels of feedback cycle that need to be considered for HTM behaviours (see Figure 6.1): the immediate feedback associated with the experiences of attempting to change and any executive reflections on those experiences (short-cycle evaluation) and two forms of long-cycle evaluation. Consolidated reflective analysis of a summary assessment of progress towards the identified goal and of any need to adjust goals and/or the strategy to achieve them and second, a similar process of reflection on past relevant experiences, which may be particularly important up to the point where the person has progressed further than they can ever remember doing so before.

Short-cycle evaluation occurs in the context of the immediate salience of current experiences, with strongly affectively charged ideas that are underpinned by those experiences potentially crowding out other considerations. This means that affectively driven arguments to re-engage in old unwanted behaviours or to abandon attempts to establish new ones may have precedence in working memory over less immediately salient, but more important long-term, considerations. As a result, strategies are needed to ensure compelling arguments for persisting are evoked, and these arguments are not open to challenge. One way of doing this is to commit to only reviewing the desirability and priority of action, plus capacity to persist, at times when the immediate risk of relapse is low. There are limited opportunities for external agents to directly influence the contents of short-cycle evaluations unless the agent is physically present or otherwise contactable in the moment.

Longer cycle evaluation is more likely to be able to be influenced by external agents; indeed sometimes they can trigger such evaluations. Long-cycle evaluation also focusses on the implications of experience, but as undesirable alternatives are typically not as strongly cued when long-cycle evaluation is usually attempted, it is easier to reflect on their long-term implications in a balanced way. Such evaluations need to have a focus on things that have changed. For example, changes in estimates of task difficulty that might lead to a re-evaluation of self-efficacy. The evaluation should also include an assessment of how much self-control and other self-regulatory activity has been required and the extent to which this has had adverse effects on the pursuit of other priorities, both life goals and challenges the OS is unable to deal with unaided. Because outcome expectancies from the attempt to change are unlikely to have been affected much, they may not spontaneously be considered when the change is under challenge; so, it is important to ensure that they are made salient so that difficult experiences do not tip decisional balance towards relapse. The overall evaluation should occur with an understanding that only arguments that remain compelling in situations where urges to relapse are absent are likely to be in the person's longer term interests, that is, where the immediate contingencies are not strongly cueing relapse-justifying arguments in ways that crowd out a rational appraisal.

The second form of long-cycle evaluation is on past attempts to change. Most people make multiple attempts to change HTM behaviours; thus, most attempts at HTM behaviour change occur with a background of experiences and expectancies from past attempts. Particularly for those without recent experience of change, relevant experiences that were not part of a systematic attempt to change, either incidentally engaged in (e.g. temporary abstinence from cigarettes due to illness), or done specifically to learn more about the challenge to be faced (e.g. seeing if you can go for 2 h without smoking) may be sources of information for the ES. That said, there is very little evidence that people actually learn in positive ways from past efforts; so, we need research to work out how past experience can be made most useful.

Making relevant knowledge salient

Decisions can only be made on the basis of the considerations that are present at the time. The framing of an issue influences what is considered because it determines what executive processes will seek (or find), while operational considerations can intrude where they are cued. Ensuring the appropriate knowledge is available is an important strategic consideration for helping to sustain behaviour change in the face of operationally driven arguments to relapse. Information can either be sourced externally or come from memory. There are three broad kinds of information that can be used by the ES to bolster arguments for change; information that can be used to argue for the change, recall of affectively charged experiences and associations that help motivate the desired change, and information that can be used to counter arguments against change. By contrast, reducing the affective force of resistance to either change or the maintenance of new behaviours involves influencing operational processes.

Delayed positive experiences of change (e.g. reduced disease risk) can only have effects to the extent that the person consciously evokes them, because on the whole they do not stimulate OS activation like negative affect does. For the ES to link such consequence to behaviour requires a belief that the two are linked. This will be easier to do when there are relevant experiences to point to, for example, pointing out the person has generally been feeling better since they quit. Where such a belief exists, the person then has the capacity to include it in internal debates about the worth of continuing the behaviour change. Doing so is particularly important at times when operational processes are generating reasons to relapse.

Having good reasons for acting and effective strategies to counter reasons for resisting is critical for behaviour change. Information is more influential when it is conveyed in ways that maximise affective force as that strengthens links to desirable action tendencies, or inhibitory impulses for unwanted behaviours. Critical aspects for generating appropriate affective force are the avoidance of negations in describing or thinking about the behaviour, the simplicity of the conceptualisation (including certainty of consequences) and the personalisation of the issues so as to provide links to existing sources of affective force. As discussed in Chapter 6, these influences are theorised to be more important than whether the arguments are framed in terms of gains or losses.

Avoiding negations in describing behaviour is important, as negations can result in a disconnect between the propositional meaning and the affective associations generated. Thus, 'Not smoking is good' is propositionally equivalent to 'smoking is bad', but affectively its opposite as it evokes good rather than bad thoughts about smoking [5], that is, what you are missing out on. This is why it is difficult to find gain framed messages that stimulate smoking cessation attempts, while loss framed graphic depictions of the harms of smoking are very effective [6–8]. By contrast, for HTS behaviours, gain-framed messages work well because they are straightforward with no negations [9]. This analysis does not mean that we should always avoid negations, as sometimes we have to use them; rather it should alert us to the likelihood that negations evoke the thing negated; so, the communication needs to be strong enough to overcome this. At times of crisis for HTR behaviours, the undesired behaviour will already be cued; so, *don't* communications that stimulate a strong inhibitory or avoidance response might be useful.

Making information personal is clearly important. However, the kinds of health risks we are concerned with are probabilistic in nature; so, any personal communication necessarily has a degree of uncertainty that need not be there for statements about populations. Thus, 'Smoking causes cancer' is true, but it has to be 'Smoking may cause you to get cancer' to be true for an individual. Thus, there is the need for a trade-off between certainty and personalisation, and which is best to choose may vary by context.

Acting on the desire to change future outcomes can never be done with certainty of the outcomes, and it is more difficult to feel certain about possible outcomes for which people have no relevant experience. More people quit smoking (or at least try) following a heart attack than based on the knowledge that smoking is a major cause of heart disease. This is because it removes from credibility a range of possible rationales for not acting, such as it won't happen to me, or it is something I can put off until tomorrow (the day that never comes). An important strategic consideration of health communication and the ways people should be encouraged to think about change is to reduce wriggle room; that is, the opportunities to raise doubts about the desired action. The further in the future an outcome is, the more room there is for doubt, and therefore more opportunities to discount the value of action above and beyond any rational discounting associated with the delay.

The ways doubt can be dealt with are different for doubts about the desirability of change than for doubts about perceived ability to achieve change. It is useful if doubts about the desirability of change can be excluded from the frame, or failing that challenged. This may involve finding reasons to believe that current discomforts will be transformed into net benefits given time, and thus discounted as reasons for backsliding. By contrast, doubts about ability cannot readily be excluded from short-cycle evaluation when difficult challenges are being faced; they need to be confronted.

It is not so much how information is presented, as how it is interpreted by the person and used at points of decision making, particularly times of crisis, that is critical for behaviour change. Ideally, thinking about change will generate affectively charged thoughts supporting the change and/or concurrently inhibit action tendencies for the undesirable behaviour. One role of communication is to frame information in ways that increase the likelihood of people being able to use it in effective ways. One way of stimulating the generation of the appropriate information is getting people to respond to questions to which they know the answer, thus strengthening the capacity to recall the information, something they will need to do when the information might be crucial for decision making.

The optimal framing of a message may vary as a function of whether it is being used by the person to support his/her attempts to change, or is being used to influence consideration of change. Further, the nature of the source, and their relationship with the person, can affect message appropriateness. More research is needed on the relationships between the ways information is presented and its acceptability to a receiver, their capacity to recall it when needed and whether it is accompanied by appropriate affective force. For arguments for change, affective force is desirable, but for arguments against change, it is desirable to find ways of countering the operationally generated affective forces supporting the unwanted change.

Arguments favouring existing unwanted behaviours will spring to mind without any effort (due to the strong action tendencies and associated associative networks that have already been activated); so, reasons for resisting will be needed. Reasons for resisting tend not to be automatically generated; so, unless the person has strategies in place to ensure their generation, the undesirable behaviour will dominate and relapse will occur. For example, just knowing that 'quitting smoking reduces health risk' is not enough to motivate resistance to relapse, there need to be strategies invoked to bring that information into consideration at the time the person is confronting a temptation to smoke.

From the perspective of a change agent, particularly ones concerned with mass influence, there needs to be a focus on maximising the likelihood that the 'choice architecture' is optimal, that is, the way the choices are presented, including whether options are made explicit. By arranging the choice architecture in ways designed to highlight the value of desired actions and reduce the salience of competing alternatives, individuals can be nudged to make the architect's choice more likely without taking away their sense of freedom of choice [10].

The occasional value of biases

Having an accurate assessment of what is involved in behaviour change is generally likely to maximise chances of success, with the exception of self-efficacy where an optimistic bias is desirable. Being optimistic about one's chances of success is particularly important for HTM behaviours where the probability of successful change on any one attempt to change is low. A realistic appraisal can create a self-fulfilling situation of failure to change. There is also a lot of literature on the power of positive thinking and how it can actually bolster the chances of success. That is not to say that overconfidence may not be a problem; in the case of gross underestimation of task difficulty and/or gross over-estimation of potential capacity, behaviour change is likely to be disrupted by unexpected negative experiences of the challenge. Optimism tempered by a reasonably accurate analysis of task difficulty, combined with a strong commitment to succeed, can prove a powerful force for success. Doubt about capacity can be useful if it motivates a search for useful additional supports to increase the chances of success, but will be counterproductive if it inhibits any attempts to change.

There are also situations where having a positive bias about benefits of change may be desirable. Humans are not well equipped to deal rationally with doubt, and concerns generated by doubt can result in an undervaluing of likely benefits. Thus, for a probabilistic outcome, they are likely to focus more on the possibility of not getting the expected average benefit, rather than on getting more. In such cases, assuming that they will get something close to the average benefit may be the best way of dealing with the doubt. However, there are situations when assuming false certainty can be counterproductive. Optimistic beliefs about the speed with which benefits will accrue can end up being self-defeating, as when these benefits do not arrive as expected, it can throw into question the whole project. In conclusion, there are advantages in simplifying the analysis of situations to make decision making easier, and to avoid biases in thinking that might prove counterproductive. However, care needs to be made in ensuring that these simplifications and biases do not result in problems.

Enhancing self-control

This section focusses on ways the ES can be enhanced by building skills to help it control or influence the OS in ways designed to achieve its goals, that is, by enhancing its capacity, especially by increasing self-control skills that are applied to HTM behaviours [11, 12]. The importance of self-control to behaviour change has been a focus of the work of Baumeister and colleagues [11, 13–15]. They tend to use the term rather more broadly than used here, where it is used specifically to refer to capacity to inhibit unwanted activities and maintain desired activities in the face of pressures to desist. Self-control, as theorised by Baumeister and colleagues, is an exhaustible resource. However, the evidence, viewed broadly, is that physical exhaustion is only one, and often not the most important reason for self-regulatory failure. Effective self-control is a function of working memory capacity; the way life challenges are framed to require similar or different responses to other challenges, or are treated as independent; capacity to be activated when required; and capacity to shift focus from issue to issue. Because of its limited capacity and the potential of that capacity to be further limited through exhaustion and/or competing demands, finding ways to use self-control more efficiently should be a focus of efforts to improve the effectiveness of interventions.

Enhancing executive functions

A recent meta-analysis by Hagger and associates [16] showed that a wide range of executive functions can be enhanced by training and that all or most forms of effortful executive function are similarly exhaustible, not just self-control. If self-control capacity could be increased in meaningful ways, it should improve behaviour change outcomes because it would facilitate efforts to resist urges to resume unwanted behaviour patterns or to overcome lack of engagement with new ones.

Recently, Houben *et al.* [17] found that training heavy drinkers to improve their working memory by practising daily for a month led to reduced drinking, with the effects sustained a month after training. Of note, those drinkers with strong pre-existing automatic associations to alcohol-related cues reduced their consumption significantly more than those with weaker reactions, suggesting the main mechanism was increased capacity to bring the automated associations under executive control.

There is a need to replicate and extend the Houben *et al.* findings. It would also be useful to determine whether improvements in working memory were achieved by just getting the participants into the habit of utilising the executive capacity they have, by improving strategies for grouping ideas quasi-hierarchically to better manage information, or by some other means. There is a long history of memory training using mnemonics that mainly act by strategic grouping of elements, and enhancing such capacity potentially allows more efficient processing, and thus in this case better capacity to monitor drinking without adversely affecting other activities. By contrast, if the effect was one of getting the person into a temporary habit of restraint, the effects might be less likely to persist longer term as restraint is unlikely to be able to be maintained long term.

The literature on exhaustion of self-control through use is in some ways inconsistent with the literature on training showing short-term effects improvements even though the amount of activity seems similar. It may be that framing executive efforts as training stimulates their subsequent activation, while framing them in ways that imply unrelated activities may *allow* them to be turned off in the new situation rather than them being exhausted, that is, as a conservation strategy. If the latter, it suggests a tendency to avoid too much executive engagement in unrelated activities when one activity requires effort. This is quite a different process to exhaustion. Baumeister [13], himself, used the example of the magician David Blaine well known for his incredible feats of endurance. When preparing for a stunt, Blaine exercises self-control in all aspects of his life, as this helps him prepare for his tasks. When not preparing he was prone to let self-control slip pretty much completely. This anecdote is not consistent with a simple exhaustion model, indeed it suggests in this case more self-control is better in the short term. I suspect this is because a blanket framing of inhibiting all indulgences may be easier to maintain in the short to medium term than one of selectivity.

This analysis suggests that a period of generalised self-control may be desirable when attempting a particularly difficult task. However, whether due to exhaustion or the build-up of other priorities, people seem to have trouble maintaining self-control long-term. The traditions in many societies, which place a strong emphasis on self-control of having festivals of excess as a way of releasing built-up tensions, attest to the difficulty (e.g. Carnivale). The shifts between such states are reminiscent of the idea of metamotivational states in Reversal Theory [18]. For HTM behaviours that are susceptible to relapse in the long term, something more than just self-control would seem to be required.

Self-regulatory exhaustion also does not account for the high levels of relapse that occur for HTM behaviours after all the hard work has been done. Perhaps there is a cumulative resistance to repeating the same self-control task too often, especially when it is not inherently enjoyable. Where self-control is perceived as disruptive, resistance to persisting in that self-control activity could build, but where the exercise of self-control is experienced as consistent with or facilitatory of ongoing activity, resistance would be less likely to build up as the activity would have been positively rewarded. This analysis implies that the repeated prevention of an urge to act will build resistance, while active pursuit of goals will not.

Improving the strength of self-control is likely only important in the early stages of behaviour change; so, it is likely to be only a medium-term aid to sustained change. The main ways self-control is likely to assist long-term maintenance is if it can be re-deployed instantaneously at times when it is needed, but where other priorities dominate working memory.

Managing and prioritising life challenges

Self-control for any given activity does not occur in a vacuum. A key, but often neglected, set of influences on the likelihood of effective action are those that are involved in managing the prioritisation of resources in the context of multiple life priorities, both those just competing for executive resources and those which may be threatened in some way by the target behaviour change. Self-maintenance functions tend to have lower priority than instrumental goals, until the system breaks down; so, they are always prone to being usurped by higher priority actions.

People having to exercise restraint in one area of their lives are often less likely to exercise restraint in others. This means that challenges in other life areas that require self-regulatory action can impact on a person's capacity to deal with a contested behaviour change.

Even during the early days of behaviour change, executive control is only exercised periodically; thus, people require the capacity to rapidly re-engage with a topic when the need arises. This capacity may be affected by the relative priority of the activity. Where it is the highest priority goal activated at that time, reorienting may be easier than when higher or comparable priorities are competing for executive capacity. To be able to be activated when needed means that the key arguments and associated experiences motivating the maintenance of change need to be highly accessible because otherwise they can be crowded out by the competing demands that typically have triggered the executive involvement. The problem of ensuring that the appropriate information is being considered is even more of a challenge at times of stress, as stress results in perceptual narrowing (more likely diverted to processing the stressful situation), which reduces effective executive capacity, and thus the amount of information that can be considered.

We cannot rely on self-regulation for extended periods and we need strategies to activate executive oversight when needed. Strategies are also needed to minimise the amount of self-regulatory capacity required and the length of time that there are likely to be regular and extensive demands on it, and to find ways of sharing executive capacity with other priorities without adversely affecting important action scripts. This suggests that long-term self-regulation may be more about vigilance, and capacity to shift attention rapidly to crises without unduly disrupting ongoing activity.

Implementation intentions

One key challenge for increasing the influence of the ES over the OS is to maximise the likelihood that appropriate ES processes are activated at times when the OS is, or is likely to be, impelled towards an unwanted pattern. The seminal work of Gollwitzer and colleagues [12, 19, 20] has shown the importance of forming specific intentions to act. They suggest that the way in which the commitment to act is framed affects the likelihood of successful implementation. Implementation intentions specify the situation in which an action is required, followed by a specific behavioural response (e.g. if I am tempted to smoke, I will take three deep breaths and if the urge is still there leave the situation). The idea is that the specification of the situation triggers the thought about the behavioural response whenever that situation arises, thus maximising the chance that it will be implemented. Obviously, if you don't think about the need to take some executive action at a critical time, it will not happen. Implementation intentions increase the likelihood that the idea of acting appropriately is in consciousness at times when demands for alternative action are strong. That is, the *if* or *when* part of the implementation intention acts as a discriminative stimulus to trigger the appropriate behavioural response in a context where it is needed, but would otherwise be unlikely to occur *spontaneously*. There is now a burgeoning literature on the utility of forming implementation intentions for discrete actions and for short-term changes in behaviour [12, 20], but more studies are needed of long-term effects and their capacity to help shape complex behaviour change.

The idea of implementation intentions was developed as a strategy for stimulating behaviour at times when it is needed. However, the technique can be generalised to include generating thoughts at times they will be useful. For example, implementation intentions can be used to increase the likelihood of thinking about the benefits of change at times when operational forces are evoking relapse.

One problem for implementation intentions is that for HTM behaviours there are often myriad situations where relapse is possible, and no one has shown that having more than a small number of implementation intentions actually helps. Creating and having ones ready and strong enough to be evoked in all possible high-risk situations may prove impossible. However, having them available for high-risk situations that are more common is possible, and the less situation-specific implementation intention around 'when I have an urge to revert to the old behaviour, I will...' may be sufficient. More research is needed on the value of implementation intentions for HTM behaviours, optimal methods for training people to be able to trigger responses when the conditions are right, and capacity to nest them quasi-hierarchically.

Implementation intentions may provide the link that allows for executive activity to be turned on at the right time, and if they were to include strategies for dealing with competing demands, may have the potential to counteract what may be a natural tendency to keep self-control to a limited number of tasks at any one time.

Enhancing self-reorientation

This section focusses on tools and strategies to help the ES better understand the way the OS works and how executive over-reaction to operational inputs can sometimes make things worse. A better understanding of the links between the two systems can feedback to reduce perceptions of the desirability of unwanted options and also remove barriers to effective action. This section also considers strategies for retraining the OS, some in ways not accessible to executive functions. The OS is retuned by, either finding itself in a different environment and thus acting differently, or by having relevant modifiable aspects of its relationship with environmental cues changed by processes of conditioning and extinction.

Mindfulness and awareness

Central to any control-based theory of behaviour is the need for executive processes to understand the operational processes that underpin their operation and the operation of themself-as-organism more generally. Executive control over operational functions can only occur where the executive is aware of what is happening. Understanding how OS processes operate with respect to HTM behaviours requires a focussed analysis of the reactions, including thoughts and feelings, associated with situations where the behaviour is cued to or desired to occur. As thoughts about basic feelings can feedback and thus result in more elaborated experienced emotions, reflection on what is happening needs to be done in ways that temporarily disrupts such feedback, or at least minimise it. This can be achieved by making the focal task of analysing feelings as prosaic as possible. Things such as locating the source of the feeling and describing its characteristics can work. This is the basis of a range of mindfulness exercises.

The concept of mindfulness is most clearly articulated in Buddhist psychology, but elements of it exist in many other traditions as well as influencing a range of contemporary theories in psychology [21]. It is important here because it represents a set of skills that can be used to show the ES how the OS operates and how the OS and ES mutually affect each other (i.e. through feedback loops). Mindfulness involves techniques that help the ES to merely note experiences, rather than try to interpret them, that is, *not* use them as stimuli for making decisions about acting. This helps separate experiences of events from the reactions and interpretations we make of them (both through the ES as ideas and perceptions, and the OS as conditioned responses). Mindfulness allows better avoidance of resistance-generated exacerbation of desire (the lure of forbidden fruit). For example, an approach tendency can be interpreted by the ES as there being something desirable, and this interpretation strengthens the OS reaction, and consequently the strength of the experienced desire. Mindfulness can help identify the non-essential nature of these links.

Mindfulness training helps us to both understand by experiencing the distinction, that the moment of awareness of a stimulus precedes the moment of initial affective reaction (approach, avoid) [22, 23], which precedes the moment when the stimulus has been sufficiently processed to be categorised in consciousness as whatever it is, which precedes any ES evaluation. This helps us to understand how each level of analysis both provides the basis for the next higher level of analysis and feeds back to influence lower level reactions. This feedback continues until there is no discord and either the stimulus can be ignored, responded to, or the moment passes and any tendencies are overtaken by new momentary priorities. The capacity of mindfulness to separate out evaluative and pure experiential aspects of experience allows for alterations in the ways executive reactions influence operational processes.

There are other ways of increasing executive awareness than mindfulness strategies. Keeping diaries is one effective way of recording activities that can subsequently be analysed to identify patterns of behaviour. Some aspects of operational functioning are not naturally available to the executive, but can be accessed in other ways. For example, recording physiological measures that index aspects of operational functioning, or counting activities (such as number of steps taken per day), can allow the executive to know more about what is happening and thus adjust strategies appropriately. Sometimes the feedback can also serve a reinforcing function by demonstrating progress towards goal attainment.

Acceptance

One important, but often neglected task for behaviour change involves understanding the conditional nature of things and of our reactions to them, and thus coming to accept experiences, including undesirable ones, and not acting in ways that accentuate them. This requires ways of challenging the often unthinking implications we draw from experiences and the ways these interpretations can feedback to influence the felt experiences. Understanding that our emotional reactions to experiences of events in the world are separate from those events is an important part of this process. Some level of this is necessary for coming to accept change, that is, coming to believe that the change is both achievable and desirable.

Two kinds of acceptance appear to be important in maintenance of change. One is acceptance of the operational reactions to events without introducing feedback loops to accentuate negative effects, and the second is to accept that past activities that were valued are no longer part of the person's lifestyle. The first form of acceptance can reduce the degree of loss associated with forgoing the behaviour and thus can act to effectively increase distress tolerance, reducing one barrier to change [24].

The second aspect is akin to overcoming grief following bereavement, and unless tackled, can add to other pressures to resume an old behaviour. Some years ago, my colleagues and I reviewed a number of qualitative studies of smoking, mainly generated to help develop more effective anti-smoking advertisements [25]. Stacey Carter, who did most of the work, took one particularly revealing quote as the title: 'Finding the strength to kill your best friend'. One woman had used this in describing her attempts to quit as having to break quite an intimate relationship with cigarettes which were her constant companion in times of stress, although she knew they were also killing her. Before finalising the report, we shared it with groups of smokers and sought their reactions. While the title statement was seen as a bit extreme, many of the smokers resonated with a toned-down version of the story, recognising a strong bond and that breaking the bond involved something akin to a bereavement experience.

If a person can come to accept that he/she is changing for good and 'say good-bye' to the old behaviour, then behaviour change is made much easier. However, achieving this is difficult, and many people need time without an old behaviour before they can come to see its loss as something they no longer regret. Acceptance is also more likely where there are acceptable alternatives. Coming to accept the core experiences and separating out what is added through cognitive elaboration can help to make the magnitude of loss appear less, and ease the adjustment to life without what was previously valued. Mindfulness and reconditioning OS reactions are two ways of achieving increased acceptance. The value of these processes for behaviour change, while theoretically important, remains under-researched [24, 26].

The value of acceptance raises the issue of the extent to which it can be achieved prior to behaviour change, or whether it is inevitably a process of long-term adjustment. Several years ago, based on the idea of there being two tasks post-change [27] of overcoming temptations and learning to become a non-smoker, we tried to hasten acceptance of being a non-smoker after effectively dealing with the short-term challenges of quitting. To be able to conduct the trial with the local Quitline, we needed to give the advisors a credible rationale for them and for their clients: we called this the two-task model, and all callers enrolling in the Quitline's callback counselling service had it explained to them. The intervention group were told we would provide some help on the second task (becoming a non-smoker), while the controls were told they would not be given specific assistance with this task. Framing the task this way had an immediate effect on the service. Based on indirect comparisons, it may have improved outcomes as it overcame a tendency for some smokers to think that the challenge of successfully quitting smoking was over when cravings were under control [28]. However, the randomised part of the intervention did not help, we now think because at the time we were trying to encourage rethinking smoking, either self-regulatory exhaustion had set in or that competing demands for executive resources swamped the consideration of these issues. That said, there is no good evidence that long-term adjustment to not smoking can be speeded up [29], finding ways to do so remains a challenge, but one which promises much if it can be achieved.

Understanding emotions and attitudes

Recognising that emotions are signs of operational engagement or need means they should be an important source of input to executive functioning. Negative emotions represent to the executive a disruption of operational attempts to manage need states, while positive emotions serve a more diverse range of functions. They can be signals to re-engage after disruptions of on-going activity, of successful achievement, or of impending success and thus of the possibility of terminating action scripts. For the most part, emotional reactions when actively involved in an activity are only experienced when the flow of behaviour is disrupted (when engrossed we tend to feel nothing or at least don't remember it). Positive experiences when natural breaks in a stream of activity occur invites re-engagement in the activity. Similarly, disruptions tend to be resisted where the experience attributed to the stream of behaviour is positive, although reaction to the disruption itself may be negative.

Feelings are signs about needs, and an important source of cues for behaviour. However, problems can arise if they are sought independent of an understanding of what produces them, that is, what they represent. Some, mainly negative, feelings signal deficits in needs, and thus should point towards actions that can meet these needs. However, if the focus is purely on the feeling, then avoidance of the situation cueing the need can lead to the disappearance of all but the strongest feelings, but the need has not been met, unless it resolves of its own accord, so can present problems down the track. Seeking feelings that signal the achievement (i.e. happiness) independent of achieving can be counterproductive, as can regularly breaking into ongoing productive activity to enjoy the feeling associated with how well it is going. This means if we follow our desires, we should not seek happiness, but the conditions that create it, and we should seek to change the conditions that cause negative affect whenever we can. However, for HTM behaviours, our emotional signalling system is leading us astray, the operational signalling system that would normally warn us about danger is telling our executive that all is fine, and activities that evoke positive feelings may be doing us harm in the long term. This is particularly a problem for HTR behaviours such as drug taking, in which we are in the continual situation of having to resist what our operational system is mistakenly telling us is in our interests (see Chapter 2). Reducing the power of these impulses to drive behaviour is central to successful behaviour change. Similarly, by failing to evoke action tendencies, the OS is telling the executive that HTS behaviours such as exercise are not worth the effort. For the executive to override the OS in such situations requires an act of faith that the analysis it undertakes is correct, a faith that is often grounded in external knowledge and/or the agreement of others.

Emotions that arise from executive activity play different roles to those that arise directly out of operational processes in relation to environmental conditions. There are two main forms: emotions that are elaborations or amplifications of OS-generated feelings (discussed earlier) and those generated through stories. The most relevant aspects of stories to behaviour change are the emotional associations with outcome expectancies, or attitudes to behaviours and related consequences. With HTM behaviours, the affective reactions generated directly by OS processes are typically discordant with those generated by the executive analysis. Research on differences between the two sets of reactions uses the terminology of explicit and implicit attitudes [30–33]. I have avoided using this terminology because what are described as implicit attitudes are conceived as being bottom-up (operational) reactions, not unconscious versions of top-down executive-shaped explicit attitudes. Attitudes are shaped by operational factors, but their essence is as affectively charged beliefs. Within CEOS, the key distinction is between beliefs that are used by the ES in analysing what actions are appropriate, that is, what should happen (the attitude), and OS-generated action tendencies, experienced as wants. This distinction is most identifiable when they point in different directions. Divergence between attitudes and urges is experienced as unease, and may be observed using the kinds of tests developed for implicit attitudes such as differential reaction times to objects linked to the attitude compared with neutral objects. Where there is dissonance between the two, the affective force for the attitude cannot be drawn from OS-generated reactions; so, it needs to come from executive activities stimulating other operational forces via the emotion-generating power of stories. Like in other forms of cognitive dissonance, the person is motivated to reduce the discrepancy between the two sets of impulses, and which will tend to dominate will be a function of their relative strengths and the strength of self-control. There is considerable evidence that for people lower in self-control (i.e. executive control), measures of urges (implicit attitudes) are better predictors of behaviour than explicit attitudes, with the reverse true among those high in control [34, 35].

Reconditioning the Operational System

One way the operational system can be changed is through processes of classical conditioning. West [36] provides a good summary of such approaches as they apply to addiction. Conditioning strategies to reduce unwanted behaviours have often focussed on the use of aversive techniques. Aversive stimuli have been used with some success but as this approach is plagued by ethical concerns, it is not widely adopted. An example of aversive conditioning is the use of the drug antabuse that causes nausea when the person drinks. It can reduce alcohol problems [37], but it does not seem to result in counterconditioning, rather in the suppression of drinking while using. That is, it does nothing much to reduce the desire to drink. This is consistent with experimental studies that show that punishment suppresses behaviour rather than changing the underlying response tendencies.

An alternative approach is to remove the reward from the behaviour, either by providing a substitute reward or by extinguishing the learnt associations. The use of methadone as a less pleasurable substitute for heroin addiction is well known. For smoking cessation, varenicline, which is a partial nicotine agonist, and the use of less psychoactive forms of nicotine reduce the pleasure associated with smoking [38]. In principle, their use while smoking should help to extinguish the associations between the act of smoking and the immediate positive effects of the nicotine. However, apart from a phase-in period of dual use, they are not typically used in this way. They are normally used as a means of supporting abstinence, and when used in this way, cannot act to extinguish the link between smoking and pleasure. Research on the use of NRT for a period before quitting shows a modest positive effect [39]. Further, there is evidence that use of denicotinised cigarettes can modestly increase successful quitting [40]. None of the above-mentioned studies were designed to maximise possible extinction effects; so, although the effects of these studies are modest, they are certainly suggestive of a potential benefit of extinguishing learnt associations.

Recently, there has been a resurgence of interest in conditioning strategies, but ones that are more sophisticated and which selectively target early aspects of the response to cues that stimulate unwanted behaviours. Wiers [35], one of the pioneers in this field, identifies three promising lines of research; reconditioning attention, emotional reactions, and action tendencies. The first of these, reconditioning attention, is of particular interest because it is something that the ES cannot do by itself, it has to be done by an external agent operating directly on attentional mechanisms within the OS.

Some of the attempts to reorient attention away from a bias towards an undesirable behaviour have used a version of a visual probe test developed by MacLeod and associates [41]. This involves presenting a pair of pictures, one of which relates to the problem behaviour, followed by a probe linked to one of the pictures that the person has to respond to (e.g. an arrow pointing up or down indicating one of two responses). Attentional bias is diagnosed when the reaction time to the probe is quicker when paired with the problem behaviour. In the retraining context, the probe is programmed to occur much more often with the neutral or control stimulus, to which the person then needs to respond. This procedure can reverse an initial attentional bias and be associated with improved behaviour, measured sometime later. For example, Wiers and colleagues have found that several sessions of attentional retraining can eliminate an attentional bias for alcohol-related stimuli in problem drinkers and lead to a reduction in their alcohol consumption [35, 42].

A similar strategy has been applied to conditioning the valence of immediate associations; that is, reinforcing positive links with desired activities and negative ones with unwanted behaviours. Houben et al. [43, 44] found that pairing alcohol with negative pictures resulted in increased negative evaluations of alcohol and reduced drinking. It is possible that some of the positive effects found for health warnings on cigarette packs operate via this mechanism.

On a related theme, the same group have shown that targeting the initial tendency to approach stimuli related to an unwanted behaviour can result in reductions in that behaviour. In the simplest form of this intervention, the participant pushes a lever away when exposed to stimuli representing the unwanted behaviour (and pulls one towards them for the control condition). This simple push–pull activity activates the basic approach and avoidance tendencies in the OS [35]. Wiers et al. [45] found that four sessions of such training for problem drinkers transformed an initial approach bias for alcohol to an avoidance bias, and in turn reduced drinking that persisted for at least a year. These are remarkable findings that need replication and extension to other problematic behaviours.

Sheeran *et al.* [12] reviewed the evidence that some of these reconditioning effects may be able to be achieved via the use of implementation intentions, reporting one study that showed an implementation intention to ignore thoughts of consuming high-fat foods was associated with reduced consumption over the next week [46].

The implications of this work are potentially profound. It suggests that a powerful way to recondition tendencies towards unwanted behaviours is to focus on conditioning lower level aspects of the behaviour rather than needing to focus on the whole behavioural routine, and that this can be done with rather innocuous stimuli. Thus, many of the ethical concerns about the use of aversive conditioning or of seemingly coercive attempts to change entire behaviour patterns are likely to be greatly reduced. If operational processes can be readily reconditioned at the level of attention and initial evaluative reactions, it will make it much easier for executive functions to make and sustain desired behaviour changes.

Targeting alternatives to the desired behaviour

On the whole, people are more interested in conserving what they have (avoiding losses) than in the possibility of gaining something new [10]; so, a bias favouring the status quo exists even outside action contexts. This is because memories of experienced benefits are more immediately salient than possibilities of what may result from something new. People's inherent conservatism means that they will be often put up with objectively undesirable conditions to maintain relationships (be it with other people, or with things) when there is a significant loss involved. The psychological mechanisms by which people get caught in exploitative and damaging relationships with other people would appear to be fundamentally the same as those that keep them caught in patterns of behaviour, including relationships with objects that are similarly destructive.

This suggests that finding ways to minimise losses and accentuate the benefits of potential gains may be important for facilitating change. Where alternatives to the unwanted behaviour exist, it will make change easier, and where the alternative precludes the unwanted behaviour, the extent of its benefits, both replacements and new benefits, will influence its likelihood of coming to dominate the old behaviour. For HTR behaviours, finding adequate replacements can be critical, at least to the extent of helping the person see the value in what he/she does when not engaging in the unwanted behaviour. For HTS behaviours, the role of alternatives may not be as central, but to the extent that the new behaviour takes up time, consideration of whether the things forgone as a result of taking that time may be important, especially where time is given as an excuse for failure to persist.

Practice

Practice is important in behaviour change because it is involved in the development of new habits, that is, the automation of behavioural schemata. The development of routines allows for greater takeover of the behaviour schemata by operational processes. It is generally assumed that practising HTM behaviours before the attempts to change them permanently are desirable. However, recent work from my group is beginning to question this. In a retrospective study, we asked smokers what they did before and after the start of their most recent quit attempt and found those reporting practising not smoking before they quit were less likely to have succeeded [47]. It may be that practising not doing something sometimes is so different to when you have to refrain always, that the experience is either misleading or it leads to exhaustion of self-regulatory functions before the quit attempt has begun. We cannot, of course, fully discount the possibility that it is due to differential memory as a result of the outcome, or that people who feel the need to do this may be those who are the most addicted. While practice is likely to be important, we need to think more carefully about what forms the practice takes.

Use of drug therapies

Psychoactive drugs directly influence the OS and may also interfere with ES functioning indirectly through influencing the operational underpinnings of executive activity. Drugs can be used as a temporary strategy for weakening OS resistance while new behavioural patterns are developed, such that when the drug is removed, the person is better able to resist relapse than he/she would have otherwise. Most drugs do not produce permanent changes in biology; so, unless they facilitate behavioural adjustment, they may need to be used long term if the removal of the unwanted behaviour is to be sustained. This highlights the need for psychologically based solutions, albeit aided by pharmacological and other aids. That said, the possibility of long-term use of substitute drugs may be a more viable solution for some. If a drug needs to be used long term, it is likely to be easier to achieve this if the drug provides its own intrinsic reasons for use, in which case it can act as a substitute for the harmful drug.

Creating more supportive environments

Interventions to change the broader environment have already been discussed in Chapter 4, so are not covered in detail here. This section considers how people wanting to change can use aspects of their environment, including their social environment and tools to facilitate change. The environment can be used in several interrelated ways: altering direct cues to action, reducing cues to act and rewards for acting in undesirable ways, seeking supports or rewards for change, communicating relevant information and/or seeking physical resources (e.g. drugs) necessary or complementary to the desired change.

Humans are social animals, meaning that our behaviour is partly constrained by and coordinated with the behaviour of others. Social factors provide the richest set of cues, both for sustaining and interfering with desired behaviour patterns.

Changing the pattern of cues to act

Reducing or removing the cues for inappropriate behaviours and increasing the cues for desired behaviour patterns can be achieved by judicious change in those aspects of the environment over which the person has some influence. Social cues can be more powerful than physical ones because of the human tendency to mimic others. It is generally a good strategy to model behaviours of those one wants to be more like, as vicarious learning (learning from the experiences of others) is a potent force for facilitating behaviour change.

Inevitably, some cues to engage in unwanted behaviours will remain as there are limits to how much people can change their environment without disrupting other valued aspects of their lives. Reactions to the remaining cues need to be dealt with, and one way is to use cues to the old behaviour to cue ES activation (i.e. as implementation intentions) or use friends to cue resistance or stimulate action.

A critical factor for creating cues to desired actions is that they occur at the optimal times for those actions to occur, for example, a prompt to sun protection near the front door, use of health warnings on cigarette packs to cue resistance strategies at the point of highest risk for relapse or having a friend come past to meet you to make sure you don't find an excuse to miss your morning run.

Rewards and other motivators

Contingent positive consequences of behaviour increase the strength of action tendencies for those behaviours, that is, they act as incentives for behaviour. The environment can be a source of rewards and other forms of incentive. Incentives can be any combination of changing the value of the behaviour (making it easier to do what is desired); changing believed consequences of the action (e.g. through increasing knowledge about likely effects); changing the context to alter the natural consequences of action (e.g. changing friendship networks to those more supportive of the behaviour) and changing extrinsic reinforcement schedules (rewards and punishment).

The last of these has been the focus of the most research. Financial rewards can facilitate short-term change, but not longer term sustained change, for a range of HTM behaviours including weight loss [48] and smoking cessation [49]. This is not surprising as it is difficult to put in place external reward structures that are maintained long term.

Social supports can provide an important source of motivation to act; so, building a network of supports, be it friends and family, or strangers met though a cessation group or online, can help keep a behaviour change attempt on track. This is particularly so where the activity can be done socially (e.g. exercising with friends) or where feedback from others may be motivating (e.g. comparing progress on weight loss with an online group). Social supports can not only have direct effects, but they can also provide additional benefits by making the desired behaviours more socially normative.

Understanding communication

CEOS theory highlights the need for communication about change to be able to trigger appropriate operational processes if it is to be effective in leading to behaviour change. This is not a straightforward process. What is communicated is an interactive function of the frame from which the message is being sent and the frame from which it is being received, modulated by any transactional interactions between the person and his/her sources. Further, the affective impact of communications may persist after the episodic aspects are forgotten, which can result in shifts in behavioural consequences. For example, in work with David Buller [50], we found that the use of strong emotive language about skin cancer led to short-term negative reactive effects on intentions to perform sun-protection behaviours, but to more desired behaviour change over the subsequent summer among those who were initially most reluctant. The negative emotional link with sun exposure persisted while the reactive elements faded.

There are three quite different forms of communication. First, communication to an audience with no real capacity for interaction, such as through mass media or books. Second, communication with others where the reactions of the person influence what is said subsequently and understanding of the messages can be evaluated in an ongoing way, Third, self-talk where the person is trying to persuade themselves about something. The kinds of communicative strategies that work in one may not be applicable in the others. For example, many forms of therapy (e.g. motivational interviewing) attempt to get clients to generate their own thoughts about motives for behaving and strategies for action. This is hard to achieve in mass communication. However, it is a powerful strategy for both having the person own the ideas, and it can also facilitate reactivation of the thoughts when needed. A more systematic exploration of the relative benefits of various communication strategies across these three forms of should prove useful.

Externalising self-control

The idea that there is more than one force operating within us is a difficult one to come to terms with psychologically, as it is inconsistent with the myth of us having a unitary identity. One way of dealing with this psychological tension is to externalise the source of what we should do onto external forces. This includes holding values about obeying social rules, including laws and expectations of community leaders (including parents). The use of therapists or life coaches is also a way of creating a context to support change, over and above any direct benefit they may provide. Having a coach, gives the problem added importance as well as the desire not to fail in the coaches eyes can act as a way of supporting commitment to the task. One particularly potent strategy is to use the structures of religion to displace all that is good and desirable (i.e. what we should do) onto a god or gods and to simplify life challenges as a continual battle between operational action tendencies (what we want to do) and the will of god.

It may be that it makes the process of reducing dissonance easier if stories are referenced to different authorities (e.g. self, powerful others, abstract deity, etc.). Thus, the family wants me to quit, but I want to keep on smoking. Externalising references can also have the effect of making it difficult to change one's mind: 'God still wants me to act that way, while I can always change my own goals'. Prayer, from this framework, is a special way of talking to yourself with what you believe that you should do re-represented as seeking to find god's will. The result is a greater normative force for action than simply working it out for yourself, by linking the *should* emotionally to what the community of which you are part wants. The use of external authorities may be for some people a partial solution to the problems created by the myth of the fully rational independent thinking individual, which can undervalue behaviour that supports societal needs when it is inconsistent with those favouring individual needs. All behaviour is in relation to the world and particularly the social world of which we are part. The myth of autonomy acts as a creative force for change, but at some point the maintenance of change will be facilitated if there is acceptance of the dynamic relationship people have with their environments, primarily through their operational systems.

The availability of what is required

The final form of environmental support involves facilitating provisioning for change (i.e. getting any required resources). These might include things such as food or drugs that change internal functioning, tools and other things that facilitate or are a conjoint part of the appropriate actions (e.g. shoes to run in, enrolling in or attending a quit-smoking course) or skills that can either directly (e.g. resistance skills) or indirectly (e.g. stress management skills) affect the likelihood of success. Some of these things can also act as cues to behave and the extent of their presence and nature can also help define what is normative. In this way, products, and more particularly the promotion of products and services, can act to shape our perceived needs in quite profound ways.

Advocating for change

The focus of this book has been on how individuals change and what they can do individually. However, one of the most powerful ways of supporting change is to modify the broader environment to be more supportive of desired behaviours. This involves advocacy into political processes and is an important part of the change story (see Chapter 4 for more details).

If we are to work to systematically change the environment to make desirable behaviours as easy as possible to engage in and, short of prohibition, remove incentives to engage in undesirable behaviours, we need to have the best possible understanding of how these policies are likely to affect individuals in their day-to-day life. This will mean going beyond research models and conceptualisations that focus on the effects of single instances of presenting stimuli to people and explore the effects over prolonged periods. Part of this inevitably will have to come from post-implementation evaluation, but as we do this more and more we should be able to build up theories that more accurately predict the consequences of policy changes. Much of my research work has focussed on increasing our understanding of the ways in which policy changes affect individuals. That said, a major motivator for this book is my increasing appreciation of the limits of social change, including normative processes, to explain the challenges of HTM behaviour change, and the lack of theorising as to how these macroforces operate through individuals to support or inhibit behaviour.

Societies (meaning us collectively) should be doing all they can to create macro-environments that are as conducive as possible to desired behaviour patterns, but this agenda needs to be pursued in the context of a deep understanding of the limits of individuals' capacities to respond to environmental cues, a sensitivity that may lead to more subtle, but effective macro-strategies.

Integrative strategies

Building a revised sense of self

In principle, if people can change their higher level goals and values (i.e. their sense of who they are), it can percolate down to affect the value they gain from many of the things they do and thus facilitate change in potentially quite profound ways. We all know examples of people 'turning their lives around'. Such transformations often seem to require some crisis to force the re-evaluation, or they tend to occur more gradually as a result of one set of changes precipitating others with a subsequent realignment of goals and values. This may then stimulate further behaviour change and/or help to sustain the changes that have been made. Large-scale changes in values can be hard to achieve as it not only requires a rethinking of many aspects of life, including some things that have been taken for granted, something that is challenging enough in its own right, but also it is likely to be accompanied by pressure from others to revert, either overtly, and/or by acting towards the person in anticipation of the old patterns in ways that encourage their resumption.

To the extent that engineering fundamental changes requires intensive challenging of the person's beliefs, there is likely to be limited capacity of self-help, and any but the most intensive counselling interventions, for providing the impetus to make such cognitive restructuring possible. Thus, it is unlikely to be a path that can be recommended from outside for most, although it should be encouraged when it does happen.

The alternative path of changing first and bringing values into line with the new behaviour is also far from straightforward. Valued aspects of the old behaviour have to come to be accepted as lost, or the functions the old behaviour served seen to be achievable in other ways. As noted earlier, attempts to speed the adoption of a new identity have so far not been particularly successful. Given that the values of one society may be considered sins in another, or in the same society at different periods, it is possibly just as well that social engineering is not so precise as to be able to shift the ways we think at will. Indeed there may be societal value in the maintenance of some diversity, and the reality that some of this diversity confers additional risks on some individuals may be something we need to accept is always going to create a basis for making major changes in behaviour difficult.

Improving recovery from setbacks

Relapse is the norm for HTM behaviours; it occurs frequently in the early days of attempts to change, but the probability of relapse remains well above zero for months or even years. In the area of smoking cessation, at least, the prevailing wisdom is that lapses are tantamount to relapse. Outcomes for cessation trials typically require complete sustained abstinence [51] on the basis that lapses are predictive of relapse. Especially for lapses that happen well after change has occurred, this may be missing a real opportunity. There should be no problem with exhaustion of self-control, and in many cases relapse does not seem to be associated with overwhelming demands from other priorities (although sometimes it clearly is); so, in some cases at least, if the person could be remotivated, their chances of recovery should be good. The challenge for change agents is that they are not there to help; so, this is a situation where the person has to be prepared to recover. Thought needs to go into ways of inoculating changers as to strategies for recovery if lapses occur to minimise the likelihood of them being converted into full relapse. Implementation intentions might be one means of doing this. Part of the challenge here will be in acknowledging the possibility of a slip in the context of a common commitment never to smoke again. However, this should be able to be dealt with. As most smokers have reached a point where they have survived the hard times of quitting [52], even a modest reduction in long-term relapse could have a marked effect on prevalence.

Optimising a script or plan for action

Plans for action can range from a simple decision to change to complex and detailed strategies. The lack of necessity for a detailed plan may be one of the reasons that aspects of preparation are often ignored in theories of behaviour change and behaviour maintenance/relapse prevention.

The key features of an action script are to articulate a behavioural goal that is consistent with one's life goals; to develop strategies for initiating action that include dealing with transaction costs (temporary costs of change) where they occur [53]; to develop strategies for maintaining change in the face of challenges and to develop strategies for coming to value the new lifestyle over the old one, which involves maximising the benefits of the new behaviour pattern and reducing any negative consequences (including losses) of the change (see Chapter 6 for more details).

Thus, a good script will have both a framework for achieving the behavioural goal and a framework for coping with the demands of achieving it. It also needs to be dynamic, with capacity to change strategies based on experiences over the course of initiating and sustaining behaviour change. Explicitly encouraging the use of coping planning as well as action planning has been shown to improve outcomes, at least for exercise [54, 55].

A script for behaviour change needs to be grounded in a self-story that provides a compelling rationale for the change and for enduring the transaction costs of change. The script need not be fully formed, but can be built up in a 'just in time' manner. Planning is not just an activity that occurs before action. Planning before action is pure preparation, but after action, it can be to prepare strategies during times of low-relapse risk to adopt in identified high-relapse risk situations, or can be on the spot planning to deal with immediate challenges. Plans may also need to be reviewed as events unfold. This means that while the broad strategy can usefully be developed in advance, it still needs to have the immediate agenda reviewed regularly: this may need to be as regular as every hour or so in the early stages of change to periods of weeks (or even months) long after implementation. From time to time, there may also be a need to review the overall strategy.

For a plan to successfully change HTM behaviour, the action script must ensure that there is sufficient emotional engagement in the change to drive action in the face of resistance and that there are strategies for neutralising or otherwise overcoming impulses to resume the old behaviour, including the management of cognitions that are created as justifications for the OS-driven urges to revert to the old behaviour. This means that the frame within which the script is built up must be broad enough to encompass strategies that have been shown to work, and to facilitate the readjustment in values and sense of self that may be required.

Commitments to change need not be absolute; they can specify any elements of the goal that are negotiable without the exercise being treated as a failure. For example, a smoker might try to quit smoking (and implicitly all forms of nicotine use), but having quit smoking, may accept the need to continue using some low-harm form of nicotine longer term. The optimal level of commitment is that which increases the chance of success more than it reduces the chances of taking any action. Which forms of commitment best do this are currently uncertain and requires focussed research.

While a good script can facilitate change, a poorly formed script can actually reduce the chances of success, either by missing important forms of help or by engaging in spurious activities that distract and/or use up self-regulatory capacity. We need to better understand what forms of planning actually facilitate change and the contexts in which they work, and what if any activities might sometimes be counterproductive.

In summary, the elements required for an effective action script include the following:

- Specifying the goal to be achieved and any waypoints that need to be worked towards, either before the change or following it.
- Being grounded in an assessment of task difficulty (including risks and uncertainty) and the main threats to success be they from the environment or from the person's OS.
- Having plans to replace or revitalise things lost or compromised by the change and/or to facilitate acceptance of the loss.
- Ensuring that the goal and plans are compatible with high-level aspects of self-concept (i.e. need for truthfulness, caring about others, etc.).
- Having mechanisms to maintain or increase motivation/level of commitment and self-efficacy; and to manage risk and uncertainty, including strategies for re-interpreting some negative experiences of change as signs of progress and thus positive rather than reasons to give up.

- Making changes to the local environment where possible to
  - Removing unnecessary cues to the old behaviour;
  - Introducing cues for the new behaviour;
  - Engaging friends and family, preferably as allies, but at least ensuring that they are not barriers to change.
- Having plans for some extraneous rewards for successes, especially where the new behaviour does not provide sufficient intrinsic ones, at least in the short term.
- Where necessary, developing special strategies for coping effectively with negative emotions, including impulse control and capacity to calm down.
- Ensuring that the script is structured in a way that triggers its re-activation when needed and which triggers the appropriate responses, for example, through implementation intentions. These should include implementation intentions for the focal behaviour pattern and for ancillary actions to deal with temptations to relapse/lapse.
- Having strategies to work towards accepting, and ideally valuing, the new behaviour in its own right, not just for the long-term benefits it promises.
- Regular reviewing, to ensure that the strategies in the script remain relevant as the situation changes. This may mean the script for long-term maintenance looks very different to that used in the early days.
- Finally, the script should not be so complex as to be unwieldy to implement at any time: simplicity is good, but not oversimplicity.

The greater the perceived task difficulty, the more elaborated the script may need to be with strategies to overcome those challenges.

As a long-term goal, it is desirable to extinguish positive associations with the unwanted behaviour in each situation that the person associates with it, either consciously or unconsciously, or to discover positive experiences associated with a new behaviour that are missed when forgone. This process will be disrupted by lapses to the old behaviour. For example, a strong and unquestioned belief that you are never going to smoke again, and that you are certainly not going to smoke in specific high-risk situations, can help this process of craving reduction enormously, largely because it provides a powerful set of cues to not smoke. This can be helped if one is able to challenge or inhibit thoughts like 'I'd really love one now'. Things the person does and thinks can magnify or minimise cravings for the old behaviour; those thoughts that anticipate positive reactions to the old behaviour can help to sustain it. The worst thing that one can do is to pine, because this strengthens the very links between the situation and the behaviour that they are trying to break. People need to convince themselves that they are *not* making a sacrifice in changing, but entering a new and better period of their lives.

The need for an action script ends when the person has acquired all the skills and routines he/she needs to persist in their new behaviour indefinitely. As the world is constantly changing, one can never be certain that this point has been reached; so, some capacity for coping with unexpected crises will always be needed. We are still a long way from finding ways to get people through this process with a low risk of failure. But hopefully some of the ideas in this book will stimulate the development of strategies that make the journey a little easier and less prone to fail.

Summary

This chapter canvasses some possible interventions based on CEOS, or more generally on dual-process thing about behaviour change. The interventions are organised into four basic kinds: (i) increasing the understanding and the use of knowledge; (ii) bolstering self-control mechanisms; (iii) reorienting the OS to be more aligned with desired behaviours; and (iv) changing the environment or context, particularly the social environment. Each of these is considered in terms of strategies the person might use in the course of trying to change, and interventions that are, or may be more effectively provided, by some outside change agent (e.g. a therapist, life coach or broader social forces).

References

1. Michie S, Richardson M, Johnston M *et al*. The behavior change technique taxonomy (v1) of 93 hierarchically clustered techniques: Building an international consensus for the reporting of behavior change interventions. *Annals of Behavioral Medicine*. 2013; 46: 81–95.
2. Borland R. Minimising the harm from nicotine use: Finding the right regulatory framework. *Tobacco Control*. 2013; 22: i6–i9.
3. Rodu B. The scientific foundation for tobacco harm reduction, 2006–2011. *Harm Reduction Journal*. 2011; 8(19): 1–22. Open Access – Review (electronic article).
4. Stead LF & Lancaster T. Combined pharmacotherapy and behavioural interventions for smoking cessation. *Cochrane Library*. 2012. doi: 10.1002/14651858.CD008286.pub2. [http://onlinelibrary.wiley.com/doi/10.1002/14651858.CD008286.pub2/abstract;jsessio nid=64FEA12CE79C95AC2618507B765C2431.d02t04].
5. Strack F & Deutsch R. Reflective and impulsive determinants of social behaviour. *Personality and Social Psychology Bulletin*. 2004; 8: 220–247.
6. Borland R, Wilson N, Fong G *et al*. Impact of graphic and text warnings on cigarette packs: Findings from four countries over five years. *Tobacco Control*. 2009; 18: 358–364.
7. Durkin S, Brennan E & Wakefield M. Mass media campaigns to promote smoking cessation among adults: An integrative review. *Tobacco Control*. 2012; 21: 127–138.
8. Wakefield M, Spittal M, Durkin S *et al*. Effects of mass media campaign exposure intensity and durability on quit attempts in a population-based cohort study. *Health Education Research*. 2011; 26: 988–997.
9. Rothman AJ, Bartels RB, Wlaschin J *et al*. The strategic use of gain- and loss-framed messages to promote healthy behavior: How theory can inform practice. *Journal of Communication*. 2006: S202–S220.
10. Thaler RH & Sunstein CR. *Nudge: Improving Decisions About Health, Wealth and Happiness*. Yale University Press: New Haven, 2008.
11. Hagger MS, Wood C, Stiff C *et al*. The strength model of self-regulation failure and health-related behaviour. *Health Psychology Review*. 2009; 3: 208–238.

12. Sheeran P, Gollwitzer P & Bargh J. Nonconscious processes and health. *Health Psychology*. 2012; **32**: 460–473.
13. Baumeister RF & Tierney J. *Willpower: Rediscovering the Greatest Human Strength*. Penguin Press: New York, 2011.
14. Baumeister RF & Vohs KD (eds.) *Handbook of Self-Regulation: Research, Theory, and Applications*. Guilford Press: New York, 2004.
15. Baumeister RF & Vohs KD. Self-regulation, ego depletion and motivation. *Social and Personality Psychology Compass*. 2007; **1**: 115–128.
16. Hagger M, Wood C, Stiff C *et al.* Ego depletion and the strength model of self-control: A meta-analysis. *Psychological Bulletin*. 2010; **136**: 495–525.
17. Houben K, Wiers RW & Jansen A. Getting a grip on drinking behavior: Training working memory to reduce alcohol abuse. *Psychological Science*. 2011; **22**: 968–975.
18. Apter MJ. *Reversal Theory: The Dynamics of Motivation, Emotion and Personality*. 2nd edn. Oneworld Publications: Oxford, 2007.
19. Gollwitzer PM. Implementation intentions: Strong effects from simple plans. *American Psychologist*. 1999; **54**: 493–503.
20. Gollwitzer PM & Sheeran P. Implementation intentions and goal achievement: A meta-analysis of effects and processes. Advances in experimental. *Social Psychology*. 2006; **38**: 69–119.
21. Brown KW, Ryan RM & Creswell JD. Mindfulness; theoretical foundations and evidence for its salutary effects. *Psychological Inquiry*. 2007; **18**: 211–237.
22. Zajonc RB. Feeling and thinking: Preferences need no inferences. *American Psychologist*. 1980; **35**: 151–175.
23. Zajonc RB. On the primacy of affect. *American Psychologist*. 1984; **39**: 117–123.
24. Carmody TP, Vietan C & Astin JA. Negative affect, emotional acceptance, and smoking cessation. *Journal of Psychoactive Drugs*. 2007; **39**: 499–508.
25. Carter S, Borland R & Chapman S. *Finding the Strength to Kill your Best Friend – Smokers Talk About Smoking and Quitting*. Smoking Cessation Consortium and GlaxoSmith Kline Consumer Healthcare: Sydney, Australia, 2001.
26. Brown RA, Palm KM, Strong DR *et al.* Distress tolerance treatment for early-lapse smokers: Rationale, program description, and preliminary findings. *Behavior Modification*. 2008; **32**: 302–332.
27. Segan CJ, Borland R, Hannan A *et al.* The challenge of embracing a smoke-free lifestyle: A neglected area in smoking cessation programs. *Health Education & Behavior*. 2008; **23**: 1–9.
28. Segan CJ & Borland R. Does extended telephone callback counselling prevent smoking relapse? *Health Education Research*. 2011; **26**: 336–347.
29. Hajek P, Stead LF, West R *et al.* Relapse prevention interventions for smoking cessation (review). *Cochrane Database of Systematic Reviews*. 2013; (8). Art. No.: CD003999. doi: 10.1002/14651858.CD003999.pub4. [http://onlinelibrary.wiley.com/doi/10.1002/14651858.CD003999.pub4/abstract].
30. Bargh JA & Ferguson MJ. Beyond behaviorism: On the automaticity of higher mental processes. *Psychological Bulletin*. 2000; **126**: 925–945.
31. Bargh JA, Gollwitzer PM, Lee-Chai A *et al.* The automated will: Nonconscious activation and pursuit of behavioral goals. *Journal of Personality and Social Psychology*. 2001; **81**: 1014–1027.
32. Fazio RH. On the automatic activation of associated evaluations: An overview. *Cognition and Emotion*. 2001; **15**: 115–141.
33. Fazio RH, Sanbonmatsu DM, Powell MC *et al.* On the automatic activation of attitudes. *Journal of Personality and Social Psychology*. 1986; **50**: 229–238.

34. Friese M, Hofmann W & Wiers RW. On taming horses and strengthening riders: Recent developments in research on interventions to improve self-control in health behaviors. *Self and Identity*. 2011; **10**: 336–351.
35. Wiers RW, Gladwin TE, Hofmann W *et al*. Cognitive bias modification and cognitive control training in addiction and related psychopathology: Mechanisms, clinical perspectives, and ways forward. *Clinical Psychological Science*. 2013; **1**: 192–212.
36. West R & Brown J. *Theory of Addiction*. 2nd Ed. Wiley: Chichester, UK, 2013.
37. Krampe H, Stawicki S, Wagner T *et al*. Follow-up of 180 alcoholic patients for up to 7 years after outpatient treatment: Impact of alcohol deterrents on outcome. *Alcoholism: Clinical and Experimental Research*. 2006; **30**: 86–95.
38. Cahill K, Stevens S, Perera R *et al*. Pharmacological interventions for smoking cessation: An overview and network meta-analysis. *Cochrane Database of Systematic Reviews*. 2013; (5). Art. No.: CD009329. doi: 10.1002/14651858.CD009329.pub2. [http://onlinelibrary.wiley.com/doi/10.1002/14651858.CD009329.pub2/abstract].
39. Lindson N & Aveyard P. An updated meta-analysis of nicotine preloading form smoking cessation: Investigating mediators of the effect. *Psychopharmacology (Berl)*. 2011; **214**: 579–592.
40. Walker N, Howe C, Bullen C *et al*. The combined effect of very low nicotine content cigarettes, used as an adjunct to usual Quitline care (nicotine replacement therapy and behavioural support), on smoking cessation: A randomized controlled trial. *Addiction*. 2012; **107**: 1857–1867.
41. MacLeod C, Rutherford E, Campbell L *et al*. Selective attention and emotional vulnerability: Assessing the causal basis of their association through the experimental manipulation of attentional bias. *Journal of Abnormal Psychology*. 2002; **111**: 107–123.
42. Schoenmakers TM, de Bruin M, Lux IF *et al*. Clinical effectiveness of attentional bias modification training in abstinent alcoholic patients. *Drug and Alcohol Dependence*. 2010; **109**: 30–36.
43. Houben K, Havermans RC & Wiers RW. Learning to dislike alcohol: Conditioning negative implicit attitudes toward alcohol and its effect on drinking behavior. *Psychopharmacology*. 2010; **211**: 79–86.
44. Houben K, Schoenmakers TM & Wiers RW. I didn't feel like drinking but I don't know why: The effects of evaluative conditioning on alcohol-related attitudes, craving and behavior. *Addictive Behaviors*. 2010; **35**: 1161–1163.
45. Wiers RW, Eberl C, Rinck M *et al*. Re-training automatic action tendencies changes alcoholic patients' approach bias for alcohol and improves treatment outcome. *Psychological Science*. 2011; **22**: 490–497.
46. Achtziger A, Gollwitzer PM & Sheeran P. Implementation intentions and shielding goal striving from unwanted thoughts and feelings. *Personality and Social Psychology Bulletin*. 2008; **34**: 381–393.
47. Balmford J, Borland R & Swift E. Reported planning before and just after quitting and quit success: Retrospective data from the ITC 4-Country survey. *Psychology of Addictive Behaviors*. 2013 (*in press*).
48. Paul-Ebhohimhen V & Avenell A. Systematic review of the use of financial incentives in treatments for obesity and overweight. *Obesity Reviews*. 2008; **9**: 355–367.
49. Cahill K & Perera R. Competitions and incentives for smoking cessation. *Cochrane Database of Systematic Reviews*. 2011; (4).. Art. No.: CD004307. doi: 10.1002/14651858.CD004307.pub4. [http://onlinelibrary.wiley.com/doi/10.1002/14651858.CD004307.pub4/abstract].
50. Buller DB, Borland R & Burgoon M. Impact of behavioural intention on effectiveness of message features: Evidence from the family sun safety project. *Human Communication Research*. 1998; **24**: 433–453.

51. Hughes JR, Keely JP, Niaura RS *et al*. Measures of abstinence in clinical trials: Issues and recommendations. *Nicotine & Tobacco Research*. 2003; 5: 13–25.
52. Borland R, Partos T, Yong H *et al*. How much unsuccessful quitting activity is going on among adult smokers? Data from the International Tobacco Control Four Country cohort survey. *Addiction*. 2012; 107: 673–682.
53. Schwarzer R. Modeling health behavior change: How to predict and modify the adoption and maintenance of health behaviors. *Applied Psychology*. 2008; 57: 1–29.
54. Sniehotta F, Scholz U & Schwarzer R. Action plans and coping plans for physical exercise: A longitudinal intervention study in cardiac rehabilitation. *British Journal of Health Psychology*. 2006; 11: 23–37.
55. Sniehotta F, Schwarzer R, Scholz U *et al*. Action planning and coping planning for long-term lifestyle change: Theory and assessment. *European Journal of Social Psychology*. 2005; 35: 565–576.

Chapter 8
USING CEOS TO ADVANCE KNOWLEDGE

This chapter provides a brief summary overview of CEOS theory and then focusses on research issues both related to what we need to be measuring, and around a better understanding of the complexities of HTM behaviours with the aim of developing better interventions; both self-help strategies and interventions from change agents to enhance self-regulatory capacities.

Key features of CEOS theory

Central to CEOS theory is the notion that OS processes are continually reactive to the context (environment) plus influences on ES conceptualisations of the situation, resulting in change in the levels of impulses to act in various ways. The framework of CEOS is about understanding the potential of people to gain greater conscious control over the way they live their lives, including how external interventions (tools, advice and support) can help them to do so. That is, it is about understanding the existing limits of self-regulation by the ES and finding ways to enhance its functioning. The actions of the ES are grounded in conscious experience and operate to influence the behaviour in a quasi-teleological manner around linguistically created goals. This creates the partial freedom individuals have to follow ideas, rather than be completely constrained by the context that their OS is cued to respond to. However, executive decisions are dependent on operational processes for their implementation. Thus, to allow the ES to operate most effectively, both in choosing appropriate goals and scripts to implement them, we require better tools to monitor, understand and where desirable influence OS processes. This is not conceived of as simply an exercise in self-control, but rather as a more dynamic process of aligning executive decisions and operational action tendencies in ways that maximise adaptive functioning.

The role of the ES is not to act, but to shape and guide the actions of the OS. Feelings, which are signals about OS states along with perceptions of environmental conditions, are key inputs that ground executive operations in the present reality (Table 8.1). This information is critical to the effective translation of ideas into action. Feelings allow the ES to consider organismic needs and states and thus the possible effects of behaving on the self-as-organism, which should be an important

Understanding hard to maintain behaviour change: A dual process approach, First Edition. Ron Borland.
© 2014 John Wiley & Sons, Ltd. Published 2014 by John Wiley & Sons, Ltd.

Table 8.1 Outputs and conscious elements of both systems

Operational System (OS)	Executive System (ES)
Key outputs:	Key outputs:
Structural support for ES functioning	Conscious within ES:
Information to ES	<ul><li>Understandings, evaluations and analysis</li><li>Stories</li><li>Ideas and beliefs</li><li>Goals</li><li>Plans</li><li>Commitments</li></ul>
<ul><li>Perceptions, both content and via effects on attention</li><li>Feelings</li><li>Associative links to ES content</li><li>Triggering of memories</li><li>Action impulses</li></ul>	
Within itself (to output)	Affective elements
<ul><li>Inhibition of action tendencies awaiting further input</li><li>Action tendencies</li><li>Action schema</li></ul>	<ul><li>Emotions</li><li>Desires</li></ul>
	To OS as inputs:
To environment	<ul><li>New concepts, and so on, to which associative links can be attached</li></ul>
<ul><li>Expressions</li><li>Behaviour</li></ul>	To OS as outputs:
	<ul><li>Action impulses</li><li>Inhibitory impulses</li><li>Action schema</li></ul>

consideration as to whether something is worth doing. Perception allows us to sense the world and thus operate in it, rather than act in response to a purely abstract concept of the world. Together, feelings and perception ground our ideas in the present reality (person in context), and under most conditions guide us to choose the ideas to implement that will be most likely to serve our purposes, and thus constrain us to act in ways that are likely to minimise risks and maximise likely benefits to both the self and the broader community. However, for HTM behaviours, aspects of this grounding are leading us astray.

CEOS has been framed broadly enough that it should be able to explain all forms of behaviour change and the conditions around which existing behaviour patterns are maintained. As noted elsewhere, it has more complexity than is likely to be needed for understanding simple changes; its strength should lie in its capacity to deal with behaviours that are difficult to change.

The CEOS framework identifies new strategies, which in principle, should enhance the likelihood of successful behaviour change, but for the most part, the potency of these has not been tested, although some show real promise (see Chapter 7, and recent reviews [1−7]).

The theory accepts that there are limits to people's capacity to change their behaviour. Some people will be unable to make changes that are relatively unproblematic for others. Individual differences, whether innate or acquired, are a reality. Among those for whom change is more difficult, the use of external aids can make it possible or easier. However, known predictors of successful behaviour change only account for a small proportion of the variance; so, the main way of identifying those who will find change hard is a history of failed attempts.

Understanding change is about identifying the elements of the biopsychosocial determinants of HTM behaviours that are most central to facilitation of the desired change. For those predominantly psychosocial or social in origin, environmental change and educational strategies are likely to be the main tools required. However, where there is a bio-psychological element, facilitating change will require self-regulatory strategies as well, and where biological aspects hinder change, may also require biological interventions.

External aids can facilitate change by making the task inherently easier, either in the short term (e.g. use of quit smoking medications), or in the longer term by providing more attractive alternatives (e.g. low-fat versions of high-fat foods). Use of long-term alternatives or replacements is fine when the alternative is not problematic in its own right, but where it remains problematic a second behavioural challenge is to eventually eliminate this form of the behaviour. In this case, the focal question is whether a two-step solution is more efficient than a one-step one, and for our purposes are either or both of the steps HTM behaviours, or will the alternative solve the problem without the need for bolstering self-regulation.

The simplest behaviour change model is one where people get information, think about it, decide to change and then act. The reality is far more complex for HTM behaviours, at least after the first failed attempt to change. The person has typically known about the problem for some time, but it is the individual's readiness to try again that needs to change before another attempt occurs. As we have seen for smoking, at least, a lot of failed attempts are typical, as well as ones abandoned before they even get started. The reality of HTM behaviour change is of a set of pre-existing determinants only generating action on a small fraction of the occasions when it is contemplated, or action is otherwise possible.

Early in the life of a problem, it is of interest to assess whether people have developed goals for change, but once these are established, the focus needs to be on efforts to implement change. Over extended periods, what should be assessed is the likelihood that the person will find contexts in which to act to achieve a goal, and the likelihood that the effort will be successful. Over shorter periods, it is possible to explore factors that determine the effectiveness of specific types of scripts, whether a script once initiated is followed through on, and if it fails, at what points failure is most likely and whether this interacts with the script type and personal characteristics. Consideration is also needed as to what influences readiness to try again following failure.

Reframing thinking

CEOS theory is designed to encompass description (or taxonomy), causation and strategies for enacting the change. At the core of CEOS and other dual-process theories is a fundamentally different framework for organising observations and relating them to theoretical constructs: the dual-process model. This major taxonomic distinction influences the way everything else is thought about. Re-framing thoughts consistent with the dual-process approach is not straightforward. In particular, it is very difficult for the human mind (or at least mine!) to position action within the OS rather than with executive decisions. It appears to me (at any rate) that where the I is placed in thinking about action is with the goal the ES adopts. Thus, for quitting smoking, if I decide I want to quit, then resistance from my OS is seen as ego-alien. By contrast if I think I should quit for ego-alien reasons, but identify with the rationalisations as to why my OS doesn't want to, I will feel as if I really don't want to and be resistant to external pressures to act. Alternatively, I can accept that when what I want is some balance between the story or justification for action that emerges from past experience and what my body tells me is desirable, I am the arbiter. At other times, I might be the source of feelings. A taxonomy of possible positions is required for systematic study. This is especially needed where there is conflict between executive and operational processes. Inappropriately assuming executive superiority when there is conflict can mislead us into trying to bypass operational considerations, rather than attempting to reorient them towards more effectively implementing executive scripts.

One example of the importance of the taxonomic framing that tends to perpetuate thinking that executive action is primary is the way attitudes are thought about within social psychology [8]. Emerging out the study of attitudes, it became clear that explicit attitudes sometimes masked different action tendencies [9–12]. These were labelled implicit attitudes, and a research tradition emerged to try to first measure them and then explore how they related to explicit attitudes. This work has proved to be a major impetus to the development of dual-process thinking, but the terminology is stuck in a different way of thinking about the world. From a dual-process approach, implicit attitudes are primary and represent associative patterns with the object and associated action tendencies, they represent how we feel about the objects particularly in the contexts in which we need to engage with them in some way. By contrast, explicit attitudes are conceived of as being a result of an analytical assessment of what is desirable, with the extent to which the OS-generated factors are synthesised into this assessment unspecified. The best distinctions from the perspective of dual-process models are ones that clearly make the primary distinction between top-down executive processes and bottom-up operational ones, and do so in ways that do not perpetuate misunderstandings about their respective roles. Thus, I don't like the term *implicit attitudes* as it suggests that they are some inferior form of explicit attitudes, and would seek a replacement term, perhaps something such as *operational inclinations*. Alternatively, if the term *attitudes* could be resurrected to become focussed on bottom-up processing, a term such as *opinions* could be used to replace it for espoused affective judgements. Whichever way the field goes, what is important is to maintain a clear separation, and to frame it in a way that it is clear that opinions or explicit attitudes are built up from inclinations in the context of executive framing and conceptualisations of their appropriateness.

Key questions to answer for behaviour change

The framework of the theory should help us clarify our thinking about the central questions for behaviour change. These are 'How should people organise their thinking to come up with the most appropriate goals for behaviour change, and what is enough information to justify the change?'; and 'What do people need to do to maximise their chances of long-term success, and how might this need to change along the journey'?, or put another way: 'What can people do so that they come to want to do something they currently feel they should do, but don't really want to'? Finally, related to all of the above-mentioned: 'How do we decide which set of arguments or forces are directing us down the right (or most productive) path, be it in setting goals, developing or implementing scripts for action, or recovering from setbacks'?

The answer to the question of deciding what is likely to be the best involves consideration of social consensus, but this can result in overly conservative decisions as social consensus is inevitably grounded in past experiences that may no longer be relevant. An alternative is to rely on rational analysis of the information available, but this will always be limited by working memory capacity, so might miss important considerations. Or we could rely on our intuitions, what feels right, but this involves an overreliance on operational processes, again overreliant on the past and on bodies that evolved to be adaptive in different conditions to those we face today, but on the other hand capable of sensing gaps in rational appraisal and in normative pressures. The reality is that the best decisions are likely to be based on some amalgam of the three sources, but living in an empirical activity and thus our ideas as to the implications of decisions we make can never be guaranteed to be right, the best we can hope for is being better off on average. This is a reality for all self-reflective systems of thought, and is all the more so for those with limited processing capacity. HTM behaviours represent an important set of behaviours where our intuitions are leading us astray; so, we need to be more reliant on social factors and rational appraisal, and work to re-align our intuitions if we are to have our behaviour serve our best interests.

The answers to the other questions are more complex, and hints about how to answer them form much of the content of this book. At the heart of the answer to how best to change is the belief that a reliance on self-control, that is, the temporary exertion of executive control over behaviour, is at best a temporary solution to behaviour change and that sustained change will only come about if the OS can be reoriented to support desired change long term. One goal of interventions is thus to hasten acceptance of change, something that requires some acceptance of loss and which is likely more difficult for those whose lives are currently not going well.

Contributions of different kinds of research

Research is sometimes divided into two broad categories: that which focusses on systems and the ways things interrelate in the real world, and that which focusses on specific mechanisms by which component parts of the systems operate. These two forms of research should complement each other, and much research has elements of both. Most of my research has been at the more systems end of the spectrum, so, I am concerned about how the various micro-theories fit together into an integrated whole (i.e. those developed out of more mechanistic studies of how various aspects affect others). The challenge of integrating micro-theories into a comprehensive model emerges from the desire to address complex multi-level problems in a coherent manner [13]. This desire is, in part, related to the differences between the ecological and internal validity of studies to understand the determinants of behaviour, or put slightly differently, the differing roles of population studies to analogue experimental studies (Box 8.1). Convergence of evidence from experiments and real-life studies gives the most confidence that an intervention can make a causal contribution to real-life outcomes. As the history of drug research shows most clearly, lot of drugs that have causal impacts on mechanisms related to disease do not end up producing the overall theorised benefit, because the reality they were developed in differs in important (albeit unidentified ways) from the more complex reality in which they are applied. So, it is with component parts of behavioural interventions. Unfortunately, there is no similar level of support for research on the systematic translation of elements of behavioural interventions into the inevitably multifaceted interventions that are delivered in real-life situations.

There is another problem with the use of conventional approaches to evidence for interventions that target executive processes. The way stories operate changes over time due to cultural factors, quite different rules to the evolutionary changes governing biologically determined processes. The evolution of ideas occurs on an altogether faster timescale than most forms of biological evolution. This means the

---

Box 8.1   Ecological versus internal validity

There are two major factors that need to be considered in assessing the strength of conclusions that can be reached from data: internal and external (or ecological) validities. Internal validity relates to the risk of making invalid causal attributions due to lack of internal control over the research, while external or ecological validity relates to the issue of causal attributions due to overgeneralisation from the specific context and details of the study to the reality to which it is applied. The research-based evidence movement focusses their efforts on the internal validity of trials; so, see the placebo-randomised controlled trial (RCT) as the epitome of good research design. RCTs answer the critical question of whether an intervention can have a causal impact on an outcome. However, while they can ensure the maximal confidence in inferring causal links, RCTs are often conducted in contexts or on populations where the results have questionable relevance to the real-world situations in which practitioners wish to apply them. They do not answer the question of whether an intervention that can work under some ideal circumstances is actually working in the context in which it is applied.

mode of interventions needs to change to keep up with these changes. An analogy can be drawn with research to develop immunisations for the flu virus and the ways a new recipe is required to improve the immunity with each new strain. This is grounded on a robust theory as to what is required and a new recipe created each year (or thereabouts), a timescale where conventional RCTs are impractical; so, we rely on the science to get a mix that does the job. So, we should consider the ways in which behavioural interventions need to be regularly changed to be congruent with changing relevant social norms and communicative styles. This requires a more comprehensive understanding of what the theorised active elements are and how they combine together, something that scientists are beginning to take seriously [14]. By contrast, the way operational processes work is much more stable, so, here the effects of research are likely to be applicable into the foreseeable future.

Measuring key constructs

The outline of taxonomy of behaviour and its determinants around a dual-process model of contested change should identify and characterise the constructs that need to be measured, being some combination of theorised determinants from the context, both the OS and the ES, as well as of the forms of behaviour of interest. Most of the concepts of interest are not directly measurable; some are only measurable via self-reports of internal states, and still others require even more indirect measures, such as physiological recordings of associated processes.

CEOS theorises that behaviour is a function of both executive and operational processes, none of which are directly observable to an outsider, but many of which are available to the person's ES and thus can be reported on to others. Self-reports can be of beliefs and attitudes (evaluative assessments of beliefs); experiences, both of the context and of internal states; and memories for past events, both experiences and beliefs. Memories are critical to all self-report; one cannot report on what is not remembered, and this is more of an issue for more distant events.

Where constructs are not directly measurable, there is a need to consider the relationships between the measures used and underlying theoretical constructs. In this section, in particular, I use the term *measure* when not concerned about systematic error (between the measure and what it is theorised to measure) and indicator, where (for the purposes of interest) measurement of the construct is known or suspected to be biased. Examples of indicators are use of such things as education level or income as measures of socioeconomic status (SES) and reaction times to associated stimuli as indicators of *implicit* attitudes. In both these cases, it is not entirely clear what they indicate, both because of vagueness in definition of the underlying constructs and the likely complexity of the relationships between them and their indicators. When we rely on the indicators, which have not been shown to be unbiased measures of the constructs we theorise, we should be cautious of how the relationships between constructs are interpreted. The associations found could be diluted by systematic error, but it could also be that the indicator is measuring some other determinant; for example, in the SES example, education level could indicate something other than SES.

This last example raises an important issue for social determinants. Social determinants are not theorised to have direct effects on behaviour. They impact on behaviour indirectly in one of two ways; first, by partly determining the range and forms of environmental cues, both social and physical, that determine the contexts in which people act, and thus both the cues they respond to and the history of responding over time; and second, they act as determinants of beliefs that people hold both about themselves (e.g. as social beings) and the contexts in which they need to act. The two need to be assessed independently, as although they can interact, the means of modifying them are quite different (environmental change vs argument).

Two other interrelated measurement issues are important to mention, both related to temporal issues. The first is whether a measure is designed to tap a construct at a point in time or to measure more tonic or stable aspects of it, and the second relates to any gap in time between when measures are taken and the outcomes they are theorised to influence are assessed (see also Chapter 6).

Relatively, stable characteristics of people such as many beliefs (including attitudes), goals and tendencies to behave in particular ways (habit strength) are important theorised determinants of behaviour. However, there are also versions or aspects of many of these that can change markedly in specific situations. The most important here are reactions to aspects of HTM behaviours when in the presence of the possibility of acting to initiate or maintain change. Measuring the more stable tonic aspects and being able to relate these to the immediate or phasic aspects is important for CEOS, in particular, and to other models of relapse prevention [15] as the interaction between the two is important for understanding the maintenance of behaviour change.

Measures need to be made at appropriate times. Even when measures are accurate (enough) at the point they are assessed, unless the constructs can be assumed to remain constant, measuring them too far in advance of the behaviours that they are theorised to partly determine contains an additional source of potential error. That is, there may be meaningful change in the underlying construct between when it is measured and when it is theorised to have its effects. The greater the delay, the more likely the construct will have changed. By contrast, if measured in the context of the opportunity to behave, it will be more influenced by phasic, situation-specific factors, making it less a measure of the stable aspect. Temporal relationships between theorised determinants of behaviours and the resultant behaviours are distorted in much current population-level research. This is largely because the intervals between measures do not correspond to the temporal relationships between the theorised elements. For example, with smoking cessation, it is common to measure intentions/interest in quitting by asking whether the smoker is planning to quit in the next month, considering in the next 6 months, open to the possibility beyond that, or not interested. In our studies, when smokers asked this are re-asked a year later, those who said they intend to quit in the next month are more likely to have reported a quit attempt than those who said in the next 6 months, although most of those attempts appear to be beyond 1 month from baseline. If this question was measuring what it overtly claims to be, then there should be no difference as the follow-up is more than 6 months later. This measure, when used over this interval, is thus more a measure of interest in quitting, rather than a measure of any specific time-based intent. However, if the follow-up was 1 month later and the intention group was more likely to have tried to quit, then treating the answer as an intention would make more sense. The point is the same question asked in a different context or given a different job to do in prediction may need to be treated as a measure of something different. More thought is needed in designing the studies to match temporal aspects of predictors to the outcomes they are designed to predict.

Measuring ES influences on behaviour

As discussed in Chapters 5 and 6, the core executive factors that influence behaviour are relatively stable beliefs or opinions about what is important and of outcome expectancies related to possible behaviour change. At the time of action, these propositional inputs interact with ideas generated from the experiences of behaving and the context to affect decisional balance, and balanced by pre-existing or new commitments determine whether executive decisions will continue to be pursued or abandoned.

Self-reports of executive processes should be considered in terms of the functions that they can play. When articulated, they are part of the way the person presents himself/herself to the world. When articulated to the self, regardless of public use, they concretise thinking and provide a locus from which associative links can spread downwards within the person. Where these are consistent with upward-spreading associations with the actual object of the belief, this is accompanied by a feeling of certainty and an overall strengthening of the associative network. However, where the existing associations with the object are incongruent, this conflict can be experienced as dissonance, and potentially a need to find a resolution (often this does not happen as events move on before it happens). Where new information evokes little or no associative network, it is unlikely to be a determinant of subsequent behaviour, no matter how compelling it may seem in isolation. For example, knowing that over 5 million people die prematurely of smoking-related causes each year evokes little emotional reaction, but knowing that your beloved Aunt Bess has lung cancer from her smoking does.

The CEOS analysis suggests that the summary conceptualisations individuals make about their beliefs represent the ways these factors are represented in consciousness and thus in decision-making processes. This means that single questions that directly tap what the person is thinking should be more predictive of his/her behaviour than multi-item measures that attempt to use a researcher-generated algorithm to combine elements, rather than to tap the implicit algorithm used by the person. Thus, the most predictive questions to ask people should be those that tap these summary beliefs and decisions. In particular, the more proximal aspects should be most strongly predictive, but as they are more dynamic, their predictive power is likely to decline over time. By contrast, more stable underlying beliefs are likely to be predictive over longer periods. Measuring these key constructs may involve no more than asking the same question, but asking for an answer that covers a longer time interval.

There are several important sources of potential error in single-item measures. First, the underlying reality that a person does not have a fixed strength of any given attitude, it varies somewhat by the context in which it is accessed. Second, there are likely differences in predictive capacity for those for whom the question directly taps a concept they use in their thinking, and for those who first need to translate the question into their frame of thinking in order to answer. Third, single items are typically assessed on 5-point scales (sometimes more), which places limits on precision. Finally, there is the possibility of lying, either systematically distorting responses or responding randomly. However, none of these problems are really addressed by the use of multi-item scales, although they do provide a greater potential range of scores, empirically they are often no more predictive, and sometimes less predictive than single items or other very short measures [16]. To understand decision making, it is likely more useful to have measures of different aspects of the summary processes involved, rather than of components that are a part of already synthesised summary concepts.

CEOS postulates that different factors may be involved in successfully achieving the various tasks associated with successful change. To some degree, our measures need to be sensitive to such factors. For example, it is hard for somebody who is not thinking of quitting to answer questions about outcome expectancies for quitting, or about their self-efficacy for enacting change. In the case of self-efficacy, the best they can answer is in terms of 'If I tried' and in this context cannot include an assessment of commitment or how motivated they feel, which if committed to trying would likely influence their assessment of self-efficacy. Also, if we are interested in factors that could motivate them to think about change, might we not be better asking about outcome expectancies for their current behaviour, rather than the more cognitively complex task of making assessments about hypothetical future possibilities? Similarly, once a person has changed, should we be focussing questioning on his/her outcome expectancies for his/her new behaviour or on beliefs about what things would be like if he/she reverted to the old behaviour? CEOS suggests that which will be most influential is a function of cognitive complexity and consistency of evoking OS- and ES-led affective reactions. This is likely to favour thinking about the current reality, and what the person is actually taking into account in his/her own thinking, but not knowing the latter in advance makes choices made on this basis problematic except within conversations where the framing can be either confirmed or negotiated.

Measures of OS influences on behaviour

There is no way to directly observe OS processes, but a range of indirect methods can be used to infer what they are. These include self-reports of feelings and of behaviour patterns, observations of expressions, recordings of aspects of the person's history, reaction time tasks (e.g. to the objects or relationships of interest or cues related to them) and physiological indicators (both measures of autonomic functioning and more direct measures of aspects of neural functioning). Of these, feelings in the form of experienced urges are probably the only ones that could be considered measures of OS tendencies, but only to the person; when self-reported to others they are subject to many kinds of error, particularly when they relate to aspects of HTM behaviour.

Self-report is the main measurement tool available outside of laboratory contexts, certainly when considering patterns of behaviour over time. This involves using conscious awareness of things such as feelings to infer operational states. One problem with feelings is that they only represent the tip of the iceberg; much of what we do and process occurs without any conscious awareness; so, at best they are incomplete. Another much worrying problem for measurement is that feelings can be influenced by ES activity feeding back to influence (dampen or heighten) the basic OS-generated affective response, distorting them as indicators of OS functioning. Further, measures taken at the time the behaviour is occurring can be disruptive: getting a person to attend to processes that would otherwise have been left to operational processes can result in disruption to performance as the information needs to be fed to higher levels of the system, which slows reactions and can interfere with lower level motor coordination. Mindfulness techniques claim to allow pure monitoring of experience, and while this seems to be achieved by some for simple repetitive actions, it is not clear if it can occur for more complex activities.

The reality is that population-based studies, reports of experiences and of past behaviour may be all we have to infer roles of OS processes. Experimental studies can be important for showing that the theorised mechanisms can occur as here it is possible to have independent indicators of their impact (e.g. reaction-time measures and physiological responses). Further, theorising from the outcomes of studies on these mechanisms can provide new insights on population-level issues. On the other side of the ledger, population-level challenges can provide questions that require experimental work to resolve. As noted in Chapter 7, there is an exciting convergence of such work and theorising stimulated by dual-process theories about how to modify OS processes, which has huge potential for developing new interventions [1, 7, 17, 18].

Measures of context

In experimental settings, the context can be fixed and known to the researcher. In population-based research, the researcher is typically reliant on the person to self-report on aspects of the context that might be important.

Clearly, people can only report on what they can remember, and memory for events is a function of their salience at the time they occurred, their recency and the context in which the recall is made, including the way the question is asked. For most purposes, reports are not required of the current context, although they can be for very recent events. More enduring elements of the person's environment should be more accurately recalled than episodic ones. These include macrodeterminants of context such as SES, living arrangements, social networks, employment status and other such things. Many of these also represent social categories, which are a part of the person's sense of self as well as being indicators of the kinds of contextual cues they are likely to confront, and the likelihood and nature of competing demands on their capacities.

Given the weak links that often exist between the indicators we have of many of the theorised determinants of behaviour, not just context, but also particularly OS processes, it is surprising that we have been able to show any relationships. That we have can be taken as a sign that we are targeting important parts of the process, albeit without any certainty that our theorisations are capturing what the underlying mechanisms are. The imperfect links between indicators and concepts leaves a lot of potential for new theories to reinterpret old findings. The science of behaviour change is still in its infancy.

Elements of a theory-driven research agenda

CEOS theory has implications for research and understanding at several levels. At the highest level of the theory, the ways it differs from alternative framings are not directly empirically testable. Evaluation needs to be in terms of the capacity to integrate knowledge from disparate areas and in the quality of research questions and new insights it generates. The aim of this section is to highlight the implications of some areas where CEOS conceptualises important phenomena in distinctly different ways to existing theories and/or makes different predictions.

Most central to CEOS is the use of a dual-process approach to better understand the implications of past experiences for future behaviour, both via conditioned operational pathways and through executive re-evaluations and attempts to exercise control. Related to this is the identification of skills and resources the person needs to be able to effectively implement a change script, and within the operations of the ES, to better understand and refine the way people script their attempts at change to increase the likelihood of success.

From a broader systems perspective, CEOS also makes some predictions about societal change and the changing nature of populations. These are changes that can only be observed over periods of years or even decades. They are not subject to discrete empirical studies, but rather require careful monitoring of trends. Understanding the dynamic nature of systems over time also provides a framework for understanding how people's reactions to behaviour might similarly change and of the implications for the ways we intervene to facilitate desired changes.

The broad framework of CEOS means that it encompasses a range of existing micro-theories within its broader canvass, as well as being incompatible with others, in whole or part. Describing the way CEOS relates to other theories provides a context for testing propositions where the theories diverge. It can also provide a framework for beginning to understand the likely limits of applicability of specific mechanisms, and thus specific predictions. If it is useful, it should provide a consistent set of explanations that is more parsimonious over its entire domain of applicability than the sum of constructs from the set of competing micro-theories that cover the same domain, although in any one area it may be more complex than any specific micro-theory as it contains elements that are not of importance within that subdomain.

Comparisons with other theories

In Chapter 3, I went into some detail on differences between CEOS and the RIM theory of Strack and Deutsch [19]; so, it is not dealt with in detail again here. The most important differences relate to the way feelings and emotions are considered, and the acceptance in CEOS that executive processes can be driven by non-rational considerations as well as rational analysis. Feelings are inputs into conscious processing of internals inclinations and need states, but are the sum of influences from operational processes coming up through the system as well as reactions to executive decisions and considerations flowing down. This means that when the ES interprets them entirely as OS inputs, it may make inappropriate judgements. This may be the price to pay for having feelings that reflect the totality of desires, something that has likely advantages in facilitating ES-generated actions when the two sources are in concordance. However, for contested change, finding ways to separate out initial OS reactions from ES-generated effects is important for understanding the implications of change to the person, and mindfulness techniques may be important in this regard. The ambiguity of sources of emotions is another source of uncertainty among inputs into executive decision making along with the inherent uncertainty of imagined futures and the consequences of change. This analysis points towards the utility of applying some of the principles of scientific evaluation to the way we think about our lives [20], a process highlighted in Chapters 5 and 6.

The emphasis on reorienting operational processes to be less supportive of old behaviour patterns and more supportive of new ones raises the issue of acceptance of change and the difficulties in achieving this. To date, no strategies have been found to facilitate acceptance. Societies use rituals as a major means of facilitating transitions from one stage of life to another. Should we be looking to reclaim the role of rituals as ways of facilitating transitions, both transitions in life and temporary permissions to indulge in otherwise problematic behaviours? If this was desirable, how could we do it in a secular multicultural society where existing rituals are not widely shared, and those that are take on many different forms? Does this matter? Can each individual choose the set of rituals they will adopt in their lives? If so, who takes responsibility for preserving those rituals and ensuring their compliance?

CEOS argues that the processes of self-regulation, and in particular self-regulatory exhaustion, are different in many important respects to the theorising of Baumeister and associates [21–23]. In particular, consistent with Carver and others [24–26], a central distinction is made between self-control and other forms of self-regulation. Apart from isolating the contribution of overall cognitive capacity (including working memory), the most important distinction, and one that falls neatly out of a dual-process approach, is between self-control and self-reorientation. Self-control involves strengthening the ES (the rider's control over the elephant) and is contrasted with self-reorientation, which involves training the OS (training the elephant to act as desired). Research stimulated by this framing is already delivering new insights [1, 7]. Further, it is argued that physical exhaustion of self-regulatory capacity is less of a problem than competing priorities, and thus a key area to focus research effort on is whether we can improve our capacity to share executive function (simultaneously or rapidly sequentially) and thus facilitate maintenance of both vigilance and capacity to respond appropriately, while minimising disruption to other priority life activities.

The work of Gollwitzer and others [4, 27, 28] on implementation intentions shows how it is possible to increase the likelihood that action will be appropriately cued, although this may not do much about freeing up executive capacity to act if it is otherwise fully committed. Research is needed to see if implementation intentions can be chunked or otherwise grouped quasi-hierarchically to allow for a wider range of implementation intentions to be remembered than a simple list would allow. Further, we need a better understanding of the conditions under which an implementation intention (or any other executive signal to act) is followed through on, or at least attempted to be implemented, rather than put aside ('Not now, I am too busy, or it is too disruptive to my current activity').

In CEOS, a key distinction in decision making for change is between the immediate contingencies (OS) and beliefs about net long-term consequences as assessed by executive processes. Unlike most other theories, complex decisions are not assumed to be made in one step; rather different aspects of a decision to change might be made quite independently and then brought together. Further, CEOS does not assume that the components of what is needed to make a decision as to the desirability of a possible goal are integrated together in a fixed order. Under some circumstances, normative issues may have the priority as theorised in the Theory of Reasoned Action and related theories, but in other cases concerns about risk might predominate with assessments of severity and susceptibility as in the Health Beliefs Model. The one fixed assumption within CEOS is that whatever longer term conclusions have been made about outcome expectancies, they interact with moment-to-moment considerations to determine what the person actually does. Which outcome expectancies end up being influential will depend on which of them are cued to be considered; for example, a person who perceives that others will not be supportive of his/her efforts is likely to focus more on normative considerations.

One consequence of the extended nature of change is the need for continuity in beliefs, both across situations and over extended periods of time. Continuity is needed to maintain the same goal and to facilitate repeated attempts to attain it. It is important to separate more tonic beliefs from their phasic counterparts, that is, the versions that emerge and change in moments of challenge. There are challenges in measuring the two separately as noted earlier in this chapter, but a conceptual separation is important as it creates the potential to integrate issues around timing of questioning in relation to effects and situational determinants of responding, including desirability effects. This distinction between the stable and situational components of beliefs is too often ignored. To help make this distinction clearer, it may be useful when asking about change-related beliefs, if the person has a pre-determined position, or whether he/she doesn't have such a position and is thus generating his/her answer to the question as it is asked. It may also be important to ask to what extent he/she is thinking about engaging in the behaviour at that moment (especially for HTR behaviours where the mention of the topic can stimulate thoughts of acting). These distinctions might also be relevant for people to consider around their internal thoughts: Does the way I think about this now correspond with my pre-existing thoughts? Such self-talk may be one way of helping pre-existing thoughts maintain precedence over the thoughts of the moment.

Because ES-generated beliefs do not spontaneously emerge in situations where they are relevant, but need to be triggered, it is possible that the frequency of having relevant thoughts may be as or more important than the strength of the belief. The frequency with which affectively charged thoughts occur is an indicator of the strength of the underlying concern about the issue. For example, if a person strongly believes that his smoking is harmful, but never thinks about it, he is unlikely to try to quit because it does not concern him in the here and now. However, even if he remains uncertain of the harm, if he thinks about it constantly, he will be more motivated to act because the possibility concerns him in the here and now. Similarly, protecting oneself from relapse requires that you think about the harms and/or benefits of staying quit at the times when you are most vulnerable to relapse if those beliefs are to have any protective capacity. This brings us back to the potential importance of implementation intentions as a strategy for increasing the likelihood of accessing protective beliefs when needed.

The balance between pre-formed beliefs and plans and the contingencies of the moment is in part dealt with within CEOS through the two main forms of feedback loops by which progress is evaluated, immediate feedback from behaving and executive reflections on progress. It is clear that the forms of evaluation that are undertaken during the experience of temptations to revert to old behaviours should differ from those that occur at times when operational considerations are not dominating working memory. This suggests that one element of self-control should be to avoid reconsidering decisions in the heat of the moment, but sometimes a reconsideration will be important; so, the person may need to create rules for himself/herself as to when re-evaluation is appropriate. Such an approach provides challenges for post-change evaluation as the possibility of the old behaviour being cued by the very consideration of the issue can make rational appraisal difficult.

More consideration may also be needed of how the executive is able to interpret inputs from the OS. We can only act to control that which is signalled to us; thus, the role of feelings is central to improving the performance of the OS. One question that needs to be asked is whether having a better conceptualisation of what various feelings and urges signal might be useful for enhancing executive influence. Would it be useful to develop a language to describe and categorise our more *primordial* urges to facilitate understanding them better and thus be in a more informed position to control them?

Moving beyond internal issues, to communications with people, there exists considerable potential for more effectively influencing arguments for and against change in ways that lead to more appropriate decisions. The insight from dual-process thinking, which is critical to persuasion, is that the OS-generated reactions to objects or concepts need to be congruent with ES-generated conceptual relationships and the subsequent affective associations they might lead to. This has led to a rejection of key elements of Prospect theory at least in so far as they relate to persuasion around gain-framed messages being superior for encouraging preventive activities [29] (see Chapters 3 and 7). It should be easy to design experimental tests of messages that differ in terms of cognitive complexity, tendency to evoke different affective reactions and gain/loss framing to determine how these influence persuasion, both immediately and over more extended periods, and as a function of current behaviour (old undesirable vs new).

The theory also sheds new light on the phenomenon of time-discounting, or valuing immediate outcomes over those that are delayed, something characteristic of much human behaviour [30, 31]. CEOS suggests that key influences on time-discounting are the imaginability of the outcome when it occurs in the more distant future, that is, the extent to which it now stimulates appropriate affective reactions and action tendencies and possible increases in the level of uncertainty of it occurring. Dispositional measures of time perspective [30, 31] may reflect capacity to imagine the future in ways that are emotionally salient. HTM behaviour changes can't guarantee the improved health they promise, and avoiding something comes with no immediate markers and thus nothing to trigger affective reactions. CEOS would predict a loss of value for any psychologically meaningful delay. It should be useful to help people fill their imaginary futures with desirable and affectively linked associations; so, they become worth striving for. For example, talking to older adults about being around to enjoy their grandchildren might be a powerful means of reorienting them towards an engagement with an imagined future. As uncertainty is another reason for discounting future outcomes, people may usefully be encouraged to think in ways that minimise thoughts of uncertainty about outcomes; for example, by focussing on the negative consequences of not acting, and on the potential of acting, rather than on the possibility that action might not achieve its desired goals. For example, worry about not gaining the health benefits of behaviour change can generate anxiety of similar magnitude to that of the original concern. An explanation of temporal discounting in terms of affective reactions rather than simply due to delay is plausible as people who hoard resources, and religious people acting for a place in heaven, seem to discount current wellbeing for future anticipated benefits grounded in very strong beliefs about the nature of that future. This could be tested by seeing if the extent of affective reactions (including uncertainty) predicts discounting better than time to the outcome.

Another area ripe for innovative new research is in the role of various forms of commitment for improving perseverance. Commitments are central to self-control models [21, 32]. We know little of the relative potency of various kinds of commitments for maintenance of change, or, of the implications of breaking them for both recovery from lapses and for strategies used on subsequent attempts. For example, is 'This time it is going to be different' enough to justify another unqualified commitment to change? Such research could usefully explore the reactions to lapses in a broader framework to include more tests of the Abstinence Violation Effect of Marlatt as an alternative mechanism for explaining low rates of recovery [33, 34] to a commitment violation effect. Does a commitment to recover help one recover from lapses? On the other hand, does allowing the possibility of a lapse make lapsing more likely?

Related to commitments are the nature and roles of plans and how they impact on the timing of attempts to change. A few years ago several papers were published, suggesting that spontaneous quit attempts may be more successful than planned ones. West [32] suggests that this relates to change often being a more catastrophic activity than a rationally planned one. That people don't constantly try to change once they have a goal is the norm, something many theories have ignored. CEOS provides an explanation consistent with West's; of change requiring situational factors to reach some threshold before there can be any thought of action, and then additional conditions such as a preparedness to act now before behaviour is initiated. More recently, the possible superiority of spontaneous attempts has been brought into question [35, 36]. While it is clear that many attempts to quit smoking occur on the spur of the moment, these overall seem to have similar success rates to those that start after some delay. Further, and largely independent of timing, the amount of reported planning is not as clearly linked to quit success as might be imagined, particularly some forms of planning made before attempts, while others (e.g. practising not smoking in smoking-related situations) seem to be counterproductive and are associated with greater relapse. I admit these findings could be because these are the forms of planning favoured by those *a priori* most likely to fail, and could still be useful, even if they don't bring the success rates up to the average. As the American humourist Mark Twain said 'Giving up smoking is the easiest thing in the world. I know because I've done it thousands of times'. The challenge is in staying stopped, a task of perseverance that requires quite different kinds of skills to being able to manage the component parts. Execution of components is the focus of a lot of practice regimes (e.g. practising not smoking in particular situations). The need for and kinds of planning and practice required to facilitate maintenance likely differ by behaviour; for example, practice may be important for building up exercise routines, but may serve little utility in shifting to lower fat foods. In this regard, maintaining HTN behaviours may be better thought of as a vigilance task where the challenge is to be prepared to act on the increasingly rare occasions when relapses are likely, and of the ability to recover if there is such a lapse.

I had hoped to analyse CEOS in relation to West's PRIME theory of motivation [32], but circumstances have thwarted me. The second edition of West book outlining a revised version of the theory only became available as I was putting the finishing touches to this volume. In it he has shifted his thinking to add a broad model of behavioural determinants called COM – B, very similar to the determinants postulated within CEOS (see Chapters 5 and 6). He has also made some attempt to link PRIME to dual process theories, but has not elaborated on the mechanisms. At a superficial level at least, this elaborated theory is quite similar to CEOS, but it is not clear to what extent the two approaches are deeply compatible. Certainly PRIME's focus on the primacy of operational (reflective) processes for action mirrors CEOS. At the other end of the spectrum, both see roles for aspect of aspects of self-identity, and in some ways his analysis is more complete than mine. West considers the possibility that a change in a long-term addictive habit might trigger major changes in a person's life, such that it effectively moves them onto a different life path. This is an important issue, but a complex one, as the extent to which a change in one aspect of a person's life transforms other aspects clearly varies across individuals. The extent of this may be a function of how beliefs around the behaviour in question relate to more fundamental beliefs and values. Research is needed to see if those for whom a target HTM behaviour is related to their self-identity need to make more fundamental and wide-ranging changes to their overall behaviour, and the extent to which this need may affect the likelihood of initiation and/or maintenance of change. I would predict that making changes strongly linked to self-identity would make initiation less likely, but if the new life path was seen as more desirable may actually help maintain the new behaviour. Change is likely to be extremely difficult where it, or the rationalisation of it, creates conflict with other important life priorities. Understanding how behaviour change integrates into a person's life is at the heart of a broad systems approach to behaviour change, which is both more broadly focussed than limited perspective rationality-based approaches and which explicitly tackles the implications of the competing forces from the OS and ES on behaviour.

Implications for reducing inequities

Disadvantaged sections of the community seem to be more prone to many undesirable behaviour patterns than their more advantaged compatriots, at least under some circumstances. It is important to understand the mechanisms of this apparent reduced capacity for change. The international tobacco control policy evaluation project is increasingly shedding light on what might be important. This study, which follows cohorts of smokers in a wide range of countries, including some of the most economically disadvantaged, is finding different patterns of association between indicators of SES and smoking-related outcomes across countries. Education does not seem to be very important for influencing basic understanding of the harms of smoking: for example, Thai peasants are similarly knowledgeable to residents of Bangkok, many of whom are highly educated [37]. Another line of research studies are showing that area disadvantage is not related to smoking cessation outcomes [38, 39], but perceptions of area disadvantage might be. There is also research showing that people with depression and highly stressed lives are less able to quit smoking successfully, despite being at least as motivated to try [40]. Taken together with the research on the importance of smoking for managing negative affect (albeit ineffectively), it appears that for smoking, at least the problem lies not in economic disadvantage but in living a life where there are less opportunities to feel good as a result of engaging in desirable activities or where stressful activities don't end up resulting in valued outcomes. Where long-term rewards are missing, people are likely more prone to activities with short-term gains, even though they may also deliver longer term pains.

Seemingly contradicting this, however, is evidence from Kahneman and others [41] using random sampling of current mood states that rates of reporting feeling good were not closely related to overall assessments of mood and life satisfaction. Kahneman [41] argues that the momentary reports reflect the truer reality. I fundamentally disagree. It is what we remember, and how we interpret our memories, which affects us into the future via executive processes. If positive experiences are had in ways that don't add meaning to stories people create of their lives, then their utility is lost beyond the moment they happen. The absorption of a computer game or being high on drugs provides little or no pleasure beyond its end, and pleasure that leads nowhere is ephemeral. By contrast, pain leading to good outcomes is seen as worth suffering [42], and is often associated with some of our most valued memories and the aspects of our lives we most value. Our kids make us angry from time to time (to time), and are associated with more negative experience, but they are also for most of us an almost unending source of joy and satisfaction. Moment-to-moment experiences shape operational responses; so, they are important to understand and highlight the need to find ways of helping people to create more meaning in their lives as a way of helping them overcome the need to engage in activities that only provide value in the moment.

Meaning can come from the strength of our own values as to what is important, but for most it is complemented at least in part by the value others see in us. Real disadvantage is not having the resources to be able to create self-stories that provide life meaning or being caught with life scripts that perpetuate misery for whatever reasons. People in manipulative and exploitative relationships (be it to an abusing spouse or health-destroying cigarettes) are often too fearful of losing the odd moment of joy and the sense of belonging to be prepared to make the change, and take on a new life path. I am hopeful that the analysis within CEOS can be used to provide means to help disadvantaged people gain greater control over aspects of their lives.

Concluding comments

CEOS theory, as described in this book, attempts to think about behaviour and behaviour change quite differently from most existing theories. It is a model of behaviour that is designed to be consistent with what we know about both control systems and human physiology. It highlights the interaction between conscious and nonconscious influences on behaviour and focusses on how a better understanding of OS processes and how they influence the ES and thus the contents of thought should help to make out thinking better tuned to the reality in which we live. It highlights the importance of considering issues of self-control separate to issues of self-reorientation or reprogramming the OS. The latter is central to maintaining change over time, while self-control is conceived of as a limited duration resource to facilitate the change.

Translated into the organisational metaphor, the challenge CEOS sets is to assist the executive to reshape the organisation, or in this case the OS such that the equivalent of staff find value in what the executive has concluded to be worthwhile and are thus motivated to pursue those objectives without undue executive oversight. However, the executive needs to listen to inputs from below as to whether it is achieving its goals, and in some cases whether it is trying to implement something that the organisation or OS is not able to comfortably manage. That is, feedback from below provides information both on work still needed to be done, and over time, whether the project is likely to be achievable.

Like organisations, individuals can learn from the experiences of others as to what is achievable, and of new ways to operate more effectively, or even to work comfortably in new ways. This is not going to result in a utopia where people always feel comfortable doing what is right, but it should result in a world where people feel more comfortable doing the sorts of things their society values, but only when they come to share those values.

The genesis for behaviour change can come from two main sources: from executive decisions as to what should be done and from environmental nudges changing conditions to favour new behaviour patterns. However, given the diversity of human needs and sensitivities, the potency of these two sources will vary, and there will always be some who find any particular path uninviting or too hard to follow (at least without some special assistance). I am not suggesting a world where everybody immediately acted as soon as any social consensus emerged, as there would be too many disasters as a result of either the consensus being wrong and all suffering similarly, or as occurs in the economic realm, of the sudden action of many creating imbalances in the system that it is unable to deal with (e.g. food distribution issues if everybody suddenly adopted a healthy diet). We don't need to worry about these things happening, although affected industries routinely exploit uncertainty. The tobacco industry seems to greet every tobacco control initiative with economic projections of doom apparently based on all consumption ceasing overnight, frightening the gullible but so far from reality as it is possible to imagine.

The goal for the executive should be to find ways of acting that satisfy OS needs while being consistent with a rational appraisal of what is desirable. This involves working to create affective engagement with what is desired and to see if it is possible to downgrade the experienced value of things that are undesirable, or if not to position them at the margins of our lives in ways that minimise their net adverse effects.

One important feature of CEOS is that the OS/ES distinction provides a framework and vocabulary for talking coherently about how these two aspects of a person interact. HTM behaviours require more complex models than those for easier to change forms of behaviour, and for discrete actions regardless of difficulty. Central to this is the task of reconditioning the person's OS to act in ways consistent with their ES-generated goals with a minimum of executive input.

Where desired behaviour change is incompatible with action tendencies, behaviour change is impossible until the ES can create contexts and experiences that generate action tendencies for the desired behaviour that are at least in some contexts stronger than competing ones. Behaviour change will not be sustained unless the competing tendencies can be kept stronger. This can be done both by creating new or strengthened action tendencies for the desired behaviour including by making strong commitments, and/or by reducing the strength of competing tendencies, either absolutely or by restricting action to times when competing action tendencies are unlikely to be at their peak.

The other major element of CEOS is the importance of temporal factors; HTM behaviour change takes time. It may be years before goals are translated into a sustained reality. Finding ways to understand this process and to shorten it is a major challenge. It will not be enough to simply look for ways to reduce rates of relapse; it should also involve trying to find strategies for leveraging off failures to facilitate future success, an area in which we are currently notably failing.

I do not believe that this presentation of CEOS is the final word, as should be clear. More thinking and research is needed as to how the theory might need to be adapted for behaviours other than smoking. I think it works well for what we know about smoking, and though not expert in other addictive behaviours, see obvious parallels. I am less certain again as to how it applies to the acquisition of new desirable behaviours, where the analysis is nowhere near as developed. I am hopeful that others will provide me with feedback on this.

Going beyond health concerns, a core aspect of the project of civilisation can be seen as attempts to bring OS impulses in line with societal needs; i.e., what is required for a good and just society, and at the level of the individual, how to have a productive and valued life. As a result, this form of theorising should be useful in other areas. I am sure it has the potential to be useful in dealing with the challenges of getting people to adopt more environmentally appropriate behaviours; however, here somewhat simpler Nudge theory might prove more than adequate. I also suspect that it has the potential for analysing problematic aspects of sexual relationships as this is an area where OS processes are poorly understood within ESs, and greater insights into the way these two sets of forces interrelate might be instructive.

To conclude, HTM behaviour change is a long-term process that begins by choosing a goal for action, followed by an often prolonged period of intermittent goal pursuit. The pursuit requires the exercise of analytical strategies to decide on what to do, self-control to maintain the pursuit of change and the reorientation of operational processes if the change is to be maintained. Change can be facilitated by a supportive environment and by effectively communicating the reasons for change and the utility of different strategies for attaining it. All this sounds simple, but it masks a reality that is far more difficult and complex. I hope this book has shed some light on that complexity.

Summary

This chapter provides a summary overview of CEOS theory and then focusses on research issues both related to what we need to be measuring, and around a better understanding of the complexities of HTM behaviours with the aim of developing better interventions; both self-help strategies as well as interventions from change agents to enhance self-regulatory capacities.

References

1. Friese M, Hofmann W & Wiers RW. On taming horses and strengthening riders: Recent developments in research on interventions to improve self-control in health behaviors. *Self and Identity*. 2011; **10**: 336–351.
2. Hagger MS. Self-regulation: An important construct in health psychology research and practice. Editorial. *Health Psychology Review*. 2010; **4**: 57–65.

3. Hofmann W & Kotabe H. A general model of prevention and interventive self-control. *Social and Personality Psychology Compass*. 2012; **6**: 707–722.

4. Sheeran P, Gollwitzer P & Bargh J. Nonconscious processes and health. *Health Psychology*. 2013; **32**: 460–473.

5. Webb TL, Gallo IS, Miles E *et al*. Effective regulation of affect: An action control perspective on emotion regulation. *European Review of Social Psychology*. 2012; **23**: 143–186.

6. Webb TL, Sniehotta F & Michie S. Using theories of behavior change to inform interventions for addictive behaviors. *Addiction*. 2010; **105**: 1879–1892.

7. Wiers RW, Gladwin TE, Hofmann W *et al*. Cognitive bias modification and cognitive control training in addiction and related psychopathology: Mechanisms, clinical perspectives, and ways forward. *Clinical Psychological Science*. 2013; **1**: 192–212.

8. Greenwald AG & Banaji MR. Implicit social cognition: Attitudes, self-esteem, and sterotypes. *Psychological Review*. 1995; **102**: 4–27.

9. Fazio RH. On the automatic activation of associated evaluations: An overview. *Cognition and Emotion*. 2001; **15**: 115–141.

10. Fazio RH, Sanbonmatsu DM, Powell MC *et al*. On the automatic activation of attitudes. *Journal of Personality and Social Psychology*. 1986; **50**: 229–238.

11. Zajonc RB. Feeling and thinking: Preferences need no inferences. *American Psychologist*. 1980; **35**: 151–175.

12. Zajonc RB. On the primacy of affect. *American Psychologist*. 1984; **39**: 117–123.

13. IARC. *IARC Handbook of Cancer Prevention, Tobacco Control, Vol.12: Methods for Evaluating Tobacco Control Policies*. [http://www.iarc.fr/en/publications/pdfs-online/prev/handbook12/index.php]. International Agency for Research on Cancer: Lyon, 2008.

14. Michie S, Richardson M, Johnston M, *et al*. The behavior change technique taxonomy (v1) of 93 hierarchically clustered techniques: Building an international consensus for the reporting of behavior change interventions. *Annals of Behavioral Medicine*. 2013; **46**(1): 81–95.

15. Hendershot CS, Witkiewitz K, George WH *et al*. Relapse prevention for addictive behaviors. *Substance Abuse Treatment, Prevention and Policy*. 2011; **6**: Advanced Access.

16. Borland R. The power of one: The case for greater use of single item measures. (manuscript under review). 2013.

17. Deutsch R & Strack F. Duality models in social psychology: From dual processes to interacting systems. *Psychological Inquiry*. 2006; **17**: 166–172.

18. Hofmann W, Friese M & Strack F. Impulse and self-control from a dual-systems perspective. *Perspective on Psychological Science*. 2009; **4**: 162–176.

19. Strack F & Deutsch R. Reflective and impulsive determinants of social behaviour. *Personality and Social Psychology Bulletin*. 2004; **8**: 220–247.

20. Kelly G. *The Psychology of Personal Constructs*. Norton: New York, 1955.

21. Baumeister RF & Tierney J. *Willpower: Rediscovering the Greatest Human Strength*. Penguin Press: New York, 2011.

22. Baumeister RF & Vohs KD. Self-regulation, ego depletion and motivation. *Social and Personality Psychology Compass*. 2007; **1**: 115–128.

23. Hagger MS, Wood C, Stiff C *et al*. The strength model of self-regulation failure and health-related behaviour. *Health Psychology Review*. 2009; **3**: 208–238.

24. Carver CS. Impulse and constraint: perspectives from personality psychology, convergence with theory in other areas, and potential for integration. *Personality and Social Psychology Review*. 2005; **9**: 312–333.

25. Carver CS & Scheier MF. *On the Self-Regulation of Behavior*. Cambridge University Press: New York, 1998.

26. Carver CS & Scheier MF. Action, affect, multi-tasking, and layers of control. In: Forgas JP, Baumeister RF & Tice D (eds.) *The Psychology of Self-Regulation*. Psychology Press: New York, 2009: 109–126.
27. Gollwitzer PM. Implementation intentions: Strong effects from simple plans. *American Psychologist*. 1999; **54**: 493–503.
28. Gollwitzer PM & Sheeran P. Implementation intentions and goal achievement: A meta-analysis of effects and processes. Advances in Experimental. *Social Psychology*. 2006; **38**: 69–119.
29. Rothman AJ, Bartels RB, Wlaschin J et al. The strategic use of gain- and loss-framed messages to promote healthy behavior: How theory can inform practice. *Journal of Communication*. 2006; **56**: S202–S220.
30. Hall PA & Fong GT. Temporal self-regulation theory: A model for individual health behaviour. *Health Psychology Review*. 2007; **1**: 6–52.
31. Hall PA & Fong GT. Temporal self-regulation theory: Integrating biological, psychological, and ecological determinants of health behavior performance. In: Hall PA (ed.) *Social Neuroscience and Public health*. Springer Science + Business Media: New York, 2013: 1–19.
32. West R & Brown J. *Theory of Addiction*. 2nd Ed. Wiley: Chichester, UK, 2013.
33. Marlatt G & Gordon J. *Relapse Prevention: Maintenance Strategies in the Treatment of Addictive Behaviors*. Marlatt GA & Gordon JR (eds.). Guilford Press: New York, 1985.
34. Witkiewitz K & Marlatt G. Relapse prevention for alcohol and drug problems: That was Zen. This is Tao. *American Psychologist*. 2004; **59**: 224–235.
35. Cooper J, Borland R, Yong H et al. To what extent do smokers make spontaneous quit attempts and what are the implications for smoking cessation maintenance? Findings from the international tobacco control four-country survey. *Nicotine and Tobacco Research*. 2010; **12**: S51–S57.
36. Murray R, Lewis S, Coleman T et al. Unplanned attempts to quit smoking: Missed opportunities for health promotions? *Addiction*. 2009; **104**: 1901–1909.
37. Young D, Yong HH, Borland R Ross H, Sirirassamee B, Kin F, Hammond D, O'Connor R, Fong G. Prevalence and correlates of roll-your-own smoking in Thailand and Malaysia: Results of the ITC-SEA survey. *Nicotine and Tobacco Research*. 2008; **10**(5): 907–916.
38. Partos TR, Borland R & Siahpush M. Socio-economic disadvantage at the area level poses few direct barriers to smoking cessation for Australian smokers: Findings from the International Tobacco Control Australian cohort survey. *Drug and Alcohol Review*. 2012; **31**: 653–663.
39. Siahpush M, Borland R, Taylor J et al. The associated of smoking with perception of income inequality, relative material well-being, and social capital. *Social Science and Medicine*. 2006; **63**: 2801–2812.
40. Siahpush M, Yong H, Borland R et al. Smokers with financial stress are more likely to want to quit but less likely to try or succeed: Findings from the International Tobacco Control (ITC) Four Country Survey. *Addiction*. 2009; **104**: 1382–1390.
41. Kahneman D. *Thinking, Fast and Slow*. 1st edn. Farrar, Straus and Giroux: New York, 2011.
42. Leventhal H, Brissette I & Leventhal EA. The common-sense model of self-regulation of health and illness. In: Cameron LD & Leventhal H (eds.) *The Self-Regulation of Health and Illness Behaviour*. Routledge: London, 2003: 42–65.

INDEX

Understanding hard to maintain behaviour change: A dual process approach, First Edition. Ron Borland.
© 2014 John Wiley & Sons, Ltd. Published 2014 by John Wiley & Sons, Ltd.

Printed and bound by CPI Group (UK) Ltd, Croydon, CR0 4YY

09/06/2025

14686002-0002